Faith *in the* Field

Faith *in the* Field

A Historical Theological Perspective on Mental Health

Sabas Hernan Flores Whittaker

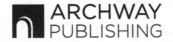 ARCHWAY PUBLISHING

Archway Publishing books may be ordered through booksellers or by contacting:

Archway Publishing
1663 Liberty Drive
Bloomington, IN 47403
www.archwaypublishing.com
1 (888) 242-5904

Because of the dynamic nature of the Internet, any web addresses or links contained in this book may have changed since publication and may no longer be valid. The views expressed in this work are solely those of the author and do not necessarily reflect the views of the publisher, and the publisher hereby disclaims any responsibility for them.

This book is a work of non-fiction. Unless otherwise noted, the author and the publisher make no explicit guarantees as to the accuracy of the information contained in this book and in some cases, names of people and places have been altered to protect their privacy.

Any people depicted in stock imagery provided by Getty Images are models, and such images are being used for illustrative purposes only.
Certain stock imagery © Getty Images.

ISBN: 978-1-4808-6276-0 (sc)
ISBN: 978-1-4808-6277-7 (e)

Library of Congress Control Number: 2018905379

Print information available on the last page.

Archway Publishing rev. date: 05/01/2018

ABOUT THE AUTHOR

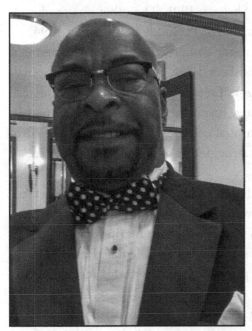

The author, Sabas Hernan Flores Whittaker, was born in Puerto Cortes, Honduras, Central America, his father a Garifuna from Punta Gorda, Roatan, mother a Caymanian of British West Indian descent. Although part Garinagu, he was primarily raised by his Caymanian born grandmother, whom refused to speak Spanish, rather allowed only English and spoke only Elizabethan, or Queens English in her home, hence he grew up in a Spanish speaking country, as a bilingual student at a very early age. Such afforded valuable opportunities to study Spanish in the public school system and English with private tutors, while practicing it regularly among his family.

His early multi lingual education, would later prove to be invaluable, and served rather well, as he disembarked, following an eight year tenure aboard sixteen different ships to pursue a short lived career as an investigator and his education throughout Puerto Rico, the US Virgin Islands and the mainland United States. His earlier Queens English mentoring became rather an asset, as he studied, read and easily understood the works of William Shakespeare, and other great classics, while ventured on a part time career as a playwright. With these being primarily, volunteer, local community, theater productions, he was able to write, create and produced 4 stage plays, 2 short films and a featured length screenplay, all to benefit homeless causes, domestic violence, AIDS and other social ills, which plagued communities in which he lived.

His early bilingual abilities, eased the possibilities to quickly adapt and learn other international languages, such as Italian and some Greek, while he sail as a teenager on board, the tug boats, cargo, tankers and later cruise ships, as a merchant marine to ascend to the rank of officer, during the 1970s to early 80's. Although his language skills would later serve, thus brought far greater benefit and personal satisfaction, years later, as he began to work in health care, as part of our dynamic US population, rapid change in demographics, where Spanish language, grew to a higher demand. He would serve as a translator for the Sexual Transmitted decease (STD) clinic in St Thomas, US Virgin Islands, and later as a psych tech, for the Puerto Rican, Dominican and other Latino immigrants residing in St Thomas. During his thirty year tenure throughout the US Virgin Islands Department of Health, Puerto Rico, Miami, Hartford, Middletown, Meriden and Newington Connecticut, with the Department of Mental Health and Addictions Services (DMHAS), from where he retired, as a Case Manager and Lead Mental Health Worker.

The author has previously written and published five books, 1 Vestiges of A journey, Xlibris, poetry. 2 Africans In The Americas, Our Journey Throughout The World, anthropology, IUniverse. 3 Away From The Field. 4 Tears of Joy Peace and Harmony While The Fire Burns Within, poetry. 5 Songs To Valentines, Songs to Love, Romance in poetry. He has lectured at the University of Syracuse, Trinity College, University of Connecticut, Eastern Connecticut State University and Central Connecticut State University. In years pass, he has also lectured and presented his poetry at various elementary, high schools, churches and community, social gatherings throughout the country.

He has also written and produced two original stage plays, Don't Look Down On Your Brother if You're Not Going To Pick Him Up, and Our Journey. One of these produced at the Warner Theater in Torrington Connecticut, to benefit the FISH, Homeless Shelters, 1991. The other was produced at the Middletown High school, as a benefit to the Middletown AIDS Buddy Network, in 1994.

Additionally, to being an author, he is a graphic artist, music composer, and an active member with the American Society of Composers Authors and Publishers, since 1991. Among his original music compositions, four full length albums, Solo Mi Corazon, Eternal Optimist, Soul Revival and Flight of The Phoenix (Tribute to Middletown). As a painter, furniture builder and sculpture, his most recent art exhibit, was presented at the ODECO sponsored conference, on the plight of Afro Caribbean and Garinagu, women economic empowerment struggles throughout Latin America, at the United Nations, in New York City.

The author, is a father of three handsome grown children, grandpa to two beautiful talented grandchildren. He now lives between Connecticut and New York City, with his beautiful talented wife, the Rev. Dr. Damaris Whittaker. Sabas Whittaker, is a former merchant marine officer, turned historian, bilingual poet, lyricist, artist, painter, music composer, and a retired Mental Health Worker, whom is currently pursuing a PhD, in ecopsychology and plant medicine, with his ultimate goal, being "an attempt to better serve."

The author proudly and dutifully gives thanks to all, whom inspired thought and shared inspiration to learned… to all with whom, he studied with, to each and all, whom never wavered, nor shied away from teaching sharing throughout the attended scholastic programs, conferences, lectures, in-services, throughout the various teaching hospitals, treatment centers, colleges and universities, where, study, work, research, quest toward knowledge, advocacy, bill-paying and justice is an everyday way of life.

Among former places of employment:

Knud Hansen Memorial Hospital, Long Term Care Psychiatric Unit.

St Thomas USVI St Thomas Hospital, PEC psychiatric ward. St Thomas USVI, 1983

The Institute of Living, Hartford Connecticut, 1985

Miami Bridge Shelter for Runaway Kids 1986

Goodwill Industries Outpatient Geriatric and Developmentally Disable Outreach programs 1985

Connecticut Valley Hospital, Department of Mental Health and Addictions Services 1986-1994

Dutcher Hall Substance Abuse Recovery Unit and Rehab Programs

Battel Hall Traumatic Brain Injury Unit (TBI)

Woodward Hall Geriatric Unit

Whiting Forensic Institute (Evening Float)

Merritt Hall, General Psych and Criminal Insane Division Programs

DMHAS Community Base Initiative, (CBI) Meriden Connecticut 1995 – 2001

Cedar Crest Hospital Acute Latino Psychiatric Unit 2001 - 2005

The stigma placed on mental illness, has not yet been fully eradicated … However, the move to equate mental illness with a physical "legitimate" illness, have resulted in a greater understanding on some aspects, as to the particular course of the disease. Sad, though truthfully so, we still have a long way left to go, but we'll keep on effectively working on it … we therefore give gratitude for your wisdom placed upon the Church and Church leaders, to again embarked together with psychiatry psychology, nursing and sociology to aid us along in this behavioral battle. We pray that our faith remain grounded, our spirit hold steadfast, while our minds glides toward finding an intermediary, a middle-ground, a midpoint, where we stumble to create a levee that helps alleviate the existent burdens, between treatment, deinstitutionalization, hospital, compassion, understanding, altruism, jail, justice, remedies and finally a cure.

We strongly hold the unbeaten helm upon these vast tortured oceans as we navigate through the wide open turbulent seas.

Crabs In A Basket Publishing

DEDICATION

This book is dedicated to the resilience of the many individuals, whom have managed to overcome the illness and now live productive lives among us ... for it is written to the memory of the number of decent men and women, whom have spent their entire lives struggling and often even dying alone, or in mental institutions throughout the world.

This book is also dedicated to all of the courageous mental health workers, who gave their time, their dedication, their love, their lives, who's bodies, at times have been the recipients of debilitating lifetime, injuries and sometimes even death, due to assaults, while attempting to admit, care for counsel, treat and minister; under the worse of circumstances, in the battlefield of mental health. As we tried to help to instill our patients, client's, dignity and respect ... to serve with honor.

I proudly and dutifully gave thanks to all, whom I learned from, to all with whom I studied... to each, and everyone of you, whom never wavered, nor shied away from teaching and encouraging me to learn, throughout the hospital teaching programs, inservices, and treatment centers where, I was able to study, work, research, learn to advocate and pay the bills.

St. Thomas Hospital, PEC psychiatric ward. St Thomas USVI, 1982
Knud Hansen Memorial Hospital, Long Term Care Psychiatric Unit. St Thomas USVI, 1983
The Institute of Living, Hartford Connecticut, 1985
Miami Bridge Shelter for Runaway Kids 1986
Goodwill Industries Outpatient Geriatric and Developmentally Disable Outreach programs 1987
Connecticut Valley Hospital, Department of Mental Health and Addictions Services 1986 – 1994
Dutcher Hall Substance Abuse Recovery Unit and Rehab Programs
Battel Hall Traumatic Brain Injury Unit (TBI)
Woodward Hall Geriatric Unit
Merritt Hall General Psych and Criminal Insane Division Programs
DMHAS Community Base Initiative, (CBI) Meriden Connecticut 1995 – 2001
Cedar Crest Hospital Acute Latino Psychiatric Unit 2001 - 2005
Whiting Forensic Institute

PROLOGUE

A Historical Religious Perspective On The Study of Mental Health.
"Facts can be taught - concepts must be imagined." Muna Swairjo

Chronic mental illness have puzzled us since the beginning of time, it has not only bewildered and confused us as individuals throughout modern times … but it have indeed challenged physical science, theology, and medicine, at times, it has also threatened divisions within families, society and the Church. Faith In The Field: A Historical Religious Perspective On Mental Health, presents a clear explanation of this debilitating disease, and successfully introduces a theological viewpoint, in which the modern day Church currently under involved, could represent a broader role in serving the outpatient population afflicted with such.

At this socially sensitive time in mankind's history I would choose to successfully take this opportunity to institute a significant synopsis on mental health issues presented through these writings entitled, *Faith In The Field: A Historical, Religious Perspective On Mental Health.* The available manuscript describes in relevant detail the history of mental health, its treatments, and religious methodologies throughout the ages. In it, we present a clear, complete history on mental health, the origins of insanity, and the obvious changes and adaptations the system has endured throughout the last 2500 years and beyond. *Faith In The Field* is an academic, historical interpretation of mental health that successfully takes readers on a journey during a period previously unknown, prior to the understanding of the illness, the emergence of hospitals, the dawn of nursing, the inception of medicines, or the introduction to rational treatment. One of my chief reasons for writing this publication is to effectively provide a moral and spiritual understanding to the field of mental health, as well as a clearer and deeper understanding between the therapeutic milieu, our overall secular and non-secular society, Church and all other faith-based organizations, interested in the field of mental health. This would in turn perhaps soften the attitudinal approach, now shared between the Church and the secular psychological and therapeutic communities, toward those whom we attempt to aid in their recovery. Another fundamental reason for this book is to help break down barriers, purposely formulated by the stigma connected with mental illness, as we educate the general public about the true facts surrounding mental illness, its origins and prognoses.

Faith In The Field, provides an in-depth analysis on the role the Church played in the field of mental health throughout the 16th and 17th century, and focuses on the positive impact the modern Church and other societies of faith could have on the mental health community, if given an opportunity. Although in previous years working with the mentally ill was seen only as a responsibility for psychiatry and the psychological communities, the thorough research conducted throughout our journey to compose *Faith In The Field,* explains how theologian, Christians and counselors within the overall faith communities have also proven success in counseling the emotionally and mentally ill. Today treatment still remains primarily of special psychological and psychiatric concern, though it is not always the highly skilled mental health professional person alone who brings out the best results. For it is a cooperative team effort, in which all concerned entities play a significant role in treatment recovery. *Faith In The Field* also indicates and dutifully explains the uncovered benefits by merging the treatment of pharmacology and Dialectic Behavioral Therapy (DBT), with inherent spiritual counseling and the benefit of Nouthetic counseling. While it also place focus on how these methodologies combined can offer untold help. *Faith in The Field* indicates how this new approach demonstrates in many cases, shared responsibility and successful results. Data collected by Jewish, Buddhist, Islamic, Christian and other spiritual counselors while briefly visiting and aiding individuals suffering with mental distress, has also benefited the academic theory of *Faith In The Field*. In part, this has stemmed from an exclusive privilege and duty that also provides us with a list of basic theologian and Christian, spiritual guidelines, and recommendations for counseling the emotionally ill. *Faith In The Field,* provides an in-depth understanding of the study on Dialectic Behavioral Therapy (DBT), psychotropic, the daily application of the scriptures, and the critical absence of God's presence in the field of mental health. Overall, *Faith In The Field* is a complete psychological, sociological, ecclesiastical, and methodological reference. According to colleagues who have read and review the manuscript, *Faith In The Field,* "it is a literary gem that should be visible in the bookcases of every Church, Faith-Based or mental health facility in the world." WG …

My particular purpose is to connect with a diverse audience and bring forth a direct dialogue surrounding significant issues affecting the mentally ill and those who care for them, from the front lines of the mental health field *and leading into the Church*. The text is scholarly researched and creatively written in a manner that unquestionably makes it accessible to all who have an interest or a need to further their knowledge of the field, the history, educational policies and immediate scientific future of the field of mental health, and substance abuse, and those who find themselves as being part of these communities.

Statistics found within its pages bear several experts testimonies of the frequency with which mental health related issues affect our communities and the Church. The literary research within this publication is designed to alert our priests,' pastors, ministers and other spiritual leaders to comprehend that they too need to think about mental health as an urgent community epidemic. Our research clearly indicates that at least one third of all women will suffer from a bout of depression that schizophrenia affects approximately 1% of our population, and that serious bipolar disease affects 2-3% of the population. This basically suggests that if we are living in a town with a population of 50,000, there will be over 1,500 people with some type of mental illness.

If there are in excess of 100 people in our church, there is a good chance that some existing members will either suffer from mental illness or have a family member struggling with such at home. When most people are suicidal, one of the first places they tend to turn to is to their ministers. Although most theologians, Rabbi, ecclesiastic ministers, or faith base leaders currently do not have any special training to deal with this complex aspect of their ministry, nor do they have a full and complete understanding of mental illness. *Faith In The Field, weaves* a therapeutic understanding of the appropriate benefit of scriptures and psychoanalysis. Therefore, allowing emergent room for rapid nouthetic, theologian counseling and effective dialectic behavioral therapeutic intervention to the severity of the illness, while at the same time applying Biblical and overall spiritual answers.

In my many discussions with individuals suffering from this illness while conducting this investigation, one of the most intriguing questions that always came up, concerned ministers and special-needs people. They often questioned about their none blind friendly congregations, while at times humoring and showing their dissatisfaction, as they asked if these congregations were also deaf friendly? They also questioned "whether a supposedly hearing impaired individual, eventually wanted to attend a particular Church?" Should the mentally ill be in Church and what kind of special needs have been allotted if they attend or were encouraged to attend? And, how can the Church, reach out to the mentally ill living in our communities? Faith *In The Field* poses questions and suitable answers to these significant concerns.

The author is also available to conduct lectures and assist Churches and faith base outpatient community treatment centers, in meeting these essential needs through a series of workshops. During a recent interview with particular women in diverse communities, I was frequently reminded that many mentally ill individuals do struggle with religious issues. They often wondered "if God love them, and if God does, then why have God purposely created mental illness?" They also asked "then why didn't God also created a cure?" Others openly questioned "whether it is a punishment from God." *Faith In The Field, effectively* provides the required tools for spiritual leaders, when dealing with these deep and meaningful religious issues by teaching a deeper understanding to the counselor and counselee, interested in recognizing and teaching that God loves and cares about them. This is one of the most powerful messages we can give the mentally ill at a moment of current crisis in their lives. However, we must have the effective tools to avoid further confusing them. Throughout its pages, we also find a complete study on deinstitutionalization, the major impact this has placed on homelessness, the increased false incarceration of the chronic mentally ill, and the essential need for the Church to become an involved intercepting agent. *Faith in The Field* is a 200,000 word manuscript, with over 600 pages of detailed information based on the author's 25 years of experience effective career in the mental health field. The informative author also provides discussion groups, lectures, and one-on-one consultation to clergymen, pastors and ministers concerned in learning and sharing this vital perspective to their congregation, as well as to lay or secular treaters.

As we reflect on when our priests, pastors, rabbi, imam and other mosque and temple leaders call upon us to come forth and approach their pulpit, or asked to get out of our seats, and move forward. When our priest calls upon us to receive holy communion, we move forward. When our pastors calls upon us on communion Sundays, we head up toward the sanctuary.

When our Rabi speaks we listen, when our hearts receives the call for us to bow, facing the East and pray, we follow and when the gong is sounded, we search in deep meditation.

In the realities of a deep religious and spiritual examination, we are following by faith and somber conviction. These are not as easy to experience and perhaps unable to even be experienced by all. Faith is almost palpable, as it reaches out to God, and to those who are fortunate enough to have experienced true faith. When we experienced true faith, it feels as if being physically embraced by God. True faith often comes to us while seeking a closer and broader interpretation of ourselves.

Not long ago if you were to ask a scientist if he believed in God, he would have directly answered you bluntly and told you, "Of course not, I am a scientist." Today, if you were to ask a scientist the same question, he would answer you quickly and tell you, "Yes of course, I am a scientist." Dr. Wayne Dyer.

THERAPEUTIC RAIN DANCE

Softly the rain started with a slow unsteady beat
while dark clouds moved across the horizon
thickly gathered and piled across the skies now covering the heavens
In the midst of her turmoil, she received a welcome breeze
to quench her dry desert thirst no longer can she dance alone on her feet

She had been locked away … some said in a much safer place
no longer tormented by the voices she had again been set free
she's now all-alone discharged to the dangers of the streets
with no place to go … she takes cover under the sheets of rain
Said she's now free to dance and to sing off key … to speak her mind
to live her life as she pleases … to take her time and take what she needs
without fear of whom planted such seed

She is somebody's daughter she has a name and a face empathize
to enter her world in prayer spiritually you'll be in a far better place
Come along dance with me perhaps we all need this time in the rain
thus refresh our souls cleanse our wounds and ease our pain
holding hands in harmony rhythmically moving their feet
melodious as the accompanied music played by the wind and the rain
she remains in therapy together the voices they've since found their our own beat

Sabas Whittaker

CONTENTS

GENESIS

In search for the beginning of the cure.
From the ashes of destruction arises the phoenix
Like an angel of the skies to fly again among the clouds of smoke
after each and every devastation to again plant and irrigate the seeds of hope
and sprinkle upon the earth, the sun now dawns a new day.
A new world forest's to spring new trees ... flowers to again bloom with splendor,
beauty of health to abound forever.

The winds, birds ... even the recycled dried leaves to again come alive
as seasons change enough for diversity to unfold and spread new streams that'll
flow into giant rivers, emptying themselves into vast oceans and bleu lakes
The seas now abundant with fish and all manner of living, as deep-sea life again comes alive
all living together as a harmonious rhythmical dance, synchronized with planet earth ... evolution
begins anew and nature moves at its own pace toward recovery

To experience the day we no longer have a need for another arm's-race
thus instead asleep quietly knowing our children are in a far better place
where our wealth and our monies fund global research that'll perhaps help rinse mental illness from
the world's face, hence we'll forever look fort toward a healthier, thus loving, caring, productive
human race

Perhaps then we'll all delve in search to safer rooms thus secured and stable men and women to live
in this new beginning where we all dwell free from stigmas jealousy and deceit.
Today I asked is this a new beginning or is it the beginning anew.
Our living God will allow it to be so ... it's been said that all things begin and all things come to an
end, thus only eternity lasts forever. Our eternal faith remains steadfast, while our Creator allow our
faiths to endlessly flow. Sabas Whittaker
Inspired by a formerly diagnosed patient with mental illness (confidential)
We must then take the responsibility to play our part and therefore, work together with the rest of the world
to create a healthier and greener planet that'll also ban hatred among brothers and sisters since we're all
God's children in full heart.

ARE THERE ANY GOOD FRIENDS STILL LEFT OUT-THERE

While free on the outside so many claimed to have cared, although half of the time they weren't even there. A few friends to share simple words to a loyalty yet hard to find nurturing and understanding, perhaps of a true loving kind … from within the confined seclusion room of an asylum for the insane to her senses, she then became … Opening her eyes to look around at the four walls enclosing thus foreign to her surroundings, trying to recollect her thoughts she quickly composed a tender song … little voices that sung again repeatedly the same words.

Where are they, when you're all alone?
You'd think they'd at least pick up the phone.
True friends I said they're hard to find, am all-alone and no one has the time to even drop a dime
It's oh so hard to walk the walk, yet easy to talk the talk and care specially, when I look and see there's no one here …

Everybody needs a loyal friend not just a gossip partner to cover their tracks to mend.
As they ran around cheating on their spouse or playing the field sometimes it seems so unreal they're perhaps too anesthetize to even feel, just like mama's cancer such selfishness thus too hard to heal.

To everyone from the very young to the very old she'll ask again and again … wondering aloud so why are people oh so darn cold, when all we need is a little love to unfold … am sure we'll all make it through until the end with a little help from a true friend. Sabas Whittaker

Inspired by an inpatient on a psychiatric ward. (confidential)

ACKNOWLEDGEMENT

This book is primarily inspired by the thirty plus years of the most amazing journey, through the experiences learned, via the time spent, working and studying the field of mental health and the wisdom with which, I have been blessed; by aiding in the recovery of those whom suffered such. It is my humble representation to humanity regardless of their faith, their beliefs or their walk throughout life. To me, it was a mandate and a calling to share in the eyes of God, to dedicate part of my lifetime work to the contribution in making of a better and a healthier world, as believers of great faith, in our quest for peace, equality and social justice. This body of work is dedicated to the memory of my good friend and fellow mental health worker, *Pamela E. Godburn* … one of the best prepared and most devoted, care-giving angels to have ever worked the field of mental health. A special thanks and posthumous dedication is also given to my very good friend, supervisor and colleague, *Marie Jassie Langley* … who was perhaps the most effective psychiatric nurse, nursing supervisor and advocate by which we'd been blessed. *"Pam and Marie, you gave with your heart and it was appreciated, your humor and sincerity always carried a smile … never once have you shown a frown or given a cruel word to our patients or clients, yet even when most of our challenges thought it was deserved."* We know that you're in the rightful place where you belong … you are an inspiration to us all … your spiritual beings lives on in our memories and the warmest places of our hearts forever … We love you!

Although there were many whom came along to help build me up, throughout the years, thus allowing me to stand upright in this field, even while being severely injured physically. I must however, always remember to thank the person, whom my intellect, interest and my humanity, gave me my first lessons, first opportunity in mental health and bestowed upon me the confidence and the intellectual curiosity in the humanities that I would someday make a good mental health worker, my instructor and head nurse, Clinicians, APRN, PhD. Toby Newman.

Also wanted to kindly and sincerely thank all whom have contributed with their prayers, inspirations, and reviews or assisted in any of the many ways with data analysis and completion of this research. Although mentioning each and everyone of you on my list, would perhaps be long enough to put together another book, so I will first start with thanking my beautiful and wonderful wife Rev. Dr. Damaris D. Whittaker, Rev. Edwin and Doris Ayala for their spiritual support and Pastor Moses Harvil, for his prayers and inspiration, to my friend and colleague, The Rev. Dr. Ethel Graham Banks and my good friend, Rev. Marvin Bryant, his wife Marie and their beautiful family, whom first aided me with their blessings, talent, their choir, their church, their generous time and their creative contributions, as I prepared to produce a play on behaviorism (Don't Look Down on Your Brother if You're Not Going To Pick Him Up. That which benefited the homeless shelters in Torrington, and was presented at the Warner Theater, in Torrington Connecticut, back in 1991.

To my good friend, global equal rights and justice fighter, activist, colleague, Professor Chengiah

Ragaven, PhD., whom believed enough in me and in this body of work, to give me a place to stand, thus afforded me the opportunity to lecture to his class on social policies, at the University of Connecticut, Avery Point campus, Groton, Connecticut and later at Central Connecticut State University in New Britain, Connecticut. There I was able to stand tall and share portions of this material, prior to it being published… thus invigorating my research confidence to learn a whole lot more about my voice via your classroom and your students. To my good friend, paisano, colega y hermano, professor Dario Euraque, PhD., whom also provided me with the space, opportunity and a memorable reception, following my book signing and lecture to his class at such a prestigious institution, as Trinity College in Hartford Connecticut. To friends and colegas founders of the Honduras Relief Committee, Ana Alfaro, Carlos Rozales (RIP), Florence McNought, Reyna, Jose, Dario, Polly, Ramon, and all of those good people, whom I stumbled upon while on this journey, despite of all the hurdles encountered, you somehow encouraged tremendously by supporting my earlier work, and also kept me grounded by positively believed in my dream. A special thanks goes out to our team of mental health workers whom kept the Meriden CBI afloat, thus moving forward, despite the arduous political struggles. Program director: Psychotherapist, Clinician, Patricia Yuskis, MS. Head nurses, Edna Williams, RN.BSN, Josie Teart, RN, Alicerine Gums, RN. MSN. Case Managers, Psychiatric specialists Margarete Wilcox, Delores Wollard, Leela Marrow, Bridgette Naemon, MSW. Jaqueline Baker, Sidney Trusty, Renette Shields, Anabel Graham (RIP), Barbara Aiello, Nancy Richards, Captain, Rev. Mark Sharshmidth, MSW, Chaplain US Army, Carole Bobb, Sterling B. McClay. Michele Daniels, Pablo Valentin, office manager Gail Ryzner. Much gratitude also goes out to Dr. Rossi and his amazing outpatient team of clinicians and psych specialist, at the Iris House.

A very special spiritual gratitude and dedication goes up to the heavens, my mentors in ethics and philosophy, esteemed professors at the various learning institutions … gentle and caring sweet soul, whom literarily took me under their wings and taught me how to fly, therefore I learned to think like a philosopher. For such I am humble, honored to have meet you … I am forever grateful.

My sincere apologies if I missed anyone's names, believe me, it wouldn't have been done on purpose … However, I purposely saved the best for last … for their aren't enough words yet created to convey my gratitude to all of my other colleagues and friends, who put aside their music, family, schoolwork, church activities, took this project under their wings, and assisted me with editing, reviewing it, thus refueling my uninspired broken and exhausted spirit, to push this project on from concept of an idea, to a manuscript, then on to a book. *Thanks to all for your kindness, your love and your inspiration.*

PART 1

CHAPTER 1

The Moral World

(Inspired by my master's degree studies on ethics at Holy Apostles College and Seminary.)

To claim validity, hence fully understand mental illness or mental health and provide rational psychological, theological, or spiritual treatment and have possible results, one should first have in-depth knowledge of the moral world.

In order to fully understand mental health and mental illness from a spiritual or a religious perspective, we should first understand the moral world and the principles of bioethics as well as the Bible, the Torah, and the Koran.

The following questions and answers will help us further understand these principles and the true meaning of ethics as well as the many ways in which they could be applied to our daily lives.

1. How do we categorize the moral order?

   In order to categorize the moral order, we must first realize that the domain for morality is autonomous and that in order to mark the terrain of morality, we must insist that morality cannot be reduced to any other aspect of our lives.

2. What kind of art is ethics?

   Ethics is the art of living well.

3. How should we define ethics?

   We should define ethics as the reflective and categorical normative science and art that deals with free human actions under the light of reason.

4. What is the meaning of metaethics?

   Metaethics, is a second order of discipline, which takes for its subject matter and not the content of any particular moral position, but ethics itself.

5. What is the meaning of nihilism?

   Nihilism, is the denial of the validity of all distinction of moral values.

6. What is the meaning of relativism?

   Relativism points to the view that in a moral matter, there are no objective truths. Thus, morality is relative to one's society and culture.

7. What is the meaning of moral realism?

   Moral realism, focuses on the view that in some sense, there is an objective moral reality, and it insists that morality provides us with reason for our actions.

8. What is intuitionism?

Intuitionism, claims that morality can be objectively true or false and that we can come to know what moral principles are, in a special way by a kind of intuition or a direct awareness of our moral properties.

9. What is egoism, and what does it tell us?

    Egoism tells, us to live to further our own interests. However, the psychological egoist reminds us that we do this anyway because it is the law of nature.

10. Describe how behavioral science works and how it applies to our daily lives.

    The behavioral science, leads us to psychology, and in psychology, we learn of aggression, sexuality, and sexual maturity. Behavioral science, also leads us into sociology, where we could examine the moral agent from the social side. Behavioral science, then leads us into economics, where it shines the light on the ways in which social justice can be achieved or the injustices wield.

11. Describe the meaning of the value.

    Values are used to rate or scale our usefulness, our importance, and our general worth. Values, are conceptions of the desirable state of affairs that are utilized in a selective conduct of criteria, as preference and justification. This is later proposed as actual behavior.

12. Describe how moral values are applied to our daily lives and their involvement.

    Moral values always involves free choice. Moral values belong only to people or persons. Our moral values touch the people within themselves, and moral values imply obligation.

13. Define the moral apriori.

    According to Sheller, values are known prior to experiences, and they have ideal states. We know them by intuition. Just as an artist sees the beauty in his painting, so can men appreciate values by direct apprehension. The moral apriori is revealed in the so-called higher feelings. For Sheller, the basic structure of the moral order comes neither from experience nor from a pragmatic approach to problems and reflections of human behavior.

14. Describe the purpose of the functional autonomy.

    The functional autonomy was first made famous by Gordon Allport, who first indicated the possibility of an activity being able to outgrow its childish beginnings and still remain vital because of a higher motive. A child is made to practice the piano even though he hates it and prefers watching TV. He obeys out of fear and parental approval, but many years later, the piano playing continues because the function has become autonomous and lives on via its motivation.

15. What is mythology?

    Mythology is the instrument in the transition of ideals. Mythology helps to overlook the facts, and it makes man larger than life. Myth makes might.

16. Describe the difference between the characteristics of the introvert and the extrovert orientation, according to Carl Jung.

    In the life history of any given individual, one of the attitudes is usually dominant. While the extrovert enjoys large social gatherings with strangers being present, he remains interested in people. The extravert is interested in people with a spontaneous adaptability. On the other hand, the introvert's basic tendency is that of withdrawal. His libido flows inward and he finds his focus in subjective factors. In a social setting, the introvert lacks self-confidence and may even appear somewhat unsociable.

17. What is the meaning of "Homo homini lupus"?

According to Thomas Hobbes, the Latin phrase means that man is a wolf to every other man and that every person fears death. This is because even when the strongest man sleeps at night, he is vulnerable to any other man with a knife. If we follow our impulses, human life will remain just what it was in the jungle: solitary, poor, nasty, brutish, and short.

18. What is the purpose of the covenant?

    The covenant helps to soften the brutal implications of men's counterproductive tendencies. The covenant brings men together to form a society by way of a social contract in which each individual surrenders part of his autonomy on the condition that his neighbor does the same.

19. Who were considered the most articulate members of the moral sense school?

    The most articulate members of the moral sense school were the earl of Shaftsbury (1671–1713), Joseph Butler (1692–1752), and Francis Hutcheson (1694–1747). Hutcheson, however, remained the most sympathetic and consistent of all three men.

20. How would the moral sense ethicists explain the moral sense? Is it a special sense, or is it a feeling, an instinct, or a faculty?

    We find that Hutcheson is rather vague in truth. The strength of his explanations rests on an analogy between the aesthetic and the moral sense. That is, between the intuition of beauty and the vision of goodness. However, we can all agree that the aesthetic sense defies rational analogies.

21. As moral agents, how would we assess the moral sense?

    In order to fully assess the moral sense, we must first call attention to the fact that there is no other place for reason. But as for it being the supreme arbiter and final authority of right and wrong, in a moral situation, we simply see harmony or deformity. Optimistically, the moral sense ethicists assumed that benevolent affections have primacy over the aggressive impulses of the human heart. Nevertheless, this primacy is not a matter of reason but of noble actions and altruistic behaviors exhibiting harmony and balance. While the selfish destructive behavior shocks us with the distorted forms, the moral sense ethicists have failed to account for the relativity of moral insight and its dependencies of the faculty and culture.

22. Who was Immanuel Kant?

    Immanuel Kant was a professor of logic and metaphysics. He was also more thorough and technical than the easygoing theorists of the moral sense schools. He managed to establish himself as the foremost proponent of the deontological school.

23. What is the meaning of good will?

    Good will is a command that is totally conformed to our duty. If the will of man were pure and holy, obedience to the law would then be a pleasure.

24. Explain the forms of the categorical imperative.

    The categorical imperative comes in various formulations. Kant was able to express the rule in five different ways. One of the two most important formulations was the *maximum*, which can be universalized as a principle that says, *if everyone is free to steal, the community will fall apart, through thievery.* The other most important formulation is the *imperative* of morality, which commands us to respect ourselves and treat others in accordance with human dignity… *do not treat others as means, rather as ends.*

25. Explain the particulars of the practical reason.

    Practical reason shows us that there is a command given to man by his own rational nature, and it comes to us in the form of an imperative. Man should act in a way according to his dignity.

The unconditional category tells us to give back what we have stolen because of "practical reason." Here we find examples in which we realize that we are all too familiar with conditioning or hypothetical commands, such as "Come on time, if you intend to get a seat."

26. What is the postulate *assumption* of practical reason?

In order to make such an assumption, we must first assume that the agent is free, because every event is a consequence of a condition that went before. While he cannot prove that he is free, he affirms responsibility for his actions. The moral agent could assume that there is some kind of life after death.

27. What is the meaning of eudaimonia?

In classical Greek, the word *eudaimonia* means happiness or fulfillment, but etymologically it, means to be watched over by good demons. Although the word *happiness* could at times be misleading, as in the case of Aristotle, whom was perhaps thinking of some kind of activity that is performed for its own happiness sake.

Q, 28. Describe the outline of the Nichomanchean ethics?

A) The Nichomanchean ethics, famous lines tells us that every art, every inquiry, and similarly, every action and pursuit, is thought to aim at some good, reasons as to why the good, is highly declared to be that, which all things are aimed. We speak of the good, but good has several different meanings. *Man is an organism with many different tendencies, for some the final goal maybe pleasure or honor, while for others it might be power and wealth, but these goods are clearly ordered as means to something higher.* We must find the good that is sought for itself a good that is never ordered like money, material goods, nor power.

Q, 29. What are moral virtues?

A) Moral virtues, are good operative habits, just as vices are bad operative habits. These operative habits are defined by prudence, which help us to find their middle ground.

Q, 30. What are the intellectual virtues, and how could they be defined?

A) Aristotle defined the good life, as an activity in conformity with virtues. Virtue exists in both the moral and the intellectual sphere, although it would seem that the moral is directed to the intellectual as means to an end and it secures control of man's appetite, as means toward some higher and more inclusive end. Moral virtues, predispose us to practice the intellectual virtues.

Q, 31. What was the need for the Neoplatonic framework and what role did they served to the early Christian fathers?

A) The Neoplatonic was a vision first formulated by Plato and later modified by Plotinus 2057 AD. Plotinus and his Neoplatonic elements in ethics, gave present day ethics, its dynamism. That which would later appealed to the early Christian fathers, whom indicated that we are to picture the universe as a vast cyclic movement of goodness, pouring out and returning to the source.

Goodness emanates from a primal source and cascade downward to the material world. Man, part spirit, part matter, longs to return to the source of goodness to entail the purification and concentration that would later enable him to ascend.

Q, 32. How would we best define and outline of the pars secunda?

A) The outline of the pars secunda, is defined in three parts. A) pars prima, which begins with God, as he is one tribune in himself, and the Creator, in the creation of goodness and beauty is poured out. B) pars secunda, tells us that we have an account, were man returns to the Epistrophe 'sources of goodness' by actions since actions have end. "Pars secunda, begins with man's last end by trying to follow the analysis of actions. We often question ourselves, what makes us human and what modifies our virtues?" We must first consider the passions to be modified by virtues of goodness and badness, for which we would have to imply an eternal standard; 'God's Eternal Law,' which comes from the mind and the will of the creator. In the second part of the pars secunda, we begin with the three theological virtues faith, hope and charity then we see how these virtues are applied to our everyday life.

C) In part tertia, we see Jesus as the remedy for sin and a guide to eternal life, through his work, which we understand that he provided to the church and the sacraments. *In order to appreciate these theological settings, we must first see that God has destined us for a goal before the grasp of reason. "No eyes, has seen what you have prepared for those who love you."* In order to pursue these goals we need teaching, because all actions are goal oriented. But in rational creatures, actions should follow the reasoned inclinations of the will, intelligent creatures do not only pursue the goal, but they direct themselves to goals freely chosen.

Q, 33.   What is your understanding of the Visio Beatifica?

A) The Visio Beatifica helps to differentiate between man's highest activities, his highest powers and his highest object. "Happiness is above all the activity of contemplating the things that are, since the object of the intellect is truth, and since God is truth himself and since the mind is directed to God." In the scripture we are told that "we shall see God, this really means to know Him directly and immediately because the role of the will is to rejoice in the good already possessed." The Visio Beatifica also indicates that the creature is completely happy and fulfilled with the love of God he now posses.

Q, 34.   What is the proximate norm of morality?

A)   While searching for the standard in an objective norm that can be applied to the trans-cultural ways of our system, we have realized that ethics is the science and art that tells us what we ought to do. This makes ethics the normative, but while the final norm of morality, is right practical reason by way of these virtues we come to realize that justice and temperance should be cultivated because they are in accord with the reason. "It is reason which tells us that certain actions accord with good order and that certain actions are neutral, while others are in direct violation of an order which we should uphold."

In religion faith becomes our guide, because of reason reflecting on its own time limitations. It sees the need for revelation on which it must reflect. Customs can be trusted, providing it appears before the bar of reason. ST. Thomas Aquinas claimed that all good men can govern their lives in the light of the 'natural law.'

Q, 35.   What credentials does reasoning have by which it qualifies as the proximate norm of morality?

A) Reasoning qualifies as the primary norm of morality by realizing that our world is contingent and only by reasoning we can assess the entire situation. Therefore, analyzing from the outside and from above and grasping with our minds all the relevant factors, past and present as ends and means. "It might be right to argue that the mind is only one aspect of the personality this is true. However, all aspects of our personality are present in the mind." a) Reason alone is public and objective, b) reason is self-corrective, c) reason is flexible, e) reason is also rational and irrational.

Q, 36.   How would you define the natural law?

A) Although it is an un-unified doctrine, it is also true that the theory rest upon certain general assumptions, the word natural and law remains however ambiguous. The natural law is an unwritten moral law, more or less the same for all men due to its foundation on the basis of man's rational nature.

Q, 37. Define the primary, secondary and tertiary precept of the natural law?

A) The primary precepts begins with a dynamic sense of our own being, because we have unfinished inclinations, tendencies and desires. But we see the need for a cohesive social order which depends on some kind of authority and at times impulses by the aesthetic. "As grown adult children, we do realize it is expected that we should respect our parents, nevertheless, we must first take into consideration that the family must be stable and cruelty toward the grown adult children must be avoided."

The secondary precept helps us to understand the logical process, while norms are made more specific, they direct us to the practical syllogism. However, analogous, it is still reasoning.

"At this time we consider the case of slavery which is immoral." To see why moral reasoning differs from scientific procedure, we must remember that in evaluating moral consequence, cultural and important previous conditioning plays an important factor. *Although Aristotle is often considered one of the founding fathers of the ethical science, he explicitly justified slavery; as did Thomas Jefferson and the English philosopher John Locke.* The tertiary precepts shows us that as we decent to the particulars the rule becomes ambiguous, while identifying the qualities and powers, e.g. a thing has in virtue principles of its secondary precepts just as they exist in virtue of its primary precepts. "The flower is attracted to the butterfly, because of its color, just as the wine is expensive because of its taste." 1) We come to the primary precept by intuition. 2) the secondary precept is enrolled with contingencies of culture and pre-training.

Q, 38. How can we define law in the widest sense?

A) We may define law as an ordination of reason for the common good, made by one who cares about their community and promulgates or proclaims such.

Q, 39. What do we mean, when we talk about the Eternal Law?

A) When we talk about the 'Eternal Law,' we are talking about the wisdom of God, as it direct all things to their proper end. *The eternal law is the supreme and final norm of morality. "No man knows the mind and the will of God directly." We have discovered the divine plan only by reflection of the world, which we have experienced.* Hence we first know the natural law which redirects man's participation in the eternal law. The natural law and the eternal law are internally connected and are different sides of the same coin.

Q, 40. What do we know about the positive law?

A) The positive law helps to make clear what could be ambiguous in the natural order of things, the positive law is a rule of action established by competent authority for the common good and promulgated by some external sign whether oral or written.

Q, 41. What is the true meaning of obligation?

A) Obligation is the first property of law. When we talk of obligation, we are referring to the oughtness or the morally compelling aspects of the law. This law comes to us as a mandate, which compels obedience. To act against this law, is to disobey it. "The binding forces of the natural law, comes from the fact that it is a participant in the eternal law." The Creator has ordered his creatures to define ends, as rational individuals, we are to participate and to cooperate in the directedness of God's plan for the whole of things.

Q, 42. What do we mean when we talk about sanctions?

A) When we talk of sanctions, we are referring to the reward for compliance and the threat of punishment for failure to comply. Sanction, is added by the lawmakers to ensure obedience. "In the eternal law, sanctions are rewards given to the faithful and the punishment allotted to sinners. In the natural law, sanctions are rather imperfect." *the weakening of the will, the experience of guilt and the discord in society.* "In the positive law, the sanctions are explicit and are usually expressed in print."

Q, 43. Who were the Stoics, and what is Logos?

A) The Stoic is a unified logical, moral, physical and moral school of philosophy. It tells us that the world order is directed by the divine and impersonal logos 'world mind' and that human reason participates in the eternal 'logos,' which orders all things to their appointed ends. *Every man is both, (a), a solitary individual and (b), a citizen of the world community and he must do justice to both.*

Q, 44. What did St. Thomas Aquinas meant by Synderesis?

A) Synderesis is a supposed natural or innate ability of the mind, which helps us to know and recognize the first principle of ethics and moral reasoning.

Q, 45. What is the meaning of Etiam daretour non esse deum?

A) Hugo Gratious, Dutch Jurist and State-man 1583 - 1650, was later considered the father of modern international laws, when he published the laws of war and peace. In it Gratious, insisted that the natural law would retain its validity, even if we assumed there is no God. (Etiam daretour non esse deum). Gratious also argued that the mind can construct a science of thought by careful analysis of definition, but Gratious looked to reason alone as his guiding light.

Q, 46. In what year was The Universal Declaration of Human Rights was declared and what is its definition?

A) Prior to World War II in 1945, there were no definitions of human rights, although several human rights principles, were codified into limited agreement prior. After World War II, the world's first truly substantial international call for human rights appeared in the charter establishing the United Nations. The charter reaffirms 'fundamental human rights in the dignity and worth of the person, in the equal rights of men and women' and established the goal for promoting and encouraging respect for human rights and for fundamental freedoms for all without distinction as to race, sex, language or religion. Revolutionizing for the very first time, human rights international concerns, and not just prerogative of individual governments. Later that same year, on December 10th 1945, the United Nations General Assembly, adopted the Universal Declaration of Human Rights, thus setting the standard for all future human rights work.

Q, 47. What are the components of a right?

A) When we reflect on the meaning of a right in both the subjective and the objective sense, we find four components. a) The subject, b), the oblige, c) the object of the claim, and d) the title. However, we must insist that the subject of these rights can only be persons. The rights of the individual maybe extended to moral and juridic beings e.g., a corporation, the army, the government and those oblige must also be persons. "A master may never own a man as a slave you may hire a person and direct him functionally."

Q, 48. Define the sources of the human rights?

A) While looking for the radical basis on human rights we questioned. On what basis is a man allowed to own property, or demand a fair trial, or to express his beliefs in public? To explain such rights, we would have to go back a few centuries, when man concentrated strongly on human rights. Like the American Constitution which contains the Bill of Rights, or go back to 1789 when the French National Assembly drew up The Declaration of the Rights of Man, which served as a preamble to the new constitution. The charter of the United Nations assumes that all men are created equal before the law and that all men enjoy basic of human rights. But what is the basis on which these statement rest? They rest upon the Natural Law.

Q, 49.   What is the difference between natural rights and acquired rights?

A) It will be our contention that the final justification of natural rights is found in the natural law. The natural law comes to us as a command. As free persons, we humans assent to the order, which is intended by the creator e.g., "We are all obliged to seek self-fulfillment, whoever wills the end, is ought to will the means; God is also the author of human rights."

Of course, we would all agree that most of our rights are acquired, but acquired rights find their origin in natural rights.

Q, 50.   Enumerate some of the titles by which a right is acquired?

A) They are seven known titles by which rights are acquired … a) occupancy, b) labor, c) gifts, d) inheritance, e) accession, f) prescription and g) contract.

Q, 51.   What is a social contract and what purpose does it serves?

A) The overwhelming majority of our rights are acquired by way of contract. A contract is a transfer of a right, so that something, which was not a right, becomes a right. What was a right, is alienated in favor of another. The contract promises and establishes an obligation in the one that is being promised.

Q, 52.   What is an onerous or bilateral contract?

A) An onerous or bilateral contract, comes to us in the form of Du ot des, or quid pro quo. "I gave in order that you give," it is an agreement upon sufficient consideration.

Q, 53.   What is a licit contract?

A) A licit contract is a real contract. The contract becomes ab initio, or 'invalid,' when one of its essential elements are missing e.g., "A man sells a car which he has stolen, the sale becomes ab initio because the car was never his to sell." The contract then becomes illicit, when it violates moral or civic laws. An aleatory contract, functions as the involvement of chance or some undetermined future events. An example of that is found in the purchase of a lottery ticket, or a visit to the casino, "they do not guaranty any winnings, but if you win, they'll pay out the money."

Q, 54.   What is a conscience, and what is its purpose?

A) In all cultures there exists a basic phenomena, we call conscience. e.g., Man may differ in the more precise details, but we are all familiar with the interior voice and all men has experienced guilt of some kind and are at times proud of themselves. We have all hesitated at one time or another because we are confused about the moral probity; "some may speak of the voice of God while others prefer the expression 'judgment of reason,' but it is the task of the ethician to clarify the making of our inner standard."

Q, 55.   What does Etymology tell us about conscience?

A) Etymology tells us that the word conscience means, a knowledge that goes along with, or accompanies an awareness of something else. "A very general awareness of the first principle of the moral order could involve two kinds of conscience."

Q, 56.   How can we apply conscience to a moral habit and what does a moral habit implies?

A) Moral habit implies that at all times, all men should be aware of an adjective moral order. "We find ourselves blaming others, accusing them, accusing ourselves and encouraging friends to live in more honorable ways; while we may disagree about cruelty, all seem to concur in that judgment of wanton 'excessive' cruelty is objectively wrong."

Q, 57. Describe how conscience works as an act and as a concrete judgment?

A) In this, case we have found that all things should be considered … an intended action, be it either moral or not. After reflecting on the relevant data of such act, the moral faculty must formulate some kind of judgment. e.g., is it morally wrong to abort a baby? "Here, we must first define the act of a conscience as judgment of practical reason and that a certain action, is all circumstances considered, morally right, wrong, or different for this subject."

Q, 58. What is the Meaning of Synderesis?

A) The word Synderesis used by St. Thomas Aquinas, is probably a corruption of the Greek word 'syneidesis,' or conscience. The development of our moral conscience takes place under the light of the 'synderesis' our conscience, which is the habit of our first moral principle.

Q, 59. How should we distinguish between the antecedent and the consequence of a conscience?

A) The antecedent conscience, forbids us and reproves certain actions, while our consequence conscience, accuses incites guilt and excite penance.

Q, 60. Describe and list the different state of conscience?

A) The list is comprised with three major components, a) antecedent and consequence, b) right from erroneous or lax conscience, c) a perplexed or scrupulous conscience.

Q, 61. What are the basic directives for conscience?

A) In order to freely describe the basic directive of conscience, we must first follow a conscience, which is at once certain and correct By certain, we mean 'definitely' correct, or in accord with objective standards. In matters of great importance, we may never act in a state of practical doubt; meaning that "we must read the law again, seek advice, or use the reflex principles if doubt still remains."

Q, 62. In what form does the final say of conscience comes to us?

A) It comes to us as free choice, or 'liberum arbitrium.'

Q, 63. Who was Lawrence Kohlberg and what stages of conscience did he focus on?

A) Lawrence Kohlberg, was an American psychologist who did research on the stages of growth by which our conscience evolves. His emphasis, were placed mainly on the cognitive in which moral decisions are explained. e.g., why is it wrong to disobey our parents, God teachings and the law? How serious is it to steal? How can we tell what one is obliged to do?

Kohlberg, was also interested and influenced by Jean Piaget and his concept of 'the moral judgment of a child,' and his aspects of cognitive and developmental psychology, but he was even more influenced by Max Webber and his theory of the idealized types. "The sociologist must be able to put himself in the mind of those whom he studies."

Q, 64. How did Kohlberg employed his studies on methodology?

A) Kohlberg employed his study by gathering material on conscience formation and by following his subjects from childhood into adult, and by questioning their behavior in a three year intervals. This enabled him to follow the level of moral subject that later helped to clearly identify and mark these stages, with the following characteristics. A) The sequence of stages is age related, B) each successive stage is qualitatively different from the preceding stage, C) each stage is more comprehensive than its predecessor, D) the stages are developed by an invariant sequence, or conventional morality.

Q, 65.   What is conventional morality?

A) Conventional morality is to a large extent culturally determined by usage or habit in the process of what we call socialization. e.g., "We all learn to follow the leader."

Q, 66.   What and how do we best define the six stages of moral growth?

A) In order to follow these stages, we must first come to the understanding of pre-conventional morality, which is identified by fear and punishment. e.g., *We all obey the law out of fear,* though our question still remains open *What is good and what is evil?* The egoistic stage, which follows the evidence of calculation; this stage amounts to a kind of deal. The good boy stage, *"in this we seek some sort of social conformity or pay off by others.* The law and order stage, which ask for social maintenance and demands for clear rules of decision making,

This law at times is subjected to external control. The contractual level, this stage displays a healthy movement from the heteronomous to the autonomy by a kind of in-depth personalization, by focusing on the conventional origins of the positive law.

That is toward a consensus. e.g., *Man was not made for the Sabbath, but the Sabbath was made for man.* The level of conscience, this stage takes us back to the absolute 'pure,' but its appeal is made to the absolute principles and ultimate values. *In order to make this appeal, we must first understand that a principle is higher than the rule, because while a rule is specific, 'do not steal,' a principle is general, e.g.,* all humans are worthy of dignity. Rules are needed, but they serve a higher purpose toward protecting the principles. We must justify each course of action undertaken. Because it is more compassionate or because it will equal the opportunity for someone, whom is otherwise handicap or physically disable to work, park, participate or compete? Should we recommend some programs for the mentally ill, because it enhances their dignity and freedom, and perhaps even foster a sense of responsibility? While rules are never absolute, ideals and principles never change. A closer example of these could be clearly examined, when we look at 'Affirmative Action' or as we attempt to advocate for better treatment to the individual suffering with mental illness.

The Need To Update Our Spiritual Faith Throughout the Mental Health Field

Throughout the last one hundred years or so, American psychiatry has shifted its field of fundamental activity from being mainly concerned with custodial care of the individual client with mental illness, to an emphasis on the treatment of ambulatory patients. In our present time, this transfer has changed to a significant concern for the immediate family, their home, the church, the school, the job, marriages, juvenile delinquency and narcotic addictions. Concurrently, institutional patterns in psychiatric care, have undergone gradual changes, leading to an open-door policy, in many hospitals throughout the country and other countries throughout the world.

When we think of the spoken word faith, we must also think of the ministerial meaning of psychological anguish, pain and relative confusion, which exist in the hearts and disturbed minds of those individuals suffering with mental illness. We must also think of their redemption and about the notable isolation, despair and depression that plague their everyday lives that further weighs them down.

When we look at sustained faith, we must first remember that we want to be loved. Each of us definitely need to understand and to believe strongly that God loves us, therefore, faith tells us that we must effectively instruct others to love God. Although its been over a hundred and forty years since the church has been practically altogether removed from the field of mental health, we pray that "the powers that be" opens their hearts and their institutional doors to once again to afford an opportunity for those individuals suffering with mental illness to benefit from the Christian and all other forms of theological counseling, by actively allowing a little more of God back into the field of mental health. Throughout the centuries we have treated, investigated and documented, what complex conditions and what special features have lead people to fall into the traps of mental illness. The church's last serious attempt to lead the march on mental hygiene, was spearheaded by a then very young, Sunday school teacher by the name of Dorothea Dix.

The core of this book, is to attempt to grapple with the issues raised by such questions, as we affectionately recognize that even in this day and age, we pose very little rational concept upon the nature of mental illness. And about what it is, what causes it and what will actually cure it, although this is true even among psychiatrists, psychologists and the mental health and psychiatric communities as a whole. This immediate admission of ignorance does frustrate and significantly impact our attitudes in the extensive field, toward the large amount of contending interpretations retained throughout the centuries about mental illness and varied key reasons for their particular purposes and treatments. Insanity, mental illness, madness, craziness or whatever other name the respected psychiatrists, psychologists and sociologists, society including the voracious consumers themselves have managed to label it with; throughout the years it still remains an elusive phenomena. Lifelong institutionalization is now a rarity. Most patients basically recover enough to be care for in their individual homes and their own communities. Community help for the mentally ill has systematically forged ahead enormously in the last two decades, nonetheless much work is still required to successfully accomplish the continuous task. Although we still do not know the exact causes for the major mental illnesses, such as schizophrenia, bipolar affective disorder (manic depression) or clinical depression, essential treatment is now available. Researchers relentlessly continue to look at genetics in an underlying attempt to successfully identify the causes. Although a definite cure may not come in our time, perhaps it will for our children and their children. The stigma of mental illness has not yet been fully eradicated. However, the collective move to equate mental illness with physical illness has resulted in greater understanding on some fronts, as to the particular course of the disease. Sad, though truthfully so, we still have a long way left to go, but we'll keep on working on it.

Abuse on The Mentally Ill Versus Slavery

When we think of chronic mental illness, we cannot successfully avert surveying the correlations and controversies the great ancient philosophers made among themselves on the significant issues of freedom versus conceptual morality. Nor should we repeatedly omit the conventional fact that in those days, non-Greeks were automatically regarded to be inferior. Therefore, if one were not of all out-Greek origins, they were instinctively either barbarians or slaves. They rendered this, while simultaneously arguing that the birthright to all Greeks, was that of free moral agents; perhaps just a limited number of intellectuals among the many were permanently excluded. This theory sends us back to philosophy and to a comprehensive examination of the interpretations of the primary, secondary and tertiary precept of the natural law. The primary precept begins with a dynamic sense of our personal being, because we have unfinished inclinations, tendencies and desires. But we frequently realize the demand for a cohesive social order. That, which depends on some interpretive sort of authority and at times is impulse by the aesthetics, e.g. *A, man pragmatically realizes that he should consistently respect his parents, but we must first take into careful consideration that the family must be stable … therefore, 'collective cruelty, must be effectively avoided and removed.'*

The secondary precept helps us to instinctively understand the logical process, while norms are made more specific; they direct us to the practical syllogism. However, analogous, it is still natural reasoning. At this time we take into consideration the contentious case of slavery, which is immoral. To generally understand why moral reasoning differs from scientific procedure, we must continuously recognize that when evaluating the moral consequences, cultural and societal previous imperative conditionings represents an important factor.

Although Aristotle was one of the founding fathers of the ethical science, he explicitly justified slavery and so did the world renowned English philosopher, John Locke who also did the same. Locke, was no ordinary character, he was then being regarded as one of the chief pioneers in innovative thinking, who besides had also made some of the greatest contributions to the literary academic analysis of politics, government and psychology. "Locke is exactly the same man, whose writings also inspired the framework to one of our most treasured documents, the American Constitution." The tertiary precepts shows us that as we descend to the particulars, the practical rule becomes ambiguous, while identifying the qualities and adequate powers … a thing have in virtues principles of its secondary precepts, just as they exist in virtue of its primary precepts. e.g., *the butterfly is attracted to the flower because of its color, as the wine is expensive because of its taste.* (a) We have come to the primary precept by intuition (b) The secondary precept is enrolled with the contingency of cultures and pre-training. While comparing the significant issues of morality, personal freedom and slavery, we cannot subsequently and repeatedly omit the similar ways in which stigma, the inhumane, ill treatment, poor living conditions, the critical lack of understanding, poverty, and the overall dehumanizing conditions that have continuously been placed on the ordinary lives of chronically mentally ill individuals throughout history.

Be it whether in large state-run facilities, community outreach centers, or private nonprofit secular and religious outpatient clinics, access to appropriate quality of care should adequately exist and remain rather available at all times for those with such needs. In interpreting the critical description among the primary, secondary and tertiary precepts of the natural law, as productive representatives of a moral and civilized society, we must first educate ourselves around the predominant significant concerns of mental health treatment.

Moreover, we must intelligently learn to willingly accept individuals suffering with mental afflictions. We have constantly learned to accept the cancer patients, the diabetic, the emphysema patients, or those suffering with abnormal heart condition, etc. My personal opinion is that we do not point at, nor talk about individuals seen on a regular basis out in the community porting insulin administering waist pouches, nor towing, pushing their portable oxygen tanks and other medical breathing apparatus.

Another fundamental reason behind this study, stems partially from frustrations witnessed among family members while trying to care for their loved ones and how such lack of thorough extensive knowledge of mental illness hampers treatment and care. These frustrations tend to spill over and emanate among the immediate caregivers, while trying to communicate their experiences and optimistic suggestions to overzealous, partially educated or carefree supervisors and limited number of rather unconcerned treatment team members. Such frustrations grows and tends to conventionally lean more toward a pessimistic and an unrealistic attitude, particularly toward those clients that have placed obstacles, unintentionally hampering their individual care, or considered resistive to treatment and strenuous to deal with. It is probably important to recognize from the start that the contemptuous attitudes of some mental health care providers have also been a significant obstacle when developing effective services for this patient population ... particularly these functions, which have for long been alternately romanticized and stigmatized over the years. Most people are repelled by the chronically mentally ill, often times this may necessarily include even some doctors, some psychiatric nurses, limited number of social workers and even some mental health workers. A mixture of deep fear, cautious guilt and a desire to keep one's distance from them, colors collective reaction to this patient group.

The undisputed truth of the particular issue is that mental patients, particularly those diagnosed with borderline personality disorder and the chronically psychologically ill does not always behave 'well.' This is examined from a variety of social and psychodynamic perspectives, they act poorly and their bad behavior unexpectedly put themselves and others at risk. They unexpectedly place others at risk, due to their deviant behavior, this is particularly found on the part of loved ones, or when they constantly produce an excessive amount of stress to those involved with their individual treatment. By this we obviously mean that any parent would be critically distressed by the sight of their daughter wandering around the neighborhood naked and openly talking to herself. Equally would they feel about a son who's been reportedly seen downtown eating out of garbage cans, repeatedly being involved in local bar brawls, or being apprehended shoplifting and thrown in jail? Although it is less readily acknowledged that for a therapist, it is far less, however, still distressing for them to have a patient wandering around hallucinating in the front lobby of the mental health facility. Or to have a patient knocking out other patients, assaulting staff members and repeatedly going into locked seclusion or mechanical restraints.

Trying to Find Reasoning Behind Historical World Mental Illness

Throughout Western academic traditions, the Greeks first tried making common sense of mental illness, or historical madness by firstly enhancing alternatives and basically requiring interpretations. In our academic analyses on Greek mythology and the Homeric epics, we will surely encounter the remnants of archaic attitudes towards the mentally ill and their deeds. Throughout these we will see where ancient Greek heroes go mad, some are driven wild, others become beside of themselves with heated fury, revenge or enormous grief. Although these myths do not present insanity in the collateral terms that were later pioneered by classical medicine and regulatory philosophy; their heroes neither possesses psyches comparable to that of Oedipus in Sophocles' play, still less to that of Hamlet nor Sigmund Freud.

As we carefully study and reexamined the ancient epic, at first glance, we might see that the individual's mentality it represents definitely offer its inherited characters no sensitive, reflective inner self or a mind of their own. We instead see it grappling with what many of the reliable experts in the field would call it at first glance, "the choice of life." Homer's heroes are alternatively more like puppets, temperamental players at the starboard mercy of significant forces, fundamentally from beyond and beyond their applicable control of gods, demons, fates and furies. Instead these myths, obviously shows us that they each have their own destiny as warriors, kings, sons, daughters, fathers, etc. They also possess powerful physical bodies for executing deeds. Homer tells us far more about their deeds than their deliberations. Their fates are decided to a large degree by instructions from above, often revealed to them through insights or dreams. These mythological characters were often cursed and pursued by terrible powers, which successfully punishes, avenged and sometimes destroy by driving the demented to suicide.

Though not fully descriptive, however, a relevant process of mental pollution and purification drives many to physical destruction. Throughout all of this, the inner life with its confusions of fundamental reason and conscience of afflictions of mental strife is certainly not yet seen as the vital center of immediate attention. Nevertheless, the contemporary mental landscape and its symbols were now emerging as the highest point of Greek civilization in the fifth and fourth centuries BC. During this era, Athenian thinking about the psyche would develop to set the pattern for out minds and insanity in the Western mind and would remain present ever since. Greek philosophers energetically set about subjecting nature, human society and collective consciousness to fundamental reason. Their definite aim is to primarily tame anarchy, widely establish reasonable order, and conventionally impose self-discipline. Rationality then became a definitive part of the noblest faculty in man, where logic and the theoretical cosmic order could still be generally perceived, and therefore, help to state a deeper understanding toward the ill nature of man. In ethics we further see and could clearly understand how reason could also be realized in order to attained through self-knowledge and open the doors to a broader and deeper understanding of human nature itself and thereby control our lower animal urges within, 'homo lupos homini.' Therefore, philosophy was then established as the most essential component toward understanding reason. Although most Greeks did not deny the practical reality to the irrational, as a matter of fact the very adulation they presented to the fundamental reasons successfully indicates their acceptance and high admiration for the mysterious forces of enthusiastic passion, typical destiny and fate which reason strongly opposed. By the same token, other schools of Greek philosophers, the stoics in particular, clearly exposed the irrational as a problem and considered it threatening and shocking, while in fact arguing fundamental reasoning should combat. They never lost their terror for the primordial forces, possessing the mind and often toying with human destiny or their admiration for the enthusiastic passion and fire, which seized geniuses and artists, lighting up visions of the divine. However, from Plato onwards, they descriptively defined how the madness of the irrational was the gigantic rock placed in the pathway of human dignity; and the contradictive parts between the rational and the irrational. Seemingly showing how the rightful sovereignty of the rational, could become fundamental to both and how their moral and scientific vocabulary, flow through them, to ours.

Philosophy enabled the Greeks to reflect upon madness with fundamental reason, by which, Homer's heroes then became the conscious objects of theoretical reflection, responsibility and guilt of inner conflicts of mind that splits between and against themselves. As in a standard form of ancient therapy they devised a distinctive technique for the future played out in speech, tragic drama, art and live theater to deal with emotional conflicts and dramatic tragedies; by which the individual's drama crushed the ineluctable rival demands of unconditional love, distinguishable hate, pity and potential revenge, enforceable duty and ambiguous desire. They obviously found that drama also suggested passages of genuine resolution and as they learnt to roll-play, they promptly adapted to using theater as cognitive therapy. These ancient Greeks were of the opinion that mental illness, or madness could be attributed as a condition of sickness of the static soul as expressed by the arts and they developed a quite different way of treating it medically. When confronted with epilepsy, which was then considered to be a sacred disease, their scientific doctors of the Hippocratic tradition, daringly denied the fact that it was a supernatural miraculous visitation from above. In an opposing manner, they strongly asserted that it was a physical illness and a product of the common powers of nature.

The ancient scientists then suggested that all abnormal maladies and all types of mental illness could also be claimed and treated by natural medicines. Confirming then that these explanations could later draw upon physical causes affecting other organs, such as the heart, the brain and the blood; as well as their spirits and often even the individual's bizarre humor. They then insisted that these cures should rely upon regimen and medicines for the scientific treatment of temper, mania, and melancholy were diseases intelligible interconnected to the human anatomy and pathology. Although, perhaps the classical thinkers were not quite clear in defining, nor solving the nature of mental illness for future generations, however, by elevating the mind they valued reason, order and cosmic intelligibility. The point being is that through their attempt on making man the measure of all things, they also made mental illness human.

Although the Greek legacy in the end never managed to solve the riddle of the Sphinx's, nor the divide between the psychological and the somatic theories of madness, throughout history both theories have had their attractions and their setbacks. However, the culture of medieval, Latin Christendom absorbed both of the Greek alternatives to madness as a moral trauma, and madness as a disease. The early Christianity also placed these two alternatives within the cosmic Christian system of Divine intervention, by which it therefore imparted a higher significance to both. Early Christian theology of course, also managed to view mental illness in quite a different light, thus far alien to the once centered ancient Greek philosophy. And from such point onward mental disorder was checked off as the war for the possession of the soul, as the 'psychomachy' waged between God and Satan, or good and evil. Therefore, medieval theological minds, regarded mental illness as religious, as moral, as medical, as divine, or as the exact diabolical line between good and bad. Intern, the Scientific Renaissance nor the Enlightenment minds of such era would succeed, thus, yet still fail to crack the mystery of mental illness … for which they were no significant scientific medical breakthroughs. To best frame such, it could be said "there was no Newton in the field of insanity, and definitely no Copernican revolution in the psychiatric arena, boasting upon the discoveries of the secrets that lay within the human mind. Through the Middle Ages and far beyond, people with mental illness rarely had any special, formal provision. Refuges, or hospital were almost, but unknown and stigma was already heavily burdened. A few number of homes for the insane were set up, a few asylums appeared in fifteenth-century Spain, around the same time the Bethlehem Hospital in London, began to specialize in caring for people suffering with mental illness. Some monasteries accepted what was then known as the 'odd and lunatic.' Mostly, however, lunatics were looked after, or neglected within the family and kept under the watch of the village community.

Most were simply allowed to wander the streets. Some state throughout the union, undertook limited welfare functions, yet the old intermingling of lunatic with people at large, possibly preserved some residual sense of common human dignity. This perhaps intervened with enough sociological binding force, to prevent a fostering of a 'them and us,' thus creating a division, which would have essentially alienated the 'them' as human beings, or perhaps even as a race apart. However, this gratitude could best be given to the early Christian teachings, which perhaps helped to maintain some sense of seeing the person suffering with mental illness as a fellow human being, a creature made in God's image and with equal feelings as all other believers. The early preachers then also insisted that "if all men were sinners, then the distinctions of the world and its outward trappings of rank, wealth, education and success might in the end count for very little in the eyes of God. Moreover, the early Christians also sought out special circumstances to form and justify their beliefs by which to form a positive value upon mental illness. "Insanity," they argued, "might of course be God's punishment for crime," as they pointed to the case of Herod's madness to exemplify. "But madness could also be holy, and seen as a faith founded upon the madness of the Cross." They then insisted that, "a crusaded against worldliness, which lauded the innocence of the infant, valued the spiritual mysteries of contemplation, asceticism and the mortification of the flesh and prized faith over intellect, could not help but see gleams of godliness in the simplicity of the fool or in ecstasies and transports of life." The Enlightenment endorsed the Greek's faith in reason and the enterprise of the age of reason, gaining authority from the mid-seventeenth century onwards, was to criticize, condemn and crush whatever its protagonists considered to be foolish or unreasonable. Therefore all beliefs and practices which appeared ignorant, primitive, childish, or useless came to be readily dismissed as idiotic or insane, evidently the product of 'stupid thought-processes,' or delusion and daydream. And all that was so labeled as such could be deemed inimical to society or the state. Indeed it was then regarded as a menace to the proper workings of an orderly, efficient, rational society. Around this time the early distinction, which the Greeks had drawn between unreason and between fully rational members of society came to weigh increasingly heavily. The growing importance of science and technology, the development of bureaucracy, the formalization, the flourishing of the market economy, the spread of literacy and education, all made their contribution to this nebulous and inexorable process of prizing rationality, as understood by the right-thinking society, who had the power to impose social norms. Solidly proving and convincing that abnormality among our society, could indeed provoked anxiety. The insane, they argued, is as likewise towards savages and slaves, but first seeing them as quite alien from themselves. Throughout the early part of the seventeenth century, a similar process of redefinition surfacing within walks of Christianity itself, tended to deny the validity of traditional forms of religious madness.

The Reformation and Counter-Reformation ages made great play of the reality of religious madness, some of it being good, which was viewed as being directly from God and manifested in ecstasies or in prophetic. However, they also saw most of it being evil and originating from within the reach of the Devil, these of course obviously focused and pointed toward witches, heretics, ill thinkers, etc.

From Greek Philosophers to the Early Christian Perspective on Mental Health

Throughout the centuries, we have treated, reasonably investigated and documented on the complex conditions and unusual features that have lead people to fall into the traps of mental illness. The unalterable essence of this book is an attempt to specifically deal with the issues raised by those relevant questions, while basically acknowledging that even in this day and age we pose very little rational concept on the fundamental nature of mental illness. Despite countless researches and innovative advances in treatments methodologies, still very little is understood about what it is, what affects it and what will actually cure it. This accurate and well documented fact among respected psychiatrists, psychologists, the mental health and psychiatric communities. This vague admission of ignorance does frustrate and color our attitudes in the field, toward the large amount of competing interpretations held throughout the centuries about insanity and varied reasons for their causes and treatments. Insanity, mental illness, madness, or whatever other name the psychiatrist, psychologists and sociologists societies, including the consumers themselves, have managed to label it with; and throughout the years it remains still an elusive phenomena.

Of course, even psychiatrists and psychologists when interviewed would readily affirm that it seemed a shared-common sense proposition to label The Reality of Mental Illness, as the title for a recent defense by psychiatry for psychiatrists. In turn, they also admitted and swiftly defended the fact that it was done primarily, as a political and social act, rather than as a mental health treatment tool or a medical principle. Psychiatrists Martin Roth, Jerome Kroll and others later also defended the act, by similarly arguing that before the label being set, it was possible to think of mental illness in terms of a manufactured illness. Around these same times, Dr. Thomas Szasz, a practicing psychiatrist and university professor of psychiatry, would later write and publish his first book *The Manufacture of Madness*. In it, he argued, "every society and every generation gets their particular classification of mental illness and the amount it deserves and that it is, but just a weaker form of cultural construct." This clearly opened the door to a series of controversies among leading psychiatric communities and even among the reliable psychiatrists themselves who openly questioned the very basic objectivity of their studies, (as to whether or not 'mental illness was truly a significant disease and a form of cognitive mental illness. Wondering afterward, if it should be compared to and treated as one would the diabetic cancer, cancer and other chronic physical human maladies?) On the other hand, others were far more critical, arguing as to if it might be regarded essentially as a badge pinned on particular individuals subjectively defined as bundles of symptoms and traits? Together, they later struggled with the fact while trying to preliminarily determine whom, among who at the bottom of human society were severely different or odd? However, the open questions remain, thus unable to clearly define the inline by which case, is that bottom-line, in which, we could accurately call the mentally ill individuals confused. Is it merely because we have an opinion, or because we found them confusing, or disturbed, essentially because we declare them morally disturbing? At this time, advocates for the mentally ill, moral ethicians and sociology professors quickly pointed out to the mental health communities if they obviously determined such, because they considered the act itself to be a rather disturbing possibility. Arguing afterward that the mad is strange yes, but does that meant anything more than to say that they are strange to us? They later compared and questioned, whether we ever stop to think about the fact that we might particularly also be strange to them? So, after all these years and all the studies, the obvious question of what insanity actually is, amounts to be fully understood and yet remains to an open and extensive debate.

Short of discovering the gene that causes schizophrenia, the controversial issues among these communities will not come to a conclusion any time soon.

The cardinal point now, is that we should keep in mind that although we have always tempted to appear superior to those afflicted with some forms of mental illness. Although our inquirers of different types of strangeness' retains its enigma, hence to this day we must lastly admit that stigma remains readily apparent. To have obviously find and descriptively define strangeness in behaviors, we must effectively work together to ultimately abolish the prolonged - lasted stigma. These issues, which have typically featured within the fractured dialogues that arguably goes on the masses or the quiet reserves between the mentally ill and sane individuals, to whom such illness is disruptive and as strange as that of one being in a foreign country.

Each society makes, but few arrangements for coping with peculiar people whose judgment and cognitive behavior is weird, disruptive or dangerous, from that degree mental illness forms a universal fact of life. But the different ways such peculiarities are described and judged, tends to differ quite profoundly from society, relatively to society, from era to era and from symptom to symptom etc. Here we encounter an element of irreducible relativism rather. Throughout the European Western cultures of today, relatively treat mild mental and emotional illness as neurosis, or what was previously commonly known as nervous breakdown, etc. It is we no longer regarded as organic, but rather, merely as a functional product of excessive worry and tension. In most cases, it is often treated broadly in an outpatient setting by basic means such as psychotherapy. However, we find the exact opposite to be true with this in China and other societies by the particular concurrence of respected physicians and patients alike, broadly comparable disabilities, are described as being cultural priorities due to neurasthenia, a principal diagnosis once common, but now extinct throughout most of the West. This is considered essentially as a disease of the body itself. The contrasting diagnoses and treatment follow from divergent socio - cultural priorities. While in the individualistic Western culture, mental illness though mild, it is relatively legitimate. Because we believe we have a right to fulfillment and happiness, we also believe we have a right to complain, when we are miserable and a right to indulgent, redress. By the same token, in the much more inflexible and communal societies of the former Communist East, Latin America and even throughout the vast part of African American society, on the other hand, to confess to such weakness, would be regarded as shameful and self-indulgent, and would forfeit claims of sympathy and attention. Hence the somatization and the presentation of symptoms in physical form linked to an organic diagnosis by contrast, it gives credibility to the sufferer.

The English author Samuel Butler in his Victorian novel "Erewhorm," make relative alternatives to clearer reversal particulars, when he creatively recorded that "crime was universally seen as a disease, but being ill was also seen as being criminal." These instances point out something frequently visible in the discussions, due to the particular fact that the universal language, overall ideas, treatments and associations surrounding mental illness do not have scientific meanings that are fixed for longevity, but are rather limited resources, which are individually used as a vehicle by the various parties for all intent and purpose to properly fit such time. One of these latest situations could be frequently seen when examining the case of borderline personality disorders, opiates and other substance abuse disorders, or by simply following the vast, extensive list of all the other personality traits.

Too Much of God Has Long Been Removed From These Paupers Palace's

So What Is The Clear Separation of Church and State?

As professionals in the field, we obviously have deep intellectual understanding on the meaning of psychiatry and stigma. Although we have considered ourselves rather enlightened about such, at times we too have shunned any major involvement of the church and our commitment to this group. Many of us currently working in the mental health field, have presented claims of commitment and at times appeared concerned about the wellbeing of the mentally ill, but the reality clearly reflects otherwise. We do not encourage prayer, or meditation among the patient population, or among ourselves when dealing with difficult clients. We will instead embark on never ending struggles and fight for the best deal that'll benefit, us, ourselves and our families, rather than fight for a better treatment for our clients, often times, we invoke petty struggles to revoke their therapeutic gains.

Instead of hardly ever concentrating our efforts on improving the care for the mentally ill, we spend countless hours battling within our institutions fighting for the best psychiatric wards where to work, with the less challenging clients. For the best suited schedules to fit our lifestyle, best shifts, best benefits, best overtime sites, best access for promotion, etc. Although some mental health workers and nurses, whom provide direct patient care, might suggest a spiritual connection and prayer to a particular patient, if administration is ever informed, these individual treaters, could be targeted and treated with disrespect, total disregard and perhaps even disciplinary actions. Therefore, often times, Christian, Jewish, Muslim, Buddhist, spiritual faith grounded mental health workers, often find themselves forced into trying to benefit in other ways, because since they are in many ways ignored, as their suggestions and advocacy toward better plans of care and treatment for the clients, is showed to the side. In otherwise, many have ascertain to have become morally de-compensated and their efforts totally unrecognized. They therefore will compensate as best as they can, albeit rather selfish terms, since such is utterly encouraged. In many instances during my tenure throughout the 1980s, 1990s to early 2003, if the word 'God,' was ever mentioned or prayer was ever suggested in the same breath of mental health treatment, one was often disrespected, seen as delusional and perhaps even considered a fanatic by their peers.

Therefore, the mental health field, is perhaps the only profession, in which neither doctors, nurses, social workers, nor mental health workers are ever considered veterans, regardless of how long one have spent working in the field, how many lives they have saved, nor how much and how, well they have contributed and performed in the field. After being accredited for saving five different suicide attempts in less than a year by their peers, a Christian colleague, "wondered if we would ever be considered heroes despite our performance and how many lives we have saved, be it single handedly, or collaboratively?" The answers to him was a resounding no. He then wrote to administration to voice these concerns, as he'd been recommended and he was later forced to resign. Perhaps no being considered deep enough as an issue that could further hamper care, if pondered long enough, one could suggest that this happens primarily, because we have removed too much of God, of our faith and of our belief in God, out of the system under the banner of separation of church and state. Therefore, we remain spiritually drained or anesthetized to pain and too selfish and too eager to take away earned credits from each other. Throughout the field we stumbled upon supervisors, head nurses, staff nurses and more importantly, though sadly so, even the mental health workers, trying to claim credit for unaccomplished work, in order to fill in that void, while trying desperately to fill that empty vessel that often overflows with self-pity and anger toward our fellowmen, because we have eagerly removed God's presence from the field.

I clearly remember once listening to a conversation that took place between a mental health worker and a psychiatric head nurse on a unit, the mental health worker appeared to have had a deeper insight regarding the treatment of this particular patient, whom had been diagnosed with, Borderline Personality Disorder, (BPD). Although throughout the conversation, the nurse had been in full agreement with the mental health worker's therapeutic insight, nevertheless, a few minutes later, when the supervisor appeared on the locked psychiatric unit, doing her rounds, the same nurse, presented pretty much the same plan of care, only this time she expressed it as if it had all been her idea. She had totally disregarded and failed to even acknowledge the mental health worker's name. This selfish politically oriented, upward mobility attitude, clearly runs from within the commissioner's offices, all the way down to the most recently hired mental health worker on the roster, and right back up through the ranks. Of course, there are many exceptions, but the overall purpose remains unethical, ungodly and borderline selfish just the same. Therefore, it is not uncommon to find burned-out and tired employees showing up to their worksite, often times unproductive, unconcerned and burdened down, soaked, with poor or bad attitudes. Their primary goal, is no longer to provide best plan of care or even participate as a team player, but of rather being to accumulate as many hours in overtime, because such reflects in the percentage points toward retirement's three best years. Of course although this is not the norm, it is done often enough to hamper care and cause stressful frustrations among those whom are actually trying to provide and improve the level of patient care. Often times, one could lead themselves into believing that such attitude, is at times spilled out by some caregivers, due to their becoming physically, emotionally and mentally anesthetized after experiencing such behavior throughout the years. Perhaps, they have simply lost their ability to believe in a stagnant system and have refused to continue given or have nothing left in them to give. . Although, we must keep in mind that the system trickles down and therefore, reflects and recognize that mental health workers, nurses, rehabilitation therapist and social workers and all those responsible for providing direct patient care, are often being equally 'mistreated, and ignored.' Instinctively we have conditioned ourselves to benefit in one-way, or another, otherwise, there would be no compensation coming from hospital administrators or the mental health commissioner's offices. This practice also takes place in the areas of seniority or tenure, and is frequently abused within the realm at the level of supervisory and the game of favoritism that some supervisors, managers and program directors put into practice, when promoting, or hiring for key positions throughout the system.

We have often times, come across under-qualified and unproductive individuals sitting in comfortable positions, which were probably gained based on seniority, or by whom they might have known throughout the system. Moreover, while still not possessing the knowledge, credentials, experience, or qualifications to perform such. This happens regardless of these being key positions throughout the department that could otherwise disrupt, enhance, prevent, or interfere with a patient's level of care and the system's plans to care for and care with.

However, we must not ignore to give the credit which is owed and been long overdue to the hard working psychiatric nurses. Quite frankly, I have found that some nurses whom perform their duties in the mental health field are far more diplomatic than some people holding key positions in offices throughout the United Nations. Although, such comparison might rather appear as a joke, though such assumption is somewhat close, and are not saying this just to create a smirk, nor simply because I have nothing-else to write about. During my long twenty plus year career in the field, I have been fortunate enough to work side by side, with some of the best in the nursing profession, in over eight psychiatric hospitals and impatient treatment facilities throughout the United States. My humble opinion, is that most psychiatric nurses should give themselves big thumbs up and a huge pat on their shoulders for a job well done, following the successfully completing of each and every shift. "Of course that is if they're allowed to go home and are not forced, or mandated to work a double, or overtime shifts, due to the alarming shortage in numbers." The reason for my saying this is that in addition to performing all of their nursing duties and responsibilities, pertaining to their psychiatric patients, they must also contend with, or deal professionally with other staff issues. This, which could sometimes mount to becoming an even bigger challenges, than that of treating their psychiatric patients, since they cannot simply tell their staff to go to their rooms and cool off, offer them a pill, or suggest they talk with their clinician's nor their therapists the following day. In addition to all the fore-mentioned duties, they must also deal with random changes in administrative policies and procedures, and the large volume of paperwork each shift.

Although we must keep in mind that as professionals and paraprofessionals, our frustrations increases more within the realm of difficulty, by which we find ourselves, while trying to work around individuals with behaviors and negative attitudes. It is however, historically documented that due to shortages and difficulty in staffing, large state hospitals and institutions customarily placed the care of most patients in the hands of undereducated and underpaid aides, often times, without the immediate supervision of professional staff. This practice, although now in lower numbers, still remains alive and well; thus, giving those less educated and ill prepared a greater voice, power and absolute control over the lives of the mentally ill persons. Though it seems clear that over the years, professional mental health workers, have profoundly shaped the types of treatment and available access to treatment, but the prevailing attitude toward the mentally ill still predominates. Arguably, we must still point out how this lack of education, godliness, lack of spirituality and human kindness, further prejudice's these prevailing attitudes by raising its ugly head to reach out and interfere with patient treatment.

These behaviors, are often displayed, embraced, condoned and even performed by those whom ought to be more understanding, because of their level of education and training. That, which yet fails to show, thus instead is further perpetrated. This attitude should arrive in the form of a 'free will and as a free moral action,' rather than by fear of losing a practitioner's license, status or employment. The point being that the act must first come from the will and that it should remain in the will, as stated in the natural law and under the light of reason. Perhaps one could argue that education, in many cases may help to change minds, although it changes not our hearts. Therefore, we should remain altruistic, and morally and spiritually upright, humanly connected, and even more importantly, remain honest to ourselves. Perhaps just a little bit of God in to the overall system and a little more of our faith could help push these possibilities far beyond were man alone, have for so long failed to reach.

A Clearer Understanding of Our Faith, Within Our Faiths

When we think of the meaning of faith, we must also think of the grave significance of anguish, and about the pain and confusion that is preexisting in the hearts and minds of those individuals suffering with mental illness. We must also think of their redemption and about the loneliness, despair and depression that plagues their daily lives and further weights them down. When we look at faith, we must first realize that we all want to be loved. Each of us want to know and to believe that God loves us no matter what! Faith, faith tells us that we must teach others to love God!

As we reflect on when our pastors, rabbis, our imam, ministers, and other spiritual leaders call upon us to come forth and to approach their pulpit, when they ask us to get out of our seats, and move forward. When our priests and our pastors call for holy communion, we move forward and when our Rabbi speak we listen. When the call is heard from the mosque, to bow our heads, bend forward facing East and pray, we follow and when the gong is sounded, we follow in deep meditation. In a closer and broader interpretation of ourselves, this means that in the realities of deep religious and spiritual examination, we are following by faith and somber conviction. So these are not as easy to experience and perhaps unable to even be experienced by all. Because faith is almost palpable, as it reaches out to God, and to those whom are fortunate enough or chosen by way of true blessings to have experienced true faith, it is as if they are being physically embraced by God. But faith isn't always that easy, even for those who desperately seek it. Although some people hunger for spiritual certainty, yet something hinders them from experiencing it. They wish that they too could taste that kind of freedom, but obstacles block their path. Objections pester them. Doubts mock them, and even when their hearts want to serve God, their intellect keeps them in their seats. So when we hear the call, still sitting in our seats, we look around, wondering, whom else is going to move up front before we do, our inner intellect is perhaps holding us back.

It could also well be that that same inner intellect, is moving us forward for business and personal reason, which have nothing at all to do with our faith. Therefore, we know that intellectuals truly believe that faith is incompatible with their intellect. Many have questioned, whether it is possible to be a thinker and a believer and still manage to follow our faith? Meanwhile other intellectuals have openly argued their beliefs, while trying to ascertain that reason and faith, are opposites that they are two mutually exclusive terms, and that there is no reconciliation, nor common ground. However, we also have those whom have concluded that "faith is a belief without or in spite of reason." Nevertheless, there are many other intellectuals, scholars, whom sees faith as a natural response to the evidence of God's self revelation in nature, human history, our scripture, resurrection, peace and everlasting happiness. Because of these and many other reasons and beliefs, we defend the fact that our faith is not built on a razor-thin foundation of wishful thinking and make believe. Through our good work, God indicates to us that our faith, is consistent, with reason and not contradicted to it. Furthermore, it is grounded in reality and not distracted from it, therefore, throughout the centuries, faith have always been able to stand up against scrutiny. My belief is that "faith could perhaps also be measured through our intuition, meaning that persons whom truly have faith, perhaps also make for better and well-adjusted individuals." But this is just my belief and my opinion. However, we do realized that faith, is important in our day to day lives, since it alters our decision making. It also helps us deal with difficult situations and sort out challenges and other problems. The reality though, regardless of ones inability to agree, we could agree on the deepest level that faith is beyond description. So in reality, our sectarian belief shouldn't really come in to play, and religion shouldn't even matter to us, as much as our deep spiritual faith should. The point I'm trying to focus on here, is that as faithful believers, our primary beliefs tells us, that we are all guided by God to follow the same five basic principles:

That is a, God does exist, b, God is all good, c, God is all powerful, d, God is all wise, and e, that evil do exist. Although we do realized that many skeptics believe that all of these statements cannot be true, but logically it is possible and not hard to prove.

We could then debate each of these individually and argue the fact that since God is all powerful, God is omnipotent and can do anything, since God is all good, then God wants to do good, since God is all wise, then he knows what is good and if we are correct, with our feelings and our beliefs to God, hence, such diminishes the existence of evil.

The following chapters, explains with further detail our clear argument to the skeptics who, still insist with disbelief the understanding significance found within faith and reason. Faith is a trust commitment to what we think and believe is true, though most Christians do realize and would agree that Christianity differs from individual to individual. To some, it might be because God speaks to our hearts and produces convictions. To others it might be that of a more intellectual approach and evidence of our explanation, which leads us to the same conclusion, in which, neither comes to faith until, we make that act of trust. That commitment to what we believe is true and when we examine faith under these categories, we then see that it is entirely compatible to reason. We find that among Christians throughout the world that even within their inner deepest thoughts, the most devout Christians knows that there is something kind of illegitimate about belief. Even while interviewing some of the most devout of today's preachers, when asked the questions, we'll then swiftly realized that underneath their profession of faith, lays a sleeping giant of doubt, if there isn't a hint of faith.

Many of the most successful religious leaders have found that the best way to deal with their doubt, is to yield to it and then conquer it with faith. And many of those who believe they believe in God, but without passion in the heart, without anguish of mind, without uncertainty, without doubt and even at times without despair, they believe only in the idea of God and not in God true living God. And this is obviously because they lack faith. Our intellect clearly refers to indicate to us that these misconceptions about faith, quickly opens doors to doubt, because they tend to create false expectations and misunderstandings about the nature of God.

Examples of these are often found in people who incorrectly believed that God has promised them something. They are easily misled into false expectations, thinking that God has promised to make everyone wealthy if they simply exhibit sufficient faith. These people quickly fall pray to doubt, when an illness, or bankruptcy looms. So in order to arrive at an accurate view toward faith, we must first clear out the theological underbrush by defining clearly what faith 'isn't,' then list some of the concerns and misconceptions surrounding what faith really is. We somehow have the tendency of mixing up faith with feelings, although in some cases they go hand, in hand, but they are not one of the same. A clear example of these is easily found within those individuals, who tend to equate faith with 'a perpetual religious 'high.' And when the high wears off, as it inevitably those, they began to doubt whether they have any faith at all. Of course, this does not mean that there isn't a strong connection between faith and feelings, but these dimensions are measured through the individual's temperament and their convictions. We must realize that some of us are not wired to feel very much, although we have strong convictions, some of us tend to be emotionally up and down, but this should not be confused as a fluctuation within our faith. An example of this is found when examining the mothers love for her child. A woman becomes pregnant, nine months later, she gives birth she then brings a beautiful child into this world, and then takes it home from the hospital. A few weeks later, the child awakens late each night screaming, needing his soiled, dirty diapers changed and fed, since he's also hungry. The new mother, wakes up each night tired in the middle of the night, places her bare feet on the cold floor to then run into the kitchen and fix her loud, screaming, hungry, crying little baby their bottle. She then feeds and cleans up the stinky messy baby. Does she get a thrill out of this, each night? Does she love doing it? Does she stop loving the child when they're dirty, hungry and screaming? Of course not, we must first keep in mind that the measure of her love isn't based upon the fact that she felt good about doing it, but that she is willing to do it, regardless of even when she isn't feeling particularly good about doing it. We also find such vivid examples between spouses and even good friends.

This could be seen as 'recta ratio agibilium,' (things that must be done). We have to have faith! We ought to have faith, we must have faith! This is what we have to learn about faith, because faith isn't always about having positive emotional feelings toward God, or life and that is a clear misconception. Some people believe that faith is the absence of doubt, but this is also not true, faith isn't the lack of doubt either. Within our Bibles, we read scriptures about the man who went before Jesus with his demon-possessed son and asked Jesus to heal his boy and Jesus said to the man that all things are possible to those who believe. The man's response to Jesus was quite powerful, when he said, "I believe, but would you help me with my unbelief?" So here we see that doubt and faith do coexist and that we can have doubt even when we believe. We find this in the Old-testament, also as study Abraham, who clearly believed, but at the same time also had his doubts. In a sense doubt can actually play a positive role toward our faith, but we must realize when to use caution, to follow a guidelines, between doubt and that corrosive, eroding negative doubt. While growing up as a boy in Honduras, I remember people from the various churches heading to homes to pray for their sick and when asked how that person was doing, they would reply, "oh, don't worry, they'll be fine because we just prayed." However, I also remember their devastated frustration when the person wasn't healed. This is perhaps because their theology, was somewhat misguided and unexamined. It had never been challenged by doubts or thoughtful questions. Doubt could have perhaps helped them to develop a substantial and a more realistically base of faith that by which, they would have trusted God in the face of death, as well as in the face of healing. So, to those whom still do not believe that doubt could actually play a positive role within our faith, this might be a good examples.

Several years ago, while attending a catholic seminary, where I was conducting research on ethics, I attended a lecture and heard a visiting Rabbi said "I am against any religion that says that one's faith is superior to another. I don't see how that is any different from spiritual discrimination. It is almost like saying that we are closer to God than you, or your people!" Although I was perhaps the only lay-student present there that evening, as I looked around the room, all of the priests, church clergy, seminarians and other very serious looking theological students, dressed up in their distinctive, respectable church garb and others in official looking clergy collars, heads bowed, quickly taking notes. I was of course wearing my simple pair of jeans and a green corduroy blazer. I later attended another lecture conducted by a Christian theologian who stated, "Moses could meditate on the law, Muhammad could brandish a sword, Buddha could give personal counsel, Confucius could offer wise sayings, but none of these men were qualified to offer atonement for our sins to the world; but Jesus! Therefore, Christ alone is worthy of this unlimited devotion!"

The Hindus belief is to accept all religions to be that of truth and that the real sin, exists only in calling someone else a sinner. This belief parallels itself with the term being recognized now by theologians, as "spiritual dictatorship." To shine a clear light and grasp a deeper understanding of such a view, we must first go back and research the writings of Martin Luther and the dreadful rumors, which surfaced, fueled and darkened a period in history, this, such being, the Christians hatred toward the Jews. During these awful times, still recognized today, as being "one of the ugliest blights in Christian history, out of such, came anti-Semitism," of course it is ironic since Jesus himself was a Jew and the long awaited messiah for Israel and the rest of the world. Each and everyone of Jesus's disciples, were Jewish and Jews also wrote almost the entire New Testament, all but the book of Acts, which was authored by Luke, who was a physician. According to history, most Jews did not thought of Jesus as a messiah and their refusal to accept such, simply transformed them as foes of Christ into the minds of Middle-Age and Reformist Christians. Add this to the fact that Christians, had been also taught that Jews were to be held responsible for the crucifixion of Jesus, and we have a lethal component of serious Christian anti-Semitism that'll last throughout the ages.

There was an overabundance of false rumors surrounding the Jews during the Middle-Ages, and throughout the Reformation periods, which added even more hatred toward them. They blamed them for poisoning the wells that caused the Black Death of the late 1340's.

They were also accused of desecrating Christian sacraments, of privately conducting sacrificial deaths and of tampering with Christian scriptures. Although these rumors were all false, they were incendiary enough to fuel, hate anger and resentment toward Jews, nonetheless. Although this was all against Christ's teachings, and although, Jesus himself, forbade such, by the time Martin Luther, came around and though in his earlier years he was considered a 'Philo-Semitic.' Obviously he love the Jews at the beginning, though he knew of some of the rumors and tried a mass conversion, in which they would all embrace Jesus as their messiah, but became irritably in his older years and wrote very ugly things about the Jews, when they all didn't convert. Although some scholars believed that Martin Luther, carried these ugly views about the Jewish people all throughout his life, but it wasn't until in his later days. Recent scholars believed that he did this out of frustration, although it still doesn't justify the fact. His statements were so horrific that Lutherans of today repudiated them and of course all Christians of today have rejected them in one way or another. In reality, I believe that true Christians cannot be anti-Semitic and that such should be rather unthinkable of any true followers of Jesus.

In contemporary times, evangelical Christians have often been some of Israel's greatest friends and the greatest attitudes we know see in many of the churches is nothing but respect toward the Jewish people. Although throughout history many horrible crimes against humanity have been committed by men hiding behind the Christian faith. The largest and most recognizable of these, being the Holocaust and of course chattel slavery.

Today, Christianity still bares blame for these horrendous crimes, given the fact that many Jewish people still firmly believe that Hitler was a Christian. Reason as to why we strongly suggest caution, when mixing up cultural Christianity and authentic Christianity. During the rise of the National Socialist Party, Hitler managed to wrap himself up around Christianity and the teachings of Martin

Luther. In somewhat of a demonic sense, one could argue of it being a cleaver and ideological ploy that unfortunately work. Though in retrospect, we look back today to reexamine what really happened and at what such high price.

Throughout the mid 1600's, many Jews believed in a certain individual, whom claimed to be their messiah, but of course, he later converted to Islam. This dashed their aspirations and since then they have thought and treated this individual as a fraud. His name was, Sabbatai Zevi, 8/1/1626, 9/17/1676. Today, in similar fashion, we believe all Christians see Hitler, as a fraud. As an evil individual and as someone, who wasn't even anywhere near Sunday school, never mind the teachings or the understandings of authentic Christianity, nonetheless proclaim himself that of a representative of true Christian teachings or a messiah. Although it wasn't until recently, back in 1998 that the Roman Catholic Church, finally issued a public apology to all Jews throughout the world for their "shameless errors, failures and refusals' toward aiding the Jewish people during the Nazi Holocaust. Cardinal John O'Connor of New York, later that same year also expressed abject shame and sorrow for anti-Semitism in churches throughout the years. About a decade earlier, Pope John Paul II, had also visited the concentration camps around 1979 and on the eve of Memorial's Day weekend 2006, Pope Benedict XVI visited Auschwitz concentration camps. This time carrying with him, an open, written apology, directly from the German people, when he stated, "as a son of the people of Germany, I've often ask God, why He remained silent during the unprecedented mass crimes of the Holocaust." During prayers, he later added "by destroying Israel with Shoah, they ultimately wanted to tear up the taproot of the Christian faith and replace it with their own invention" (Shoah is the Hebrew given term for the Holocaust, during which the Nazis killed over 6 million Jews. Although Pope Benedict's father was an anti Nazi, The pope himself was enrolled in the Hitler youth brigade, as a teenager. As a young man, he also served in the German army during the last months of the war. Pope Benedict, however, failed to comment on the controversy surrounding the war time Pope Pius XII, who's ethics are still being questioned and accused of doing nothing in his power to aid and prevent the deportation of the Jewish people to the concentration death camps.

The church, however, has yet to issue an apology for the huge role they played in dissemination and total destruction of our enslaved African ancestors, the African continent, and the genocidal destruction of our Native Americans, i.e., 'Indian' territories and their way of life. Given the fact that slavery and the cruel treatment of Blacks and Native Americans, were also handed down by the Church. It was not only handed down, but the overall Church practically breathe out of such evil. Man rejects God neither because of influence, or intellectual demands, nor the scarcity of evidence. Man rejects God because of the moral resistance that forces him to refuse to admit his need for God. But man uses the name of God to systematically empower himself and cause endless destruction to God's own creations. So be aware how and whom we blindly follow. There is now even a new term created for those who follows blindly and believes without doubt. The old familiar terms was 'fanatic and extremist,' the new term is now appropriately called 'true believer mentally.' And it refers to those individuals, with bright smiles and glassy eyes who never have a doubt in the world, those who always think everything is wonderful, everything is great. One often wonders what happens to their inner relationship with God and their faith when things like this occurs. And of course, we have the extremist, who follow these ideological dreamers into destruction, those whom would kill in the name of religion and those who blows themselves up and kill thousands, in the name of what they believe is God.

Some of the Facts, Behind the Great American Deinstitutionalization

Deinstitutionalization is the term which has been given to the policy of shifting severely mentally ill people out of large state mental institutions, followed by closing down these institutions, in order to shift monies to other areas or simply appear as political smoke screens to opposing political parties. According to research, our observation and that of several experts account, it could easily be said that deinstitutionalization, remains a major contributing factor to the mental health crisis that currently exist. Deinstitutionalization began gathering steam throughout the United States around mid1950's, with the widespread introduction of chlorpromazine, a medication, that later became commonly known as Thorazine. Considered back then, as one of first and most effective antipsychotic medication at the time, Thorazine received national and international momentum, approximately 10 years later, the federal Medicaid and Medicare Act was enacted, thus allowing individual Americans the right to medications, mental health and medical treatment. However, due to its toxicity and debilitating physical side effects, today long-term chronic psychiatric patients have been known to cringe simply at the mentioning of this awful medication by name.

Deinstitutionalization yields a two part injury: a) the moving of the severely mentally ill out of the state institutions, and B) the closing of part or all of those institutions. The former affects people whom are already mentally ill.

The latter affects those who become ill after the policy went into effect because hospital beds had been permanently eliminated. The magnitude of deinstitutionalization of the severely mentally ill qualifies as one of the largest social experiments in American history. In 1955, there was a total of about 558,239 severely mentally ill patients in the nation's public psychiatric hospitals. In 1994, this number had been reduced by 486,620 patients, to 71,619. It is important to note, however, that the census of 558,239 patients in public psychiatric hospitals in 1955 was in relationship to the nation's total population at the time, which was 164 million.

Another strong moral foundation for the deinstitutionalization argument, was based on the principles that the severe mentally ill individual, should be treated in the least restrictive and humane setting. This, was further reinforced by then President Jimmy Carter's Commission on Mental Health. During this time First Lady, Roselyn Carter's ideology rested on "the objective of maintaining the greatest degree of freedom, self-determination, autonomy, dignity, and the integrity of body, mind, and spirit for the individual, as they participated in treatment and received services." This in fact could be seen as a praise deserving goal for some in society and perhaps for a good number of deinstitutionalized individuals, the dream was at least partially realized. However for a substantial number of chronically mentally persons, deinstitutionalization, has been a colossal psychiatric nightmare. Considering the facts that for too many, their lives are now virtually devoid of either dignity or the integrity of body, of mind or spirit. The back then popular term "Self-determination" widely used and coined to help spearhead the march back then, today it simply means that the person has a choice of soup kitchen, police brutality or garbage can. And "least restrictive setting" often turns out to be a under a bridge in a cardboard box, a jail cell, or perhaps a terror-filled existence on the streets plagued and harassed by both, the real and the imaginary enemies within their heads.

The Rapid Political Failure of the Secular Community Base Initiative Projects

During the late 1980's to mid 1990's there was a massive increase push, geared toward the deinstitutionalization of all psychiatric hospitals, the state hospitals in particular. The news then surfaced that Norwich State Hospital, Fairfield Hills State Hospital and the Connecticut Valley State Hospital, all three of the psychiatric state hospitals in Connecticut, were scheduled to close their doors for good and the state, had yet to implement a comprehensive plan or device a policy, suited for the patient treatment to at least remain in a humane way … it was total chaos and madness. Inside the hospitals and out in these large and very concerned communities. Meanwhile, the staff of these hospitals pulled out their hairs, wondering what was concurrently going to happen to all of these people, state politicians fought hard to try keeping it from leaking out to the public. Therefore, committees were organized among the hospital staff to advocate for the client's wellbeing and at the same time prevent catastrophic layoff's that would have resulted in unsafe and severely ill individuals being poured out to the streets. These committees, were rather successful in achieving both of their targeted goals, to accomplish the successful implementation of the States Community Base Initiative's 'CBI,' comprised by all well experienced and dedicated longtime mental health workers and nurses. Although two of the major state hospitals in Connecticut afterward closed their doors and the third being the largest and more centrally conveniently located also began to orderly transition and discharged chronically ill individuals into these CBI programs to help cushion the impact on both the community, the individual consumers and their families. Throughout the prior months and years, union, state and community work hard collectively at implementing these programs, together, we were all very proud of them, trusted that they'd work as a nationwide model, because of their significant function. It was a wonderful idea that proved its effectiveness almost immediately. These statewide CBI's, located throughout the cities of Hartford, New Haven, New Britain, Meriden, New London and Torrington, provided human dignity for the individual patient, while offering us caregivers, case managers, therapists, and the overall treatment team, an opportunity to ably teach them to again breathe free and live like human beings. To enjoy the little things in life that we so took for granted. Simple things, such as going to a movie theater, regularly attending a church services of their choice, going to a dance, visiting a park and participating in the local community activities, budgeting their monthly allowances, and allowing themselves the pleasure of eating in a restaurant once a month. Licensed, registered dieticians monthly visits, contributed tremendously with preparing learning about proper diets and aided us and their home attendants with their individual meal preparations. Meanwhile regularly community mental health groups, helped them rebuild social skills and maintain productive relationships. Considering that just the fact of simply owning and operating a television set and a microwave oven of their own was a challenge that often reawakened paranoia or sat them back to a delusional state of being, promptly requiring medication change or an increased dosage.

Although this might same mundane to the average persons, but these were significant affairs to these people, common task, chores and simple things that some of them had been able to accomplish on their own, in excess of 20 years, due to their being locked away in restricted and highly safety therapeutic environments. We were ambitious, had high expectations and we genuinely believed in the success of these programs. I personally believe that we were actually making history and to this day, I still strongly believed in what we did! We truly trusted and had full faith in our team, ourselves our therapeutic milieu with the clients and how working together, we could successfully assist these people to develop and effectively attained their objective goals toward recovery and independent living.

Once these programs had been implemented, and up and running, I was offered the opportunity to choose anyone of the programs, since I was one of the few bilingual seniors, I spoke, read and wrote Spanish, and these programs, were all mostly located in primarily inner city minority areas, with a high Latino or Spanish speaking population. Since given the choice, I choose the Meriden program, which had the most senior and more experienced two of the most, fair minded, goal oriented and dedicated psychiatric head nurses I'd known and worked with throughout the past eight years in a restrictive in an inpatient setting. A team which consisted with other well qualified staff, equipped to organize groups, implement transitions, understood punctuality, more importantly, the ability to work individually or collectively. Many of these team members were fully involved in the church and made church a center part of their lives. Although at the time I wasn't, but I found it rather important and were able to equate this toward their being more dedicated and responsible. It was also a much closer ride to home.

Prior to fully agreeing to the position, I had also made a previous assessment to quickly realize I'd made the right decision. As I studied the other programs, I then realized then that less than seventy five percent of the staff, was very much committed to professional type of care, growth and progressive development needed to accomplish such task and that about three percent did not know or didn't really care what they were doing. Although few, were somewhat prepared to approach as a team player and even fewer were determinedly willing to learn. Overall still believed they might have in the long shot tried to do their best, but many of their program directors were underqualified, afraid to take any chances for fear of losing their jobs, they were also under trained. Furthermore, the state had stop providing in-services or upward mobility training for community base employees. Nevertheless, there was also that one percent that persistently remained egotistical, self-centered and with an attitude of self-commitment. Stubborn to follow or implement a team approach, to instead settled for childlike behavior and rather ready to hamper client's treatment, in order to have a negative effect on a particular case manager's work, rather than participate as a team player, dedicated to see that all of our patients thrive and successfully accomplish their ultimate goal.

A case in point that clearly comes to mind, being that of a thirty something year veteran of the state Department of Mental Health and Addictions Services, intrusion with a newer and more educated employee's therapeutic approach. This young case manager strategically developed a comprehensive treatment plan, where twice a week, he took these particular clients, whom displayed awkward social deficits to the laundromat, allowing them do their own laundry independently, while casually engaging in socialization with the general public. .

The much older employee although, possessing not more education than a thirty-two years-old high school diploma and perhaps a few hours of in house training, had been promoted to supervisor, with the authority, which provided her capacity to block his valid approach. Of course, they'd also been some previous back and forth, and she unquestionably unable to, or just simply refused to necessarily perceive the therapeutic value, designed within this treatment plan. And after separate attempts of complex manipulation and discriminative interventions, the only effective measures of structural sabotage, was to complain to the program director about how this particular case manager "continuously placed their client at risk by leaving them unattended out in the community, while he took off on break." Of course, the program director apparently had difficulty being fully assertive, they also failed to appropriately by not measuring the growth nor implementing a new therapeutic approach that would've perhaps served all best. Unfortunately the program director neither, understood the emergent need for such plan of care and proceeded to automatically make it a blanket policy to ban such practice, without fittingly examining it any further.

Seven long years later, this client was still in essential need for someone to help him with his laundry. The selfish and ungodly attitude of that one person, whom had elected to sabotage this plan of care, would unnecessarily cause this particular staff to throw his hands into the air and give up, so the little progress the client earned was unexpectedly lost. Fortunately, he was later prescribed a home health-assistance to assists him once per week with laundry; but sadly, it was at the expense of our collective tax dollars and the possibility of his independent status.

This drastic scenario, is not unique in and of itself for the critical record of similar practices went on until the programs were later privatized and handed over to the political donors in the private sector.

As caregivers, we commonly encounter frustrating and stressful situations, while trying to determine, the real extent of our knowledge about the availability of development among each individual patient. One of the main challenges, often times encountered is about the obvious difficulties found, when making a suitable definition. Not long ago, most treaters were of the opinion that a particular, comprehensive definition could've eased relative confusion, when redefining community treatment. However, as we actively concentrate from one program to another and from one particular person to another, we quickly see that each appears to have its own, peculiar definition, about whom would undeniably benefit and who might not. Frankly what this basically suggests, is that utterly different, but overlapping patient populations are being fostered under chronic illness programs. An instructive example that easily comes to mind is that of the regrettable shortcomings of the Community Base Initiative programs, *CBI's,* throughout the states. These reputable promotional programs, were initially set up as a twenty-four hour supervised apartment programs. Such apartments were pre-chosen for consumers due to funding criteria. The programs were primarily designed, for a more assertive and far less restrictive, organic patient population, who'd recently been discharged from psychiatric hospitals. One of their chief requirement, was that they belonged to a particular catchment area.

The goal, was to effectively educate and foster independent-living and not to simply warehouse, nor further institutionalize anyone. Besides, the idea designed behind these programs, was to encourage and adequately teach these clients to execute daily tasks, with minimal assistance, with their ultimate goal being independent living geared toward a successful outcome.

Initially, it was an impressive idea, geared to the development aspect and appropriate input that stemmed from the consumer-clients themselves; certainly, by this, we basically meant these being clients - consumers with less severe and prolonged mental illness. They were to voluntarily participate in the program's development and perform at a maximum level, in a client driven and

Interpersonal, skills building, support system of services, rather than to persistently remain dependable and untrained toward life's basic social aspects. Nevertheless, social workers, hospital officials and program directors, subsequently overlooked their intended purpose and immediately began referring acute, untrainable and severely ill, chronic clients, most of whom would've benefited in great part if discharged to rest homes, or specifically selective group home services, thus not to undoubtedly prevent, in any way the growth and development of those for whom these valuable services were intended. Although the staff collaborative belief's was focused on an approach toward a more concise treatment, which would have been to develop two comprehensible and unmistakably different models of programs, while keeping in mind the transient level of education, academic qualification and training of each designated staff member, regardless of the client's catchment area. In my opinion, they were supposed to set an approximate timeframe for gradual transition, with a specific data format in place that could have easily measured each client's individual progress. This approach would have respectfully, provided each client involved in such treatment, an incentive to work toward specific targeted goals.

Program directors, were to also follow what was previously a clear definition of their program's policies, such as the comprehensive sharing and transferring of clients, case managers and counselors, if therapeutic relationships among clients and case managers failed to develop within a specific time frame. Taking into a careful analysis, consideration to evaluate and reevaluate that trust and bond had been attained, between individual clients and their primary therapist. Keeping close attention to recognize that these were the most significant tools in developing therapeutic relationships and that such, is not an ordinary overnight process. Although it does provide solid, long-term solutions. This new approach, when suggested, was however, largely ignored, and the multiple diagnosed, chronic, severe psychiatrically, medically ill clients, were continuously thrown into the communities, without an efficient method being fully set into place, to effectively provide adequate treatment. However, the whole system was being profoundly viewed and influenced by political issues. The central focus would soon be placed on medical interventions, which, in many ways determined the way the program was generally regarded.

Since most hospital's current interventions were medical, it became difficult for therapists and case managers alike, to think about chronic illness, as anything other than a clinical problem. At the time, there no longer appeared to be any questions, regarding cases we received and those reviewed, ignored, was also the bizarre behaviors, which the untrained public, was now seeing wondering around their communities. Although appropriate consideration of these significant concerns should have been coming from a health care perspective, in some instances, the fundamental problem of each individual, was being skipped over in order to arrive at rapid-elusive, cure solutions that was measured in adulterated numbers. This was unacceptable, but rather promptly and reluctantly understandable, given the circumstance that public and political pressures for quick solutions progressively continued in the wake of mass de-institutionalization the system faced.

The allowable relocation of long-term mental patients from hospitals to the community resulted in a large number of socially disabled individuals, continuously being thrust into communities that were neither fit, nor willing to essentially understand, nor assume their care. More than any other single factor, the failure of de-institutionalization as an effective method, geared to improving the quality of life for the mentally ill, unnecessarily created a vast urgency to find suitable solutions to the unresolved problems of chronic illness. Once these community base initiatives were set in place, noted improvement and gradual progression, came upon the horizon for these individuals. Nevertheless, the lax attitude coming from those responsible for policing it, left much to ask for from the staff, which in turn left much to offer to those whom we served. Progress was left unmeasured; the staff was thrown out into these newly implemented programs to learn on their own. The easy access to drugs and alcohol and the impoverished neighborhoods, where most of these programs were set up, made it a bit more difficult to successfully managed and achieve maximum success. However, despite all these strenuous situations, goals were routinely set and goals were essential attained. Many of these clients in our programs achieved progress and a quality of life they and their families had perhaps never thought was possible. Although no credit or recognition was ever given to any of the staff involved in such great effort and to name them all would perhaps mean writing a specific book.

Many of these client's whom had previously been unable to remain out of hospitals for any considerable length of time, suddenly remained discharged and functioning well in their community for up to after seven years. Some clients had been able to go back to school and further their education, others, steadily obtained and maintained fulltime employment, some had gotten married and by way of one to one, family groups and therapeutic coaching, learned to keep a family and successfully live independently. In one particular case, an individual client completed his high school, went on to a university, where he studied and majored in computers, taught at a local community college, and successfully opened his own computer business. He later landed a prestigious job with an out of state computer company, earning more than $150,000 in annual salaries. This had never been seen nor previously heard of before. Not even Clifford Bears, had attained such success and accomplishment in a very short while.

As a team, we were all rather proud to finally get the opportunity to point out this very important point of our clients accomplishments to the 12 member panel, representing a delegation from the state's commissioner office, the scheduled meeting held between state hospitals human resource offices, advocates for the protection of the mentally ill and fellow union members. The panel refused to admit to any failure on their part, although they came to an agreement on the significant progress, our team had managed to achieved, with these difficult clients. Nevertheless, still they insisted on replacing our team with an independent, privately operated outfit. This of course wasn't much more than spoils of war. A multimillion dollar payoff that had perhaps been negotiated and offered up by the incumbent governor to the multinational corporations, whom had financially supported his bid for a second term. Perhaps, simply to poke the union brass in the eye, since we had been fighting him on his promises for better health care for our recently discharged individuals. We were certain, it had nothing to do with better treatment, mental health or health care at any level. The simple fact that these transitions were taking place secretly, very underhandedly, at such rapid pace and without offering the consumers any adjustment period, raised an enormous red flag. We almost immediately realized that it was being done behind a massive corrupt political move, orchestrated by the Governor's office and that although the overall concept looked very good on paper, it was however, realistically baseless from a therapeutic viewpoint. It also offered the clients and their families no alternatives. During the meeting, we reminded members of the panel that working with chronically ill clients, could be considered somewhat as the workings of an oncologist that we, could only treat their illness, with whatsoever tools we might have available at the time. We could not recommend a cure and often times, some clients needed a significant amount of time to develop trust with their therapist before they could even begin to point to any great significance.

We in addition cautioned and reminded the panel that often times, these individuals could regress and act out in overt and bizarre fashions if this trust is immediately interrupted. An example, would be that of seeing themselves losing their therapist and their complete support system overnight. This move, could've perhaps been seen, as a rather smart political maneuver, if measured from a politician's viewpoint, however, if examined from a therapeutic standpoint, it was rather selfish mean-spirited and borderline cruel. Again this obviously showed a lack of concern and benevolence toward those less fortunate within of our communities.

We should keep in mind that this panel was assembled by the commissioner on mental health offices under a direct order of Governor John Rowland, whom was later convicted on political corruption, served one year, got out, and was caught again bribing another politician, was rearrested, once again charged and again found guilty and is still doing time in federal prison.

Now let us just pause and collectively imagine, thirty five chronically ill patients losing their complete support system all at once. This basically meant that their case managers and the entire body of the staff, whom they'd known, effectively worked with, frequently seen and trusted, each and every day for the past seven years, who'd been their lifeline, out in the community, was suddenly abandoning them all at once. This was not only an outrage and a blighting case of abuse and political shenanigans, rather it was also an abuse of the trusted and binding relationships, established with these clients, and the community. Many members in the community, thought it was rather risky, and should have been officially considered a significant public safety issue, a problem that should have been looked at more closely, but again it was missing a chief ethical component, it was actually missing the godly approach. The meeting later concluded and we had clarified issues regarding the privatization of all four CBI programs throughout the state. Even though the state panel at first believed that we were there fighting to keep our jobs, although this wasn't actually the case. Our designated union negotiator, continued reminding them that regardless of today's outcome, we still maintained permanent employment that we had jobs security, protected via our bargaining union contracts, emphasizing that we would obviously be transferred to work in other facilities throughout the department, where we would perhaps work far less, with far less responsibilities and perhaps some of us might even gain promotions, with higher pay. And he was right! We continuously reminded the effective panel that we were not fighting for our jobs, thus rather simply advocating for our clients' rights that they may uninterruptedly continue receiving the exact same services and humane treatment once transferred to the private sector.

Most of us had been around the system for a very long time, and understood full well, via relevant facts that privatization could easily mean, cutting cost, by turning around and employing far less qualified, dependable individuals to do mediocre job for a lesser pay, compared to that of ours, by virtue of their experience, education, etc.

Additionally, we had a moral obligation, and that we were going to stand our grounds. Our difficult and arduous struggle for the rights of these severely ill clients, was primarily set on the basis of faith. Throughout our journey, we have experienced firsthand, how the chronically and criminally insane population, their spouses, their children, siblings and other close family members, often bare a tremendous financial and emotional burden for the care of their disabled. While many of them still have the potential threat of becoming criminals, many of them ultimately cost the public significant amounts of money. And many could be easily identified by sight, because of their bizarre dress, posture, behavior, mannerism, etc. Many aspects of their behavior and some of the social problems they create, are upsetting and destructive and should be viewed as such. We, the case managers, and the psychiatric nurses of the state run Community Base Initiative, employed at the newly organized

Meriden Independent Living Community Program, proved effectiveness within ourselves by being able to effectively keep over forty of these people out of the hospitals for an extended amount of time, which lasted over seven years. Nevertheless, we were also able to ensure their safety, assuring that they learned skills for independent, daily living and specifically prevented them from becoming a public or social burden in their communities. We did this primarily by continuously encouraging them not to draw public attention that could further increase more stigmas upon themselves and to appear presentable, to dress well, and that this would in turn, help to decrease unwanted stigma. We also encouraged and fostered social outings and cultural gatherings that enabled them to dress appropriately and to feel better about themselves and to further elevate their self-esteem. Though not all of our clients were able to learn daily living skills and a small percentage of them did not possess the intellectual ability to learn how to budget their monies and prepare their own meals, therefore, these teachings themselves became a challenging task.

Ever so gradually some of these individuals came around and after two years of intense coaching, groups, teachings, etc. They eventually learned how to purchase appropriate foods, prepare their own meals and follow a simple diet plan. Although some of them remain unable to grasp these concepts, it didn't meant, they shouldn't have been treated humanely, since they all equally deserved and received the best of care available. Although we should not delude ourselves from the real nature and volume of the problems involved when caring for this patient population, especially when caring for them in a community setting. Nevertheless, 90% of the group of patients for whom we cared remained cooperative and compliant with their individualized treatment plan following part of our program expectations that included learning how to administer their own medications as prescribed and responding to following all therapeutic interventions.

They also attended all scheduled individualized treatment and group-oriented activities, with their therapists and were on time to all medical appointments with their psychiatrist and psychologists. Some of them did it without reminders. Meanwhile others were unable to learn how to eat properly during social activities, or while in restaurants during outings, or had difficulties simply learning how to use a microwave oven. They did not cause any social disturbances, nor did they display destructive behaviors to private, public, nor state property. Neither did they threatened, or caused bodily harm to themselves, or others. We neither allowed them to become innocent victims of public hostility, indifferent to humiliation and social exclusion. We also tried to maintain total confidentiality among their neighbors. One great aspect to admire about these client's, whom we worked with, is that for the seven and a half years they were in the program, not once had we seen any two individuals get into a physical fight and rarely did we noticed them involved in a form of verbal disagreements among themselves.

Nor did they engage in gossip, rather they showed compassion, sympathy, empathy and an overall understanding for one another. It was a challenging seven plus years, but we had met our objective goal. Throughout this time spent, I learned to admire and respect the mentally ill individual far more than I did some of my own colleagues. Although our society's standards and the stigma imposed upon them may indicate otherwise. Years later, some of us are still asking ourselves, how did we do it? How did we, a handful of nurses and mental health workers turned case managers, managed to accomplish such success with these clients, almost single handedly?

Did we refused to engage in the usage of punishments, or threats? The answer to this question is a simple 'no.' we had an effective treatment team; we gave choices and pointed out consequences. We were altruistic and quickly realized that these clients were human beings with a mental illness, whom had previously been institutionalized. That they were all grown adults, not our children, nor were they either stupid. We practiced a simple approach and followed a practical philosophical method, 'altruism.' We treated them as we would have liked to be treated, and in the end, it all worked out well. They in turn learnt that if they did not took their medications as prescribed, or refused to attend scheduled groups, they could rapidly begin to de-compensate and begin to exhibit bizarre behaviors, which would sequentially lead to public attention and that such would cost them to return to the hospitals. Mostly, we just provided encouragement, options and choices. Of course there were times when we might have needed a crisis intervention, or perhaps a 15-day physician emergency certificate 'PEC' to spend a few days in a medical hospital, respite bed. We also experienced a tragedy, due to a refusal of treatment that lead to a deep clinical depression, where, as therapist, I believe we dropped the ball, such lead to one of our client's to commit suicide, by jumping to his death off the fourth floor roof of the building. I believed that if paid closer attention, perhaps it could have been prevented. Sadly, this was one of the most traumatic evenings of my entire twenty plus year career in the field. Client was a foreign born, spoke very limited amount of English and wanted to be sent back home, but the state refused and he became desperate and suicidal. Although he gave no prior indications, except that he had been refusing to attend and participate in any types of groups. Instead of us planning to send him back home to his country as he'd requested, the system had made covertly making arrangements to have him re-hospitalized. In evaluating the implementation to operate these programs, we had fail to cover this area. Our hands were tied regarding repatriation, but was designed rather to re-incarcerate. This caused a tremendous impact on our clients, the staff and members in the community, whom thought about this being repeated and perhaps even fall atop one of our senior neighbors sitting out in the yard, catching some fresh air. The evening followed by having to go around the entire building, debriefing each and everyone willing to talk about the tragic incident. It was a rather long night.

In the end, however, it all worked out well for the clients and for us all. Regardless of their level of mental status, each of these individuals had their own fully furnished one bedroom apartment, with all the amenities. We fostered and provided the type of care as we would for ourselves and for our families. We advocated for them, showed them respect and treated them, just as we would've like to be treated; 'we promoted basic self-respect.'

They loved their space and their freedom and the responsibility of having their own apartment, each with a nineteen-inch, cable TV, a microwave, air conditioner, telephone, a small dinning room set, a couch, sofa, or love seat, bedroom set, set of pots, a stove, refrigerator and eating utensils. Together as a team, we searched for existing benefits and therefore, found discounts on monthly cable and telephone bills and kept abreast with the Department of Housing for affordability based on each of their incomes. We provided basic ADL's training, however, to those unable to learn housekeeping skills, we provided them with a home health aid to further assist and teach them daily hygiene and meal preparation. We also organized social outings while implementing the 'proper attire is required' policy to encourage grooming. Most Case Managers in our program, made it a point of becoming competitive, while trying to outdo each other, therefore, each of our clients, benefited tremendously. As we would in our homes, we reminded them that their apartments were their homes, therefore, anyone wanting to be let in, must first knock and request to be let in. This meant that even us, the program staff, except during an emergency, could not just marched in to their apartment uninvited. Of course, this was also clinically based. Each of these clients were proud of partaking in their recovery and rapidly showed improvement and managed to regain their dignity.

Since the focus of mental illness remained placed on medical intervention and sequentially such predetermined the way in which such illness is viewed; most current interventions remained ignored or criminalized, therefore, chronic mental illness remains viewed today primarily only from a clinical prospective.

There should no longer appear to be any questions toward such. Although researchers and their findings, have been quick to point out that out of the many groups, the one who shares the most responsibility for the plight of the chronically ill is nursing. These, have also singled out the profession as the prototype of the callous authoritarian by arguing and insisted that caregivers, must be prepared to examine their own attitudes toward patients and be aware of patients' attitudes toward them. This is true in many cases, however these researchers have also failed to provide other alternatives. And have in fact continuously pushed for the separation of church and state, when in reality this could not and should not exist among the mentally ill population, who's only remaining faith, lays between their basic religious foundation and their connection to God. We must admit, however that although skill teaching, caring, medication monitoring, resource teaching and persistence, still isn't a full warranty that the chronically ill, or institutionalized persons will remain out of hospitals, and in to the community that re-hospitalizations, indeed, do occur. And that as caregivers we can only hope that our previous work with a mentally ill individual, will enable the re-hospitalization to be a brief one, with a quick return to community living.

Regrettably, one of the major failures of the CBI's that the governor was able to capitalize on, was the significant component in nationwide police education and training toward regaining control psychotic driven out of control situations. If these ideas had been given a chance for fruition, there would certainly exist a huge reduction in police shootings and professional training toward de-escalation, regarding assistance or confronting the mentally ill, in their homes or out on the streets.

Their targeted goal for independence only lessens, when we continue to institutionalize them, be it out in the community, or in large psychiatric institutions. Although many believe that we must let them learn from their failures, in order to later make good judgments, or realize and live their consequences. Thus far, eliminate and curved growing professional interventions, which can actually be blamed for producing certain symptoms that originally, were believed to be the diagnostic criteria of certain illnesses and cultural dependence. Following this and several other studies researchers have concluded that deinstitutionalization doesn't work well for everyone and that we simply just switched the mentally from one place to another …

Meaning that instead of sending sick people to the hospitals for treatment where they could actually benefit in the hopes of getting better, these severely mentally ill individuals are now being put in jail. This lack of treatment in the system does not serve the mentally ill persons or our communities in any positive form. It is however, rather costly to taxpayers, who continues pouring money into a bottomless well.

A Perspective of The Faith Base Mental Health Initiative's Fight

The collective term, 'Faith Based Initiative, was an economic aid, proposed by President George W. Bush toward helping churches, fundamental faith oriented institutions and religious organizations, reach their targeted goals through government funding. Although many of these nonprofit organizations, now argue among themselves, when trying to uniquely determine the accurate meaning and infinite use of the word 'faith,' while subsequently, ignoring the difficult challenges they now faced with, by strongly opposing grass root organizations, determined to challenge this new initiative, under the separation of church and state. Some of their particular assertions, is a sort of a parallel bipolar opposition that often times mirrored each other. Some of these organizations primary argument, is that all benefiting organizations should fundamentally have an affiliation with Christianity, because if we consider this situation the word 'faith is rather universal. While others intensely argued that every organization, or anyone for that matter can exercise faith in their lives, because we use our individual faith, to bring about an obvious change and that every religious organization regardless its denomination, utilizes faith in their standard practice. In reality the main focus point most often heard, is that Christianity is not of the same kind of faith, because it relies on God, through Jesus, to respectfully give or react to our needs and desires, while other religions rely on different kinds of 'gods' and that some even rely mainly on the universal forces that be.

In a recent interview throughout my research, I was invited to a church in a Southwestern state, it was there that I immediately realized that some Christian churches had gone as far as to undermined the act, by raising the following arguments among their parishioners. Questioning that since Christianity, is a faith which is dependent upon Jesus, it cannot rely upon any other religion or other programs, given by secular entities to ultimately achieve success.

And that if it does, then it is no longer dependent upon Jesus and is no longer based in Christ's faith? Although many churches from diverse denominations have come together at 'the table of brotherhood to support and consistently defend this bill, claiming to the fact that "the work of God is in these new faith based programs!" That the faith based help, is God at work; because God, can do the work through whomever is chosen to accomplish such through).

Nevertheless several hard line churches still contend their principal ground by vehemently arguing that "this is all hog wash." That it is all a cop out from not wanting to rely on real spiritual faith. They have gone as far as to reiterate that "God now has many witnesses to do the work of the church and that God, doesn't need to call upon wicked people to do the work that saints, are supposed to be doing! I later requested an exclusive interview with the pastor, which I was of the opinion that it would gradually help me to further understand this particular church's minister's point of view and it was granted. The good Bishop, pastor and minister, afterward began to explain his position, by insisting that "the Church has always relied upon itself for survival and that was the fundamental explanation, as to why the impressive body of competent witnesses, were so large in many churches and around the spiritual world."

The good pastor, later added that "there is no scripture written anywhere in the Bible, clearly showing, where secular banks were used at any point to further the mission of the gospel." Going as far, afterward, as to compare the faith base initiative with "God obtaining a low interest loan out of Hell to repair the heavens, or God going into Hell to bring out some frills to decorate the Heavens." Earlier on throughout his address, he emphasized that "God has consistently provided for Gods own people and that people should look toward God to be taken care of because God does not need the Devil's money, and that if any of these churches are having financial problems, it was because they were not trying hard enough, or that perhaps they did not yet have a large enough body to effectively make it work." I promptly began to lose particular interest in following the ignorance and reactionary approach, which fueled his arrogance, when he cited the book of Acts, in Acts 4: 34, and after demanded that his parishioners "should gave and give plenty, and willingly. That they should bake plenty cakes and cook plenty of their good food to help the Church because this principle still worked." That the First Church sold things to successfully build itself that they could do it because they are the church." As he continued lecturing to his congregation he buried himself even deeper in anger, by name calling and belittling his fellow pastors and other churches, hastily concluding that "I don't think very much of these church's pastors, whom jump before they think." Accusing them throughout his sermon and boldly stating that "these pastors are motivated by their 'big heads and big egos,' merely trying to 'look big by taking on secular programs. He accused them all throughout his sermon of "just wanting to build enormous churches, with all the add-on and trimmings, such as gymnasiums, classrooms and daycare centers." I eventually wished to interrupt and voiced my concern toward the churches responsibility to education, but he didn't enable me get a word in. He then went as far as to accuse these other pastors of wanting to feel like someone powerful and of being 'power hungry.' The good Bishop sorely missed the whole point, but afterward concluded that "in either case the world is getting worse, because their churches are reaching out for secular power, rather than enthusiastically continued focusing their efforts on getting the word of God out to the lost souls." He subsequently stumbled a bit when I revealed to him that I was of the opinion that "the church for many centuries, had looked upon the mentally ill individuals as lost souls?" Throughout the sermon and during my interview he denied the fact that ("President Bush's faith based promotional programs, are not for Christian organizations, but rather for secular organizations" and that If "any church has faith in George Bush's money giving program, then they cannot have faith in Jesus.") However, he did not end his lecture at the sermon, but later went as far as to publish it on the internet. Where he after concluded in writing that "the Bible tells us, we could genuinely love one and hate the other, but we cannot claim both and that any church, who willingly accepted this faith base money is seeking to clearly claim both and that they cannot, because the President's work is secular driven." I continued with my interview and did not try to further debate any of his points, realizing after that this was just one man's personal opinion. However, I remained objective with my research, realizing then that perhaps neither him, nor any of his family members had never been involved with the mental health system and that it wasn't about him, but rather about the millions of Americans whom would later benefit from these faith based organizations that are trying hard to gather the needed funds to successfully help provide outreach programs for the mentally ill and their recovery in their communities. On a more positive note, we rather look toward the future and focus our attention to those faith based organization that are now working together for the greater good of men, women and children. On those nonprofit organizations that share love, compassion, understanding and most of all treatment and recovery through their gospel, doctrine and perhaps someday soon, through therapy and early intervention. I fail to instinctively understand how one could look at this initiative and genuinely believe that it is all President Bush's money, when in actuality it is the American people's own money? The United State of America's taxpayer's money if you may! By then, I'd also gotten a bit fed up of the words 'church and state,' when in truth, if we are talking about the African American church, we are automatically talking about the separation of church and state. One could go as far back as the initial development of the first black church, African Methodist Episcopalian (AME) church and most other black churches, including those under the UCC banner built in this country since. If you were to read and research a little, perhaps you might find proof and actual data, to witness that our churches, often had to stand up and fight the status quo and confront the state for one reason or another throughout history, primarily that of dignity and respect and the right to worship in peace. We could then move forward to the more recent and perhaps most important legislation in the history of mankind, which is 'the Civil Rights Bill' and wonder, if it was the state who fought to give us those rights we now take for granted? Or was it not implemented in the African American Church, Rev. Dr. Martin Luther King and all of the other hundreds of ministers and their Churches, whom were essentially involved in the arduous struggle and the 'marches?' I believe we should applaud those churches that developed schools and daycare centers down in their basements to ably educate our children and help provide quality, affordable childcare for working young families and single mothers trying to significantly further they education. And yes, had we not complained for as long as we did, about our deteriorating health and all of the various illnesses associated with black people's health, such, which is due in part to the lack of a good education, exercise and poor diet? So what if there is a church with a gymnasium, a trainer and a dietician? Wouldn't then we might perhaps live a little longer, healthier and enjoy happier lives for God and enjoy a more wholesome mind and body for ourselves, and our wives and husbands to appreciate? I heard another argument during this research that came into question, was the critical fact that "if the Federal Government, automatically started to give you money to fund your projects, then they might perhaps want to look at your books?" Well, yes and if there is a crook within their midst, then he might not deserved to be leading a congregation. If a church receives a ten million dollar grant and cannot show what they have done with the money, one would certainly tend to believed that they have a significant problem with or accounting issues. I recalled suggesting to this minister that I definitely believe that if any church receiving any sort of grants, should immediately hire an independent accountant. But then I believed the faith base initiative is all a 'free will and perhaps if a church is doing well independently, then they shouldn't have a need for the permanent use of public funds. This could certainly be compared to a person whom previously has a job going to sign up for unemployment, or to someone, whom already has a home trying to get on the list for a section eight housing.

Got A Few Questions About Our Faith?

Throughout history, perhaps dating all the way back to the medieval age, mental health had been somehow tied into religion and religious beliefs. Although at times, often shunned by the Churches, whom had little to no understanding in the obvious differences, between good religious madness and bad religious madness. Many where often led to believing that the individuals suffering from mental illness had either been cursed, fallen out of discriminating grace with God, possessed by demons, at best, perhaps under some kind of evil spell or witchcraft!

In recent years, a gradual shift in the wind toward the cultural and prominent religious belief, has been slowly appearing on the horizon, a gradual changed that has until recently been accelerated by the presidential 'Faith Based Bill.' The bill was introduced by President Bush during the first months of his being in the White House and signed by Congress at the close of 2001. Although it did not began to pick up steam until late 2002, it could perhaps, be considered, as one of the most positive approaches toward the treatment of mental health since Dorothea Dix's plight for the mentally ill, which historically took place over a hundred and sixty years ago.

The significant humanitarian campaign, in which she vigorously struggled, fought for drastic changes in legislation, advocated and petitioned The U.S. Congress throughout the 19th century and lasted until her dying in 1887. Or perhaps, even Clifford Beers Mental Hygiene movement that happened at the turn of the last century. In any event, it is still been almost a hundred years. Although throughout the years, the Christian church and all other religious organizations have voluntarily been involved in aiding the homeless, implementing drug and alcohol treatment centers and advocating for HIV, AIDS and many other humanitarian efforts.

Although many of these programs implemented and run by faith or religious organizations, dealt mostly with the stressors, anxieties and afflictions caused by mental illness, or are the leading critical determining factors for mental illness, they rendered it inspired by sustained conviction and their love of God. Although often times, rather blindly to the effects, or the thorough understanding of any therapeutic approach and with little, and perhaps no training in mental health services at all, they rendered it and they have done it all by faith, thus rather, straight from their hearts. Now, these newly implemented, Faith Based organizations, which have since emerged through the signing of this bill has created a new hope for the overall understanding of mental illness by all religious organizations.

Therefore, in addition to the afflicted particular individuals and their families, benefiting from this modern Christian approach, there is a renewed hope for the necessary eradication of the illness through research. My particular belief is that this new approach could besides, help to precipitate the overall understanding of the illness and perhaps, even contribute to successfully ending the tremendous stigma that is often times associated with mental illness.

Leading mental health organizations in several states throughout the country, have recently began approving generous grants to churches and other religious organizations involved in serving their communities, through Faith Based mental health programs. In addition to prayer, many churches are now taken renewed, therapeutic particular interest toward learning about the causes for mental illness, appropriate treatment and methodologies, for dealing with community mental health. Some sociologists though of this approach was a great first step, a first of a kind in modern history, adding that "if handled appropriately, in reality, this could definitely be regarded as the greatest change in mental and social engineering in mankind history.."

I genuinely believed it is a winning, win and fortunate situation for our society as a whole, perhaps we could undoubtedly say that everyone in America will benefit from this new approach; the church, the individual and the community, as well as the field of mental health through applied research. Although we first caution these organizations to not stray too far away from the understanding of the individual's illness by trying to conventionally impose their beliefs, "they will come to you in due time," to work side by side with mental health professionals. To thoroughly search, intelligently learn and successfully find different methods, in which they could weave and apply both the prominent religious, as well as the therapeutic approach to treatment and to commonly open their doors to modern workshops conducted by the experienced individual mental health care provider. One of the prosperous organizations in Connecticut to recently take on this approach and perhaps the only one in this state that came from behind its pulpit to reach out and seek professional guidance from mental health professionals in the community is the *New Life Ministries*. The New Life Ministries is a faith based organization of women of different Christian denominations that now provides tremendous support services, personal development spiritual groups and implement suitable workshops that deal with mental health issues. This organization in addition to providing services to other faith based organizations, such as the Personal Development Institute for Women, their clients whom are often pregnant women, seeking outpatient services for alcohol and drug recovery. Their main objective is to effectively provide mentoring services that'll also help to develop their faith, as well as to equip them with the compulsory tools toward becoming valuable members of society. Another successful Christian organization to recently receive a valuable governmental grant from the state of Connecticut under the banner of faith base is the *Phillips Metropolitan Church*.

With an assembly of more than 600 active members, a standing longevity for over 73 years in the Hartford community, a senior leading pastor, with an MSW in social work. Reverend James B. Walker, whom have in excess of 20 years of seniority within the church. Phillips Metropolitan is in addition to a collaborating partner with the Greater Hartford Urban League and the First Cathedral Church, to successfully implement The African Family Connection Project (AFCP). It has also recently partnered with the State of Connecticut Department of Mental Health and Addiction Services (DMHAS). With its new purpose and targeted goal, being the Family Strengthening Program Model (FSPM), to adequately deliver weekly educational sessions, concentrating primarily on at risk families, effectively granting information and support, as well as the tools and cognitive interpersonal skills that includes a strong focus on the counter impact, caused by substance abuse upon the family. In addition, this church continues moving toward developing new partnerships with other community established initiatives, such as Capital Region Mental Health the SANDS and Strive Workforce, by implementing mentoring initiatives clearly intended to actively recruit and train mentors toward supporting particular individuals in recovery, reentry into the work force. As well as to mentor and support those individuals with an extensive history of previous involvement in the criminal justice system. The church have done this through a series of teaching workshops and by assisting these individuals in how to best balance their lives and relevant employment, while integrating faith built, detailed subsequent applications. A formally submitted responds to this approach, has been greatly successful, when measured under the Hope Strive Mentoring Program, this which has now lead to an ambitious expansion of their program in a short few years.

The Phillips Metropolitan Church's mentoring program successfully continues to focus on the multiple integration of faith and overall recovery through mentoring and by paring positive role modeling, which is mainly accomplish through singular and group mentoring. According to all measured systems presently in place, Philips Metropolitan Church's approach has been very effective. Although it's only been a short time, the successive effectiveness of this approach has been shown extremely successful noticed and measured precisely in the black communities. And there are now many other churches appearing daily to take the leading leadership of this valuable opportunity that is as valuable for the churches, as well as to the virtual community as a whole. However, just as the many religious organizations incessantly continue to work hard toward accomplishing successful goals in the mental health and substance abuse treatments through progressive growth, alliances and partnerships, with local, state and other faith base institutions and community constructed organizations. There are still a large number of individuals whom still remain ducked down deep in their trenches, still ready to defend, criticize and ridicule.

CHAPTER II

The Birth of The Diagnostic Statistical Manual of Mental Disorders (DSM).
Psychiatric Nursing, Nursing Treatment and The Historic Treatment of Nurses
The History Behind The Illness ... Our Earliest Views on Mental Illness
Our Earliest Views on Mental Illness.
On The Banks of the River of Faith ... Upon The Bay Where Mental Health First Met **Face To Face**
With World Religion

The Birth of the Diagnostic Statistical Manual of Mental Disorders (DSM).

Consecutively, we have identified institutionalization, as being the chief culprit in many aspects of social disability. This is evident in the progressive social deterioration, its accompanying social isolation and in the passive behavior seen in many long-term patients, specifically in those symptoms that were once believed to be indicative of the standard course of chronic schizophrenia. Such dilemma, flashed the light and brought to the surface, the realization to the widespread difficulty in diagnosing chronic psychiatric illness and, accordingly, extending into the problem of differentiating between acute and chronic illness. Previously, even when there were little questions about an individual being ill, however, determining the type of mental illness that the individual was experiencing, remained still unresolved. Unfortunately, the real question regarding the reliability of the diagnosis and the validity of diagnostic categories in chronic psychiatric illness automatically persisted for many years. Therefore, it was obviously found that many individuals, regardless of their initial diagnoses or subsequent symptoms, ultimately ended up being re-diagnosed, as having chronic undifferentiated schizophrenia if their mental illness persisted for a number of years without remission.

During these critical times, researchers also noted an increase in the number of persons being diagnosed with this illness, according to the length of any potential contacts they've had with any mental institutions. In the following years, private psychiatric treatment centers, in an attempt to significantly further understand the phenomena on their patients, sliding back into a diagnosis of schizophrenia, they later followed an unwritten policy, in which they would no longer diagnosed patients as schizophrenics.

Other noted approaches that eventually showed significance as it took effect, where the following, if it appeared that the patient had schizophrenic symptoms, the diagnosis could temporarily be delayed in hopes that at some point, the patterns of symptoms would alter sufficiently to permit the possibility for another diagnosis.

The fundamental reason for these standard practices, also led to significant pertinent questions, regarding the validity of other diagnostic categories, such as 'hebephrenic schizophrenia,' which was an illness simulating a childlike behavior, this which is now rarely seen in this day and age. Although at one time, many individuals throughout institutions for the mentally ill, was labeled with such diagnosis. Anyone who'd ever had the opportunity to effectively enter a large mental hospital during the late 1970's, throughout in the late 1980's, could perhaps still remember, the characteristics of a smiling elderly woman, dressed in a house coat, wearing soft slippers, walking up to visitors, extending her stuffed animal, repeatedly soliciting it be admired and held by anyone who obviously noticed. Some might also remember the grown adult rolling around on the floor making strange childlike noises. Personally, I could also still remember hearing the 'old-timers' or long time hospital employees, talk about their patients, (crawling on the floors, hidden behind furniture's, and stretching out from behind them, trying to grab at the ankles of those passing nearby.) We question ourselves whether this illness really disappeared, or has there been some subtle change in the current thinking and handling of such diagnoses? Our questions, are based primarily, on the various international epidemiological studies, administered throughout the United States, Europe, Canada and Latin America. However, it is also significant to recognize that there were some cross-cultural variations in analyses and significant classification of symptoms that unquestionably made it difficult to compare the incidence and pervasiveness of the illness's, in different geographical and cultural regions. Certain symptoms, perhaps could have been related to a medical condition, a toxicity level in their system, since were unable unidentified via a simple blood test back then. Or perhaps, even a side effect exhibited from certain medications.

Since this difficulty was fundamentally recognized, there had been numerous attempts to improve the extensive reliability of diagnoses. One such attempt, concluded with a series of revisions in the standard diagnostic manual, conducted by the American Psychiatric Association and an immediately revised systemic framework, was proposed for standardizing the diagnosis of chronicity that would later become appropriate to a variety of illness categories. This conventional proposal, recognized the immediate necessity to improve the required ability for clinicians to make a differential diagnosis, between the acute and chronic manifestations in a broad variety of symptom patterns. It persistently declared that a number of illnesses, could in fact become chronic or have both acute and chronic variations and because, such, there should be a standardized criteria for any differentiation, rather than an ordinary and insignificant subject to the discretionary whim, of the individual diagnostician. It also focused and set a systematic criteria pattern that included a consideration for the duration of time of the illness and the critical continuity of the symptom. The implemented constitutive framework unquestionably stated that 'chronicity,' required a period, no less than five years without significant remission. The following decades helped propelled the advent of the Diagnostic Statistical Manual, (DSM), DSMs I, II, III, 'DSM IV, followed by the DSM V revise edition and beyond.

The standardized diagnostic manual became a sort of 'General Constitution,' A Bill of Rights, if we were to examine it from a legal stand point, rather than just from a medical, or a scientific approach. The revised framework proposed by the American Psychiatric Association, also suggested that within this time period of five years, no period should be symptom-free for more than six months, except in the case of suicide where the psychiatric illnesses themselves had led directly to their death. Thus recognizing the fact that all fatal psychiatric illness shall indeed then be consider 'chronic.' The 'framework' also suggested that chronic psychiatric illness be divided into the four categories, chronic-death, chronic-self-limited, chronic-remission, and chronic-recurrences. A complete mastery for the final outcome of the literature had to then be created, thus preventing it from becoming far less of an overwhelming task on even a limited number of facets regarding problems confronting the chronically ill for most clinicians. Prior to such becoming rather available, literature relevant to the care of the psychiatrically ill patients, was scattered throughout numerous disciplines and media. Medicine, nursing, psychology, social workers, occupational, and rehabilitation therapists, the ministry, philosophy, sociology and historians have all since contributed to the current understanding of chronic illness. The social, psychological, physical and biochemical interventions, was also considered, although, some of the literature did not clearly differentiate between acute and chronic illness or between the treatment of the initial acute episode and symptom exacerbation, as part of a chronic illness.

Psychiatric Nursing, Nursing Treatment and the Historic Treatment of Nurses

Not long ago, much of the academic literature geared toward psychiatry, was centered on the problems of chronic schizophrenia, while other authors concerned themselves with a range of diagnostic categories. Some of the literature focused on limited composed groups, such as women, children, ethnic minorities or lower economic groups. Thus, it became increasingly difficult to adequately analyze noticeable similarities, or crucial differences in patient diagnosis, symptom, or prognosis. Additionally, there was a growing body of literature addressed to the political, economic and other system issues, such as de-institutionalization, involved in the care of the chronically ill. Almost all of the psychiatric nurses encountered throughout the mental health system this day and age, in current or present practice, are caring for or have cared for patients with a chronic psychiatric illness; this is true regardless of whether they have been hospitalized or treated in outpatient community-based programs. While a large number of former long-term inpatients have previously been discharged back to communities, despite everyone's best efforts, a hardcore number of unremitted and chronically ill patients still remain in hospitals.

Many in-hospital patients and an unknown number of those whom have never been hospitalized, but who still have long-term psychiatric difficulties, are being cared for by nurses as their primary caretakers or as members of interdisciplinary mental health teams. Patients are also being treated on a daily basis, on a regular basis by nurses in emergency rooms, or outpatient clinics, general hospitals, crisis centers, as well as in community mental health centers. Public health nurses and visiting nurses also care for discharged patients and their families. Liaison nurses work between hospital and home, and nursing homes, are still being flooded with psychiatrically disabled patients.

Although, it has been previously pointed out that a great number of nurses, currently care for many chronically ill individuals, the perceptive nursing literature with reference to this type of patient care, still remains surprisingly low. Meager in treatment plan, though a large volume of which, is geared more toward policies within these facilities, rather than essential treatment. Until recently, there had been limited number of articles authored by nurses and for nurses, describing nursing's involvement and treatment with the chronically and psychiatrically ill patients, but it has been far from voluminous.

However, most of what does exists, is directed toward systems policies, or role issues and policies, rather than relevant issues pertaining to direct patient care. Therefore, frustrated, psychiatric nurses go through extensive and stressful journeys, when trying to effectively work with a newly admitted individual. The admitting nurses must rely profoundly on their staff and the remainder of the treatment team, on their perception, trial and error and on treating each patient as an individual. Although their professionalism ought to be, respected and their on the fly quick judgement decisions, quite frankly admired. Nevertheless, at times hospital administrators appear to continue to further disregard and disrespect their contribution; moreover, administration diligently remains involved in further revising or enforcing new policies. Most of which, however, is done without ever consulting the invaluable and much-required nursing resources, these outdated, ill sound practices, serves to significantly further stress out the psychiatric nurse, thereby, making their already difficult job that much harder.

Nurses in the domain of psychiatry are still constantly faced with many unanswered questions, relating to their established roles, when working with such patient population. This in fact have conducted other professional disciplines to often times wonder and even question whether nurses actually should be involved with the chronically psychiatric ill and if nurses should, then what should be their legitimate role?

Throughout the years, nurses themselves have in addition questioned, 'what can they, or what should they bring to the table, in regards toward caring for this patient group?' One wonders then, should their functions be any different from those of other mental health professionals? Are they in any way different at this point in time? What professional and educational background, has prepared nurses to do best, with these patients? As an immediate end result of this, in recent years nurses have automatically began to fight back by further expanding their careers and are now returning to school, and highly specializing in more managerial roles. This however, increases the everlasting shortage of nurses.

In the last four to five years, steady streams of nurses have specialized in designated areas, such as Clinical Nurse Specialist, Advance Nurse Practitioners, Nurse Anesthesiologists, Master Science in Nursing, clinical specialist, nurse midwives, PhD's in nursing, etc. Many nurses have also engaged in and have taken on the role of educators, emerging rather less stressed and very successful in their new careers. Reasons perhaps for which, health care reform throughout the last decade, has seen an increased visibility of advanced degrees in nurses, most of them arriving from within the psychiatric field.

Throughout the field of psychiatry, the academic concept of the psychiatric nurse practitioner is rather new and has basically been spawned due to closing and downsizing of hospitals. Nevertheless, there still hasn't been a mass-migration of APRN's, CNS's, NP's rushing back to the psychiatric hospitals, or to psychiatric, outpatient clinics. This is perhaps believed to have a correlation or the end results, stemming from the ill treatment received from some hospital administrators and their absence of understanding, and shared disregard for their staff and more importantly for their psych nurses.

Regardless of the particular fact that federal funding for graduate programs across the country has expanded and NP programs, have officially updated their CNS curriculum to a more pharmacological and scientific health management based system. In reality, it looks practically as if we were back at the turn of the last century and history was also repeating its-self. All of these changes being noted, yet administration continuously remains engage in playing political games and therefore, shuns their nurses away in other directions. One definite fact remains, the fundamental need for primary health care, throughout America has progressively become all too obvious, while the powerless mentally ill clients, remains stuck in public hospitals, shelters, inner cities, poor miserable rural areas, jails or on the street, still lacking the fundamental, badly needed health care.

The History Behind The Illness

Our Earliest Views On Mental Illness.

To understand chronic mental illness, we must first try to essentially understand its origins and at times ask ourselves the most relevant question. What is chronic psychiatric illness? Everyone particularly seems to know about it, yet no one appears to basically recognize that much about it. Although historically, it is unanimously and officially regarded as one of the oldest and more significant health issues since the beginning of time, regrettably we have disputed, lamented it, fastidiously rested virtual blame and rarely, have we tried to descriptively define it as such. *About some four thousand years back, the ancient Egyptians did not differentiate between the mental and the physical illnesses. Despite their indications, they was of the opinion that all diseases undoubtedly originated by some types of physical causes, while strongly suggesting that the human heart was responsible for mental symptom.*

Hippocrates and the early Greeks, thought as well as we do today that all illnesses is the direct end result of biological malfunctions. In the case of depression, their belief, was that the individuals were suffering from an excess of 'black bile;' such could have been seen as a 'potential, chemical imbalance.' So, the ancients weren't too far off their marks, as to specific causes, and their normative vision of mental suffering and their endless quest for medical causes were right on track.

Our Earliest Views on Mental Illness.

Early Egypt: During this time period, causes for mental illness, was believed to be 'a loss of status or money.' The recommended treatment, was to talk it out, and to turn to religion and faith. Suicide was also accepted during this period.

Job and the Old Testament: Despair and cognition, was then accepted causes for mental illness, 'faith was the recommended cure.'

Homer: Homer's belief, was that mental illness was caused by God's taking one's mind away. Homer offered and suggested no specific treatment.

Aeschylus: Believed that such cause, was due to a Demonic possession. This was the theory he used to explain mental illness. "Exorcism was his recommended cure."

Socrates: Socrates believed that mental illness was heaven-sent and not shameful in the least. He believed it to be a blessing, therefore, 'treatment was not required.'

Aristotle: Aristotle's belief, was that melancholia was the cause of mental illness. According to him, 'music was the cure.'

Hippocrates: Belief was that both melancholia and natural medical causes contributed to mental illness. He advised abstinence of various types. He also recommended a natural vegetable diet, daily smoothies and exercise as treatment.

Celsius: Celsius believed mental illness to be a form of madness, to be treated with entertaining stories, diversion and persuasion therapy.

Galen: Galen's belief, was that psychic functions of the brain were considered to be the foremost cause of mental illness. His recommended treatment consisted of confrontation, humor and exercise.

One of the prehistoric forms of mental health treatments 'cure,' was to drill holes in the patient's skull to let the bad spirits out. These 'spirits,' were thought to carry the disease that caused the illness. As history has forged ahead and we believed to have moved beyond the years the worlds view of mental illness came to predominate, and with it came the central conviction that the victim was to be blamed. Possession by evil spirits, moral weakness, and other such "interpretations" placed a stigma on mental illness and the additional responsibility for a cure on the resulting outcasts themselves. The most apparently ill, were then chained to structured walls in mental institutions such as the infamous "Bedlam" Saint Mary of Bethlehem in London, where the rest of society could conveniently forget that the person ever existed. In Bedlam, as in most hospitals throughout the world, the conditions where appalling, the sick were thrown in together with criminals and restrained with manacles and chains. The little medical treatment administered to them, was misguided and more than often barbarous. Violent patients, were beaten into insensibility, others were often bled, or purged to the point of collapse. Some spent many years under tight uninterrupted restraints, with harness made of chains, allowing them only to move up and down. There was little compassion from the outside world. This same public, was later allowed to visit these asylum on Sundays and holidays for a small fee, "similar as to how we would visit the zoos today;" this unquestionably made it a very popular pastime for the outside world to goad and jeer at the patients.

Conditions in these mental institutions were horrible. "Inmates" as they were called, were crowded into dark cells, sometimes sleeping five to a mattress that sat on dank damp floors and chained in place. There was no fresh air, no light, very little nutrition and they were whipped and beaten for misbehavior, much like wild animals. No differentiation was made, between the chronic mentally ill and the criminally insane, all were jammed packed together. Many women were committed merely for the "crime" of attempting to leave their husbands and many of them at their husband's request, in order to gain full control of their inheritance and other assets.

They were not recognized as sick people and were often accused of having forsaken themselves too remarkably, as it may especially seem, but they are a limited number of individuals whom still may harbor some of these beliefs in this day and age.

The mentally ill were charged of having succumbed to spells, incantations and of having committed many sinful offences and crimes. They were persecuted without mercy and often times burnt at the stake. The few doctors, who tried to relatively assure the authorities and the general public that the 'insane were mentally ill and sick-emotional people, whom required attention and care, were often ridiculed. Often they too faced immediate danger to their personal and professional reputation as well. During the 1700's many individuals, were being simply locked away by their families; sometimes for an entire lifetime. Poorer individuals, were imprisoned or placed in publicly funded almshouses. They received basic care, but conditions, were still undeniably bad.

Upon The Banks of the River of Faith Where Hope Forever Flows.

On The Bay Where Mental Health First Meet Face To Face With World Religion

It is estimated that throughout the mid 18th century more than one half of the Christian world reflected upon the poet, William Cowper's published writings of 1766, in which he called 'religious madness,' fanaticism and foolishness. While simultaneously he openly questioned the other half and wondered "but isn't such behavior is warranted by the word of God?" And both parties agreed. He was referring to his own religious faith, as he had recently become an adherent of the Evangelical movement, which was rapidly gaining converts throughout England. During these times religion, true religious followers and the true believers, were merely typified, as 'brands plucked from the burning.' But as far as Cowper was concerned and later declared publicly that "these feelings are not just an issue of intellectual assent to an established, documented program of proofs, doctrines and regular conventions, which could be seen as pretended beliefs. It is an ardent embracing of a lively faith, shooting out of the heart with a spiritual quest, and inner certainty." He then later argued that "this is subjective, it is also very personal and it is very experimental." The word 'experimental,' of course, was the term best preferred by the Evangelical movement during these times. "Experimental was seen then as the meaning of being grounded upon individual *experiences.*" Stating that what actually redeems and what saves the individual sinner from the sentence of the eternal perdition he so richly follows and later deserves, is not, in fact, his own faith, but the spontaneous and quite unmerited gift of Divine atonement, and salvation by grace. Because the conversion of each soul is the experience of being overwhelmed with God's grace. Evangelical Christianity, thus required not merely a pure zealous emotional conviction, but the total commitment of the believer's conscience to a framework of beliefs, which are ultimately, transcendental and mysterious beyond reason.

A theology enshrining the cosmic battle between God and Satan for the soul and the radical sinfulness of mankind, is the reality of eternal hellfire, with shared punishments for the damned and eternal bliss for the saved. Cowper, then pointed to the special interventions of Providence in guiding the pilgrim's progress. The poet went far out on the limb it was, in consequence, rather easy to call a true Christian of this caliber 'mad.' Although during such times, many Christians themselves had in fact traditionally welcomed the label. After all their defensive argument, then was that "perhaps God himself would have indeed been mad to send 'His Son' to be crucified for mankind's sake."

Most Christians then felt that perhaps, then 'the madness of the cross' had indeed been echoed in the 'patristic' and noble idea of the spiritual ecstasy of the true believer, which could itself be seen as a form of going out of one's mind or out of one senses, by literally standing outside oneself, or being beside oneself. The 18th century Christians believed that good madness of this kind, had a long and noble pedigree in Christian theology and it would remain thus strong throughout the ages. Prior to Cowper's writings and many years earlier, there was the Dutch Renaissance, humanist, catholic priest, social teacher, theologian and classical scholar, Desiderius Erasmus, 1466 – 1536. Erasmus wrote primarily in classical Latin, he'd also written and published papers such as *Praise of Folly*, concerning Christianity and the Christian world. Throughout his writings, he focused primarily on the Reformation and the Puritan revolution. In his body of work, Erasmus, also asserted that "the godly and the pious, in particular the more antinomian and contradictive of the 'saints,' were considered to be widely in touch with divine voices and the ability to witness visions in dreams, and utter prophetic truths. He also attested that "above all, Christians do have the ability to see the hand of God in everything."

Of course, during such times, there also existed a culturally grounded knowledge and beliefs toward bad religious madness.

As in many modern day cases still existent today, it was widely believed back then that Satan is always striving to take possession of the weak and tempted sinners, and that those possessed by temper, duly manifested their own marks of senselessness. It was believed back then, as it is today that those who cursed, got drunk, whored, committed idolatry, broke the commandments, fell into despair and took their own lives (suicide back then was both, a deadly sin and a crime). Christians and faith followers, was warned frequently to be aware that the devil is wily and cunning and he could at times, easily insinuate himself into souls under the pretense of being the 'Word' and the Will of God own self. Many Christian authors of that era, wrote penitential diaries and spiritual autobiographies, describing their personal encounters with Satan. Following these publications, the nineteenth-century Austrian author, Christopher Haitzmann and his British contemporary George Trosse, also recorded their encounter and temptations with the Devil years later. During these times and throughout the history that follows, other lesser known people throughout history, also reported how they too, had languished under the fatal conceit, after believing that they were in the process of receiving divine commands, in their heads and in their dreams. Many others, reported on encounters, signs and manifestations, only to awaken in the nick of time to be disabused, therefore, discovering that the Devil had in fact found them. Though their reports differed, they all concluded to often be thrown head-over-heels into crisis, but would eventually come to differentiate between the diabolical and the divine. Throughout Heitzmann and Trosse's writings and published works, we are able to see that both of them provided us, with illuminating points of comparison and contrast. Their valuable historical documentation provides us with detail account of their lives, part of which, is filled with terrifying experience and spiritual crises, assailed and troubled, with visions and temptations, yet they both later recovered to present happy endings.

Nevertheless, the process of crisis for the German Catholic, is revealingly far different from that experienced by the puritan English author. Johann Christoph Haitzmann, was born in Bavaria between the 1640's and 1650's, he was a painter of poor and humble beginnings, whom primarily dabbled in depicting demonical paintings. Haizmann case, have been researched, taught and deeply studied, researched and written about in psychology and psychiatry, throughout the twentieth century, by Freud, Gaston Vandendriessche and many others. Although he had no prior written history about him and nothing else was actually known about him nor his family background prior to introducing himself in the late 1677, to the pastor of Pottenbrunn, Austria. At this time, he was almost to the point of drowning in despair, when he met with the pastor that day after church. He told him that he had succumbed to 'fits' on August 29th and that these symptoms had continuously plagued him throughout a number of days. He was then immediately referred to the ecclesiastic officials and went before them as a supplicant. The officials first question, was to ask if he had had any prior connections with the Devil? Haitzmann then broke down and confessed. He revealed that nine years earlier, right after the death of one of his parent he had become "depressed, hopeless and in despair; unable of even being able to earn a livelihood." He told the body of ministers that while strolling through the woods one day he had been approached by someone, whom he thought "was the Devil in disguised as a burgher, walking a big black dog. And that ever since such day, 'temper' had lured him with a pact." Haitzmann then added that nine times he had been approached and to each he had refused, but that he had eventually, succumbed to temptation and at the end of nine years, he had resign himself in mind, body and soul, to Satan's power. Stating that, "the nine years are almost up and I am now awaiting his doom." The ecclesiastic officials interviewing him, documented that Haitzmann, was in a state of faust-like, "a charlatan, whom is highly successful, yet dissatisfied with his life, which lead him to make a pact the devil, exchanging his soul for unlimited knowledge and worldly pleasures," or simply agony of the mind. Haitzmann then assured them that the only chance he had of inducing "Satan to yield up the pact, laid perhaps within his obtaining a pilgrimage to the Blessed Virgin Mary at Mariazell." He was immediately referred to the pilgrimage and given a letter of introduction.

Haitzmann arrived at Mariazell early in September 1677, and immediately submitted himself to three days of continuous exorcism, expiation, atonement and prayer. Haitzmann, then wrote that on September, 8th at midnight, while praying at the holy shrine, the devil appeared to him in the form of a dragon. He stated that he then made a flying leap and snatched back the pact. Haitzmann, latter described in his writings that "once rescued by this miracle, his melancholy ceased and he was cured." Perhaps the penitent included pledging to join the monastic community at Mariazell and in gratitude for his cure he painted a series of nine pictures, setting out his satanic temptations. It is believe that all of his paintings still survive to this day. Shortly thereafter, following his discharge from the convent, he went to stay with his sister in Vienna. But within a month of his being discharged, he was once again molested by the Devil, this time, undergoing a fresh set of seizures, which wreaked havoc on his body, with such great physical pain, as to induce paralysis. The seizures continuously plagued him, until early into 1678, during this period, Haitzmann was again assailed by a series of apparitions. These initially appeared to him, offering all types of worldly temptations of the deadly sins. He then documented that while in a trance-like state of mind, he would at times see himself seated in famously feted lavished halls, surrounded by gorgeous seductive ladies, dressed in all their finery. Adding that throughout these dreams, people would try to lure him into the lap of luxury, promising him power and wealth beyond the dreams of avarice, and persuading him to renege on his religious endeavors. Haitzmann recalled in his writings that when he was approached by these devils in disguise, he had to actually struggle to summons up the strength to call upon the Holly Mary and Joseph, thereby banishing them and reawakening himself from these trances.

Although sometimes, these apparitions would suddenly change and he would then be shown visions of blessed austerity of simple ascetics in abstention and hermits, leading pious existences in purity, which would then torment him and call him a backslider. He would then be commanded to forswear the paths of wickedness and reminded of his unfulfilled religious vows, while being told to do six years penance in the desert. Haitzmann wrote that he would then, see himself confronted once again by damnation and by the flames of hellfire, which engulfed him, as punishment for continuing to walk the ways of the flesh, then evil spirits would reviled and chastise him with wet ropes. Under such tormented agonies, Haitzmann would again collapse, returning to the convent at Mariazell, once again as a perpetual sinner in May 1678. This time, he would make yet another confession and he would finally reveal that all along there had been a second pact with the Devil, acknowledging then that this last pact had been written in ink, because the first had been signed in blood. Once again these 'Holy Fathers' conducted exorcism and again they were successful, Haitzmann remained at the convent and was later baptized, as Brother Chrysostomus, until his death in 1700's. Finally realizing, perhaps that he could only be assailed by the Devil if he was in his cups. His contemporaries, many of whom considered him to be a mad man. Although such term during those days carried a markedly different meaning for different people. e.g., "An out-and-out skeptic in these matters such as Thomas Hobbes, who thought that all claims of immediate personal contact with God or the Devil, were by definition, fictions or crazy delusions and marked as diseases of the head." He therefore, argued and publicly ridiculed these, stating that they lacked scientific, plausibility and had no authentication. The majority of educated men of that period also publicly accused Haitzmann of fraud, while others went as far as calling him religiously derange.

Back then, this was considered a serious diagnosis, associated with otherworldly powers, reserved for those individuals, whom the Devil had taken possession of their will and the understandings of their soul. In 1621, Robert Burton then published his immense and influential *Anatomy of Melancholy,* thus further describing the interpretation between the religious despair and strife, which prevailed during the age of Reformation and counter-Reformation, in precisely those terms. (Although most Protestants of that era's belief, was that followers of the Roman Catholic faith were '*ipso facto,*' or infected with that kind of madness anyway.)

What is clearly noted during the studies conducted around this period, is the utter absence of the term 'insanity' and any other similarities, or terminology within the language that pointed to any type of illness. Researchers later examined Haitzmann's historic writings and other important written documents and commentaries about his case, during his time spent at the Mariazell's convent. They carefully examined documentation written by the clergy and confirmed that Haitzmann indeed, had suffered with melancholy, but nowhere was it suggested that his visions of Satan, was a form of sickness, unreal hallucinations, nor even vague hints of diabolically induced madness. Rather these, indicative documentation showed that Haitzmann, was simply possessed. However, it was simply agreed that both God and Satan had visited him, with contending good and bad visions and was treated, not by confinement in a madhouse, but by the formally sanctified ecclesiastical ritual of exorcism. During these times the Roman Catholic Church deeply believed in the miraculous success of the casting out of demons. In a marked contrast to the beliefs surrounding the crisis suffered by Haitzmann's English contemporary, Rev. George Trosse. Rev. Trosse, 1631 – 1713, was an English, nonconformist minister, whom is best known for his biographical accounts of periods of mental illness, he experienced during his younger years.

Here, we clearly see that Trosse's episodes, bear many points of resemblance, in terms of madness, albeit, of course, although not organic, but devilishly originated. It is, furthermore, utterly at odds with the shiny finish, inevitably placed upon the events in Lower Austria by the modern psychiatric commentator. More than 200 years later, Freud, perhaps quite possibly intrigued by Haitzmann's Austrian, Vienna connections, took on the challenge of reexamining Haitzmann's case in 1923. To do this successfully, Freud, first underlined and focused on the fundamental interpretations of the experiences that transformed throughout the years. Realizing then that during the eighteenth and nineteenth centuries, Haitzmann's despair, would have been typically viewed as a hypochondriac, with all the symptoms of a victim with organic maladies and plagued by constant auditory and visual hallucinations. Freud, then thought that the unsatisfactory resolutions themselves had been superseded in his own day, and that any psychological explanations, relating the consciousness to the unconscious, by which these had at least taken their rightful place. Freud also added that "ironically, the ancient demonological interpretations, actually shared much in common with the psychoanalytical accounts." Indeed, Freud was unaware of further ironical possibilities and stated then that "it could be said that the demonological theory of the dark ages in which he lived, had in the long run justified themselves." Concluding in his findings that both the demonology and psychoanalysis stressed the priority of turmoil in the consciousness, rather than resting content with lazy suppositions of mere organic disease. Freud also stated that the superstitious theory of the 'dark ages' had presupposed and assumed these 'maleficium' forces possessing from without and from above. Modern psychiatry, later reexamined this same case and saw such disturbances, as triggered by forces within, welling up from below.

Modern psychiatrists also concluded that reason "the religious neuroses of several centuries back, should be seen as the type of neurosis that is seen among children, because it is easier to crack than the complex organically disguised neurosis of latter days." Freud thus believed that Christian demonology, had stumble upon yet ultimately mystified the true nature and cause of disturbance. He indeed thought that such mystification lay bare and proceeded to show how the theological language, was a sort of code, recording all the hieroglyphic clues in a strange tongue, which would succumb before the right translation device. Of course Freud had no hesitation in labeling Haitzmann a case of neurosis. Freud believed that the key to understanding such type of neurosis, laid in the understandings of Haitzmann's attitude toward the Devil. Of course, Freud, being Freud also believed that Haitzmann's Devil was instead "a father-substitute and that Heizmann's unconscious had fantasized the notion of the pact with the Devil." Freud then argued that such had been the only legitimate means of expressing his profound, passive homosexual longings for his own father. Freud continued reaffirming that the death of Haitzmann's father was the cause of his melancholy and his inability to work; concluding then that Haitzrnann's compact with the Devil, offered him an outlet and a twisted kind of marriage with his father. Throughout his arguments he also stated, "it had lasted for nine years, because if one read years as a screen for months, it determined the length of time, for a baby's gestation period, before the actual birth." Of course Freud perhaps did not anticipate resistance to his readings, which were after all devoid of any supporting evidence. But Freud's critiques then argued that "if Haitzmann truly had erotic longings for his father why didn't he express them openly?" Freud then proceeded to defend his theory by insisting that perhaps it was shockingly terrible to contemplate or to imagine any kind of homosexual ties with one's father.

Adding then that such could entailed retribution by castration and contended that it was utterly impossible for Haitzmann to consciously confess to his father's-longings.

The theory was later challenged as being wrong and totally off-beat in, Daniel Schreber's *Memoirs of My Nervous Illness,* in which, he openly challenged Freud's theory by asking, then that "if for these reasons, not the father, but the Devil had indeed embodied Haitzmann's wishes and once displaced these had become a dread?" Throughout other writings Schreber continued questioning and challenging him, arguing "but wasn't it peculiar to simply pick the devil as a father-substitute, as a love object?" "Not a bit of it," Freud replied, "and for several good reasons," he then stated "one being that the Devil, as portrayed by Haitzmann in his paintings possessed many of the macho features for the sexually desirable." And the other reason, Freud then concluded, "the Devil admirably served as a symbol of deep ambivalence for Haitzmann, alike those a son would feel towards his father's, mingling fondness and submission, with hostility and defiance, thus creating tensions between the longing and the dread." According to Freud, Haitzmann's ambivalences, were supported by the portrayals he painted of the devil, showing him with prominent female secondary sexual characteristics, particularly the large breasts. Freud also claimed that this was a most unusual presentations of the Devil, hence a psychologically significant way of representing Satan. Adding that "in fact, these could have been the projections of Haitzmann's feelings of femininity, therefore, giving the Devil the attributes of tenderness, would had further help to defuse the fear that this, his 'father-Devil,' would prove a castrating threat." Freud's critics later confronted him publicly by insisting that "it is clearly seen that his bizarre fantasy to spin, truly makes demonology seem like a sweet reason." Schreber contended his theory by arguing that Freud's, was "built upon evidential quick-sand."

Further more, he insisted, "we don't even know despite Freud's confident supposition that if Haitzmann compacted with the Devil soon after the death of his father, because the historic text was originally written in Latin and it says 'parens,' which could just as easily mean his mother or indeed even another closer relative." Schreber concluded that we have not the slightest scrap of independent evidence connecting Haitzmann's relationship to his father. Furthermore, he insisted, Haitzmann's depiction of an ambi-sexual Devil, was not in reality an aberration of the painter, but was rather confirmed to longstanding artistic conventions. That in those days, the Devil was commonly presented as a double-sexed monster, part man, part woman, part bird, part fish, a creature whose ability to terrify, lay precisely in transgressing all the proper boundaries. Moreover, he continued, what is especially peculiar about Freud's account, is the ambiguity of its presentation of demonology as neurosis. Earlier on Freud had argued of Daniel Schreber's analysis, insisting that it was "precisely then, when Schreber's unconscious came to insist upon its longing for the object of its homosexual desires that Schreber had collapsed, because of the irresolvable conflicts such desires sets up." But the opposite seems to have happened with Haitzmann. His diabolical pact with his father-substitute, does not make him guilty, thus rather makes him prosper; yet for some peculiar reason he falls into crisis just when, at the end of nine years, he is finally about to give birth to his father's baby. Daniel Schreber was the chief justice, to the Dresden Courts of appeal, whom later suffered a nervous breakdown and was treated by Dr. Paul Flechsig at the university psychiatric clinic at Leipsig. Throughout most of the Christian world during the Victorian era, he spent caught between the rules of Freudian theory, the implausibility of discrepancies and proliferation of saving-clauses invoked; for him it was surely became a bit much.

The number of critiques toward Freud's interpretation grew larger throughout the years, in particular the ones mounted by psychiatrists Ida Macalpine and Richard Hunter. Although both were of distinctive schools of psychiatry, they both had quite different set of psychiatric postulates than that of Freud's oedipal assumptions.

They were diagnostically at odds with Freud's usage of the word neurosis in this particular case. Critics later labeled their published work *Schizophrenia* 1677. They had realized that the root cause of Freud's mistakes, lay in seeing the Oedipal phase as "father-son rivalry" as cardinal in generating the conflicts, which erupted in neurosis such, as Haitzmann's. As a result, they argued that Freud sought father-figures and suffered father-induced crisis and of course, finding them in himself, he found them everywhere. Hence, in this case, he read the Devil as a phallic superman, as a projection of Haitzmann's father, and saw Haitzmann guiltily in love with the Devil.

Macalpine and Hunter, later noted that Freud's own theories of ambiguous father-son relations, developed soon after the death of his own father, therefore, maybe Freud's tale about Haitzmann tells us nothing about Haitzmann and everything about Freud. But what is remarkable, Macalpine and Hunter pointed out, is how unlikely of a 'superman' Haitzmann's Devil actually is. Contrary to the expectations set up by Freud, in none of the nine paintings does he have genitals of any kind? (as Freud disingenuously notes that this Devil has no female genitals, but does not point to the absence of a penis). Indeed, Haitzmann's Devils is as much female as male. What this truly signifies, they argue, is that Haitzmann's neurotic fantasy derives not from repressions stemming from the oedipal phase, but from pre-Oedipal psychic stirrings produce long before the infant is aware of gender differentiation, produced at a time when the child might see his ambisexuality as normal.

At this stage when the infant consciousness is pre-sexual and pre-phallic, it is primarily concerned, with life and its origins, and sees new life babies being engendered, not by the successful resolution of sexual conflict, but of oneself or quasi-magically. Hence the androgynous nature of the devil, pin addition to Haitzmann's fantasies of feeding and being fed, and the clear importance of mother-figures to him, not least the fact that he goes to healed at the shrine of the Blessed Virgin Mary.

It should be noted that Macalpine and Hunter's writings gives more respects to the evidence, than Freud's does. However, their preoccupations with Haitzmann's alleged fantasies of gestation and repetitious concept of nine, together with their fixation of the breasted devil, are no less of a prejudice bias or a 'parti pris.' Above all, their very attempts of shining the light upon Haitzmann's own psyche by the analysis of such tiny and inconclusive scraps of evidence, seems a pitiful, abandoned 'sad' forlorn, foredoomed and condemned enterprise. Haitzmann was worried about temptation, being evil, being doom. Therefore, saddling Haitzmann with gender ambiguity, gestation fantasies and dilemma over creativity, tells us no more about him than does the claim that he was fixed on his father. All these psychiatric techniques of isolating figures like Haitzmann, putting them on the couch and diagnosing their problems can indeed become positively perverse. Doing so only withdraws attention from the social, cultural, institutional and linguistic environments, which gave all their actions meaning. *And what Haitzmann's life-story does reveal very clearly, is not his personal psychopathology, but rather the assumptions and procedures routinely deployed in that society to make public sense of the trials of life and the notion of God and the Devil, the involvement of the Church, the realities between Heaven and hell, the goodness of good and the badness of evil, etc.*

In their own practice psychoanalysts does not believe that they have to show why their patient have a need, indeed a neurotic, or a need to fantasize the very institution of psychotherapy, as a defense displacement-projection of their own troubles. It is as a cultural given of modern society.

Although researchers still argue, stating that "no more do we need explanations of Haitzmann's own therapeutic resorts, such as the devil's, because Haitzmann simply subscribed to the givens of his own times." Freud then throws down a new challenge questioning "if a person does not believe in psychoanalysis, or even in the Devil, he must be left to make what he can of the painter's case." Perhaps, but doesn't that pose a great problem? What Haitzmann did, and said he did, was not uncommon back then. Poor isolated folks during such era, were widely believed to commune with the Devil to provide them with a source of strength, albeit, as ambiguous one as it may sound, but such practice still exists today. Although in lesser numbers, but to the female, as the witch's resort to diabolical powers and magic potions many of them still result to using religious symbols and 'saint' figurines to guide them. The idea of selling their soul to the Devil though perhaps a 'faust myth,' was in one way or another a story familiar to all, a tale, a spiritual diagnosis Haitzmann could present to the church's authorities knowing that they would then be able to make sense of his troubles and his needs. The battles Haitzmann saw in his visions between the temptations of the world and the duties of renunciation lay central to Christianity itself.

The best sense that we could possibly make of Haitzmann's case is thus to say that it should be seen not as one of individual psychopathology, but as one reflecting collective beliefs, long embodied within the Church's institutions. He is not a great personal puzzle, but rather a representative figure in a standard scenario. It is not unlikely that one of the factors, which made Haitzmann's rescue possible, was precisely the fact that he was not labeled 'mad, neurotic, nor schizophrenic' and thus not treated or looked down at of being aggressive, full of danger and anxiety as a 'parlous case.'

Rather through his own admissions of being bedeviled by alien, evil forces outside himself, he was readily absorbed within structures of remedy. It may be noteworthy if we choose to follow through Freud's own comparison that Haitzmann ended up happily in the convent, tormented by the Devil only when drunk, whereas Schreber endured nine terrifying years in the asylum, suffering acute isolation, primarily because none of the psychiatric authorities would give the slightest authentication to the term "religious persecution," in which he himself experienced his psychosis. *In reality we could in fact note that the effectiveness of religion and faith, as a set of beliefs and practices for handling grave personal crises is clearly seen in Haitzmann's case.*

This is also visible in studies conducted on the practices of the seventeenth-century parson-physician, Richard Napier, as Napier personally, called upon the angel Raphael for medical advice. It surfaces also in the life of George Trosse. George Trosse, grew up in Exeter at the time of the Civil War, he wrote his life story between 1692 and 93, when he was in his early sixties. It was in the classic mould of Puritan spiritual autobiography, as best epitomized by John Bunyan's Grace *Abounding the Chief of Sinners.* The genre told a story of youthful indifference or sinfulness, an unthinking rebellion against God, leading to satanic temptation and even possession, culminating in crisis. The providential outcome of this was, however, eventual conversion, and a mature life spent, walking in the paths of righteousness. As Patricia Spacks has stressed in her *Imagining A Self,* the Puritan autobiography is by definition a success story. What made Trosse *Apologia* distinctive, though not unique, is that his crisis took the form not merely distinctive of an acknowledgement of sin, wickedness and debauchery, a traumatic emotional experience, the rebirth of a regenerated person, the sinner reformed, but rather of a full-blown episode of insanity, involving medical treatment and confinement.

Trosse regarded his religious madness, not as a fashionable theorists of his time, the age of the scientific revolution increasingly did such, as a physical disorder, producing wild symptomatic delusions, but as a literal psychomachy, a fight between God and Satan for possession of his soul.

George Trosse was born in Exeter England in 1631 to a wealthy prominent Anglican family of well connected, political royalist's lawyers of Presbyterian standpoint. A patriarch ripe, in years, Trosse later denounced his youth as an absolute Sodom of sin. In his writings he tells us that throughout most of his youth he had been a very "Atheist and a dreadful enemy to the Puritans, who had followed every cursed, carnal principle that fired his lusts." Enticed by a an elaborate traveling desire for riches, and live luxuriously throughout the world, he chose to venture abroad as an apprentice merchant so he could enjoy to his fill "the pleasures of the unregenerate world, the lusts of the flesh, the lusts of the eyes, and the pride of life." Like most young men and women of today, in thrall he followed his mentors, with a blind mind, a foolish fancy, and a graceless heart and was led into great sins and dangerous snares. Living amidst the abomination of poverty in France and Portugal, he neglected all religion, and instead followed the paths of drunkenness and sexual dalliance, thus indulging into the most abominable and unclean acts of fornication. He got sick and came back home to recuperate, but while back home in London, a spell of business led him to toy with a relative, whom was engage to a merchant abroad. "So lost was my life at this point that even through periods of near fetal illness wouldn't led me to think on death and perdition, or on the merciful providence that spared me." He eventually returned to his home town, as a notorious and persistent sinner, still fighting against all the commandments, suffering from drunkenness and the depravity that had blinded his mind, and hardened his heart.

He sinned, he recalled, "as a Devil and a raging fury," though of course he had given no thought to his own abominations. At last, in the lower depths, a crisis arrived. After one particular gross bout of drunkenness, at which he flopped more like a hog than a man, he awoke the next morning hearing some rushing kind of noise and seeing a shadow at the foot of his bed. "I was seized with great fear and trembling," he later wrote. He heard a voice asking "Who art thou?"

Sure it must be the voice of God, he contritely replied, somewhat remorseful "I am a very great Sinner, Lord!" Trosse fell to his knees and prayed. The voice proceeded. 'Yet more humble, yet more humble.' Trosse then pulled off his stockings, to pray upon his bare knees, as the voice continued to place demands. He then pulled off the rest of his clothes and laid flat on the floor. The voice then warned he still wasn't low enough, Trosse found a hole in the floor where a plank had been removed and crept inside the hole, praying there on the bare dirt, while covering himself in dust and mud. The voice then commanded him to cut off his hair, it was at that point when he finally awakened and came to his senses anticipating that the voice would tell him next to cut his own throat. A spiritual illumination had suddenly dawned. The voice wasn't that of God's but rather the Devil's. Trosse later wrote that 'he knew he had greatly offended, and finally heard a voice, which he took to be the Holly Ghost telling him "thou wretch, thou has committed the sin against the Holly Ghost." These sins he feared he had committed, which had led him to fall into despair, these voices had used to torture and torment him by leading Trosse to believe that sins against the Holy Ghost were unpardonable. Trosse wanted to do nothing, but curse God and die. "My head became filled with a babble of clamoring voices, making a torment of my conscience."

Trosse was then able to formulate and visualize that in his own wickedness to a peculiarly sinful thought, induced by his malicious will the notion that in his own hopeless, wretched, damned state, he could himself actually torment the Almighty and unchangeable God through this blasphemy of desperate enmity and hostility against God. Possessed by further voices and visions of gremlins and great claws appearing on the walls and so forth, he fell into an utterly distracted condition.

Fortunately, through his family connections, he had good friends who knew of a successful physician in Glastonbury, whom were highly esteemed and very skillful in such cases. His friends managed to get him there by pure force, although he was strapped down to a horse, he fought and resisted with all his might, believing that he was being dragged down into the bowels of hell. Trosse later wrote that while on the journey, voices taunted him by asking "what, must you go yet farther into hell … Oh dear fearful and dreadful soul?" and later recounted how the Devil had finally taken full possession of him that day. As they arrived to the sanitarium, the voices got stronger and he quickly identified it with being in hell, and quite literally regarded the chains and shackles as instruments of ritual satanic torments and torture. His hallucinations and delusions were so vividly that he began seeing fellow patient, as his executioners. Eventually, though long after seeking revenge and rebelling against God, Trosse began to grow more tranquil, resigned and composed. This was largely thanks to the doctor's wife, Mrs. Gollop, whom he regarded as a very religious woman, who soothed and prayed with him. "Although at first, these encounters were no more effective than a drop of water spilt upon the rocks," he wrote, "but gradually they began to take effect and his delusions, distractions and blasphemies eventually began to subside.

Prior to his being discharged he wrote back home "I bewailed my sins" and was thought to have recovered enough to return to Exeter. Regrettably he proved to be no better than the proverbial dog to his vomit, returning back to his old ways, with motivated recidivation. This time however, the battle with the Tempter, was at least more in the open, however, he still pursue lewd and lascivious actions. While on the other hand, he applied to godly ministers, such as the famed Presbyterian Thomas Ford for guidance in removing his great load of guilt. Self-trapped in this renewed torment, he was carried to the Glastonbury physician once again.

Once there Trosse again ragged against God and thought himself in hell, still believing that he had sinned against the Holy Ghost. "But the doctor reduced me again to a composedness and calmness of Mind." Trosse again concluded.

Still his regeneration and conversion were not complete, although he now possessed religion, yet his faith remained pharisaical and hypocritically based. Trosse frequently backslid into unspecified folly of extravagance and was persuaded to return for the third time to Glastonbury. He later wrote, "finally and this time permanently God was pleased, after all my repeated provocations, he restored me to peace and serenity and gave me back the regular use of reason." While reflecting to the fact that the main source of his cure and conversion had been Mrs. Gollop; "she has been the prime instrument both of the health of my body and the salvation of my soul." Trosse was now a man reborn. He went off to study at Oxford. He was now powerful enough to overcome the demonic dreams of the Devil's temptation with God's assistance, he assured himself that he was called to the ministry at the great ejection of 1662, which lead to the expulsion of old Puritans from the Church of England and became a Nonconformist. He spent the rest of his career as a dissenting minister in Exeter, sometimes undergoing persecution and occasional imprisonment for his conviction.

He looked back on his life and penned his autobiography, with a very clear-cut concept of his religious significance in madness and wrote that "reason, was walking in harmony with God and that madness was that state of mind, when the soul, possessed or obsessed by the Devil, railed in blasphemy against the Almighty." At first Trosse seems to have had no concept of positive holly madness, but he later realized that such madness, was thus a desperate, negative condition that played a vital function in the redemption of souls, because it brought a sinner's evils out into the open and into a state of crisis that provided a prelude to recovery.

One might say that Trosse was a fortunate man, supported by friends and a helpful asylum, which came to believe himself redeemed and finally assured of his ability to distinguish the true voice of God from the temptations of the Devil. He never looked back, but for many sincere believers after seeing a sign of God's voice, the providential finger remained obscure. They were uncertain whether the dreams they dreamt and the voices they heard were God's, Satan's or merely their own sick delusional fantasies. The dilemmas over what was true and what was merely deceptive inner experiences, created immense chaos, chaos not just for the individual, but also for entire congregations and for society at large. Therefore, remaining uncertain as to whether those smitten by outward marks of religious madness, were truly saints, the worst of sinners, or just sick. Partly for this reason, for many the whole concept of Christian madness, ever ambiguous, came under a cloud. Expert opinion-leaders and tolerant eighteenth century theologians argued in the rational sense the "surely divine wisdom would not use such an uncertain and dangerous medium for revealing God's word and God's will to God's people? Surely in God's mercy, would not subject believer's consciences to such excruciating torments and allow the devil to delude?" Increasingly it appeared more likely that such tormented souls, were truly possessed neither by God nor indeed by Satan, but rather by misconception, disorders or malady. Those who ranted and raved in the name wailed out in church, or fell into fits while listening to sermons, were increasingly seen as objects of pity. They were sick; they needed treatment. They were in the grip of religious melancholy.

Religious melancholy was the diagnosis commonly pinned on the Methodists and Evangelicals, who formed a rising force in mid-eighteenth-century England. The phrase 'Methodically mad' became something of a catchphrase among those whom, by simply attending service, made it all too commonly to threw themselves into fits by what was then, known by the antireligious movement as "Welsely's hellfire preaching," who attested that sometimes these preaching's even drove followers to commit suicide. They were contemptuous of the canting Wesley's and Whitefield's, whom they stated fanned such hysteria. Little wonder why William Cowper is later quoted in his biography suspecting that his "own mode of faith would have been thought to be mad." In which he stated that not only was he a close friend of John Newton, one of the most emotionally and volatile of all the early Evangelicals, also noted, Newton as being notorious for 'preaching people mad. Not only had he undergone a full conversion experience. But he had actually undergone it, rather like Trosse, while in a madhouse, recovering from what even he admitted was a terrible bout of insanity. Cowper's immensely sad existence was stained with mental disturbance of the melancholic kind, as he put it best when he wrote, "the thread of his life had a sable strand woven into it."

He suffered five distinct severe breakdowns, during some of which he tried to take his own life. The first came while in his early twenties, the last set in when he was sixty-three and it dogged him throughout the end of his days. Between these episodes, the black mark of despair, was rarely far away, managing to stay at bay with forced sociability, application and activity. For Cowper, writing a verse was not merely just a creative process, but rather a quintessential occupational therapy to stave off the idleness, which led to melancholy. His disturbance was never a poetic fiction, it never smacked of the *modish penseroso persona,* so common among super-sensitive artistic souls, suffering from the English malady in that age of syrupy sensibility. Rather it communicated itself, through his letters, poems and autobiographic recollections, about his most terrifying and crushing burdens, which often culminated into a profound desire of never to have been born. It overwhelmed him with anguished feelings of hopelessness and abandonment, a cast-iron certainty of being damned, as told by his close friend Samuel Johnson, who in his own words compared it to, "a sense of being sent to hell and punished everlastingly."

Attempts have been made from various twentieth-century viewpoints to diagnose Cowper's condition, some sounding more like the ancient Greek philosophers, rather than modern day practitioners. James Hendrie Lloyd, tried to resolve the whole problem in a few words, when he wrote. "The case is probably best described as a form of circular insanity, with alternating phases of profound depression and mild hypomanic reaction. Without distinct intervals of complete sanity, it was a constitutional psychosis." R. R. Madden thought that the answer laid in his stomach and speculated that "Cowper may have suffered from some organic disease, akin to dyspepsia," also arguing about "what else would have made Cowper complain so much about his digestion? And that if doctors had simply put Cowper's stomach to rights he would have been spared the agonies of the soul." Others remain puzzled about whether "some embarrassing physical defect had created the shyness and solitary attitude that plagued and made him feel like a lone tree on a hill." Early in the nineteenth century Charles Greville obliquely recorded that Cowper was an apparent hermaphrodite, although there are still some debates, about whether Greville knew exactly what that term meant. However, what we do know is that Dr. William Heberden reported around that time on the case of a man who had castrated himself and that many of the facts found within the report fit's Cowper's description. The hypothetical presence of some abnormalities of his sexual organs, which where possibly self-inflicted, could have perhaps account for the fact that when Cowper became engage to be married, he rapidly plunged into another insane episode and the engagement was immediately called off. Although to this day this remains no more than a speculation.

Isolation and abandonment, may well have been connected with his childhood distance from his parents. His mother, whom he remembered as being one of the most indulgent, died when he was six years old. He was soon sent away to school, and never seems to emotionally get close to his parson father. Indeed Cowper specifically recorded an anguished childhood episode in which his father got him to read Montesquieu's *Lettres Persanes,* which contains arguments favoring the legitimacy of being suicidal. Cowper recalls that when he attempted to refute these ideas, his father did not back his efforts. One may surmise that Cowper perhaps feared this meant that his father would not object if he were to kill himself. Cowper's stepmother hardly receives mentioning throughout his writings, by which we could assume his difficulty in making close attachments. Perhaps due to the result of a lack of his early childhood close bonding, when he later fell in love as a young man, he experienced difficulties. The first and only time being with his cousin Theodora and he was mortified when her father vetoed the relationship, though we're not certain why. But it does confirm to Cowper's fragility and inspirations of intimacy. The evidence also suggests that Theodora herself later grew melancholy, ending up in a state of maudlin novel and confined to the very same lunatic asylum, Cowper himself had once occupied. Hearing about this, Cowper was grief-stricken and wrote. "Oh that the ardor of my first love had continued." He later became engaged again in his early forties to the widowed Mrs. Unwin; historians of the era wrote that "she was a woman he habitually likened unto as a true mother to himself." They also believed that Cowper himself saw a connection between his later grief's and some childhood want of intimacy with his parents. The evidence do not showed us that Cowper ever blamed his parents or other relatives for his morbid melancholy.

In fact his relationship with his elder brother, John grew close and supportive, according to his *Adelphi,* which is a pious story about two brothers that tells us of how John had been the agent of his rescue and ultimate conversion, when he had run mad and how he had succeeded in converting John, before approaching his deathbed.

However, one particular letter loosely suggests that some links existed in Cowper's mind, between family father and stepmother, and immediately went on to say that "these losses lowed in short order by his own loss of spirits." Cowper himself overwhelmingly understood his own sea of troubles of his mind in terms of his religious life, as a believer's quest for assurance of salvation in a world of sin ensnared by Satan. Cowper's insanity is a tale of two quite distinct, chronologically sequential, spiritual experiences, the first being an account of ultimately good religious madness and the second a saga of bad madness. The first we are familiar with from a memoir he wrote in the late 1760s, almost at the halfway stage of his life. This was a narrative following the pattern of the classic spiritual autobiography. It portrayed the hero sinking ever deeper into the slough of sin, falling into Satan's clutch, undergoing crisis and finally becoming a convert to the truth, thanks to saving grace. (It was not published until after his death.) For the Cowper of this tale, madness was a providential medium and an instrument of regeneration. But the terror and despair of his earlier crisis would return, multiplied, deepening him into a series of further crises from 1773 onwards, as inky depression and conviction of indelible doom took possession of his whole existence. We know about the mad bouts of these years, letters he wrote at the time (and even more so, if frustratingly negatively from letters he didn't write. Between 1773 and 1776, the normally almost unrestrained Cowper seems to have written no letters at all).

Only a brief spiritual journal towards the close of his life, written about his descent into hell survives, his last five years is all but unremitting depression and marked by an almost wholly silence. Cowper, believed that for him existed two types of madness, a madness which is mastered with a meaning in a providential scheme and the madness that is insupportable and incomprehensible. Cowper's first madness was a prelude to his Evangelical conversion and having a clergyman for a father, despite going to Westminster School, but chose to grow up, as he tells us in his *Memoir,* "a little better than a pagan." He had realized from young that God made continuous attempts to show him the path of true religion. When he was terrifyingly bullied at school, he learned to cope with the problem by having a text from the Psalms leap into his mind. "I will not be afraid of what man can do unto me," but as he grew older the divine lesson was soon forgotten. When as a youth he had proud and profane rebellious intimations that he might be immortal in the flesh, but then believed God smote him mercifully with smallpox and with a consumptive disposition, as manifestations of God's powers and of man's frailty. Cowper recalled the lessons were lost on him, he grew up in total forgetfulness of God. The first time Cowper fell into profound melancholy in 1753, he was then in his early twenties, his shallow young companions, warned him about his religious exercises, discouraging by letting him believed they made him morbid. He then took a short trip to Southampton and was soon recovered. Although no wiser than a heathen, Cowper attributed his cure to the change of scene and the sea air. Appearing more realistic in his later years, he recalled in his *Memoir* that "it was the mercy of providence, which worked its recovery." Cowper then frittered away his time and his talents in his twenties as a young man-about town, living at the Temple, going through the charade of the study of law.

Divine intervention was again revealed to him after he narrowly escaped injury in a shooting accident, falling debris from a building barely missed his head one evening, still he took no heed at the time, remaining hard-hearted and indifferent. Eventually, in 1763, financial crisis loomed and he needed employment and income. His uncle, Major Ashley Cowper, controlled some patronage in the appointment of the clerkship to the journal of the House of Lords and Cowper solicited the post. He secretly wished for the present incumbent's death and the man died shortly after, Cowper was removed of remorse and guilt. Unselfishly adding later in retrospect, "it pleased the Lord to give me my heart's desire and in it, an immediate punishment for my crimes." As a result of politics, it then transpired that Cowper could not after all be appointed unless he underwent an examination before the Lords. He studied to acquire the skills needed for the post, but grew ever more convinced of his own utter incapacity; increasingly trembling at the prospect of the examination, which he saw as a judgment, Cowper became paralyzed with fear. He had to escape, but how could he? He then used madness, he says, "madness was the only way out, but at this point Satan was far upon the scene. The Tempter insinuated the idea of suicide into my head." He then recalled how his father had never dissuaded him from suicide and an apparent casual conversation with a stranger in a tavern, further convinced him that suicide was a legitimate course of action. That the fact of the act might have been sinful, never even crossed his mind. He bought 'laudanum,' a tinctured opium, with all of the opiates alkaloids, including morphine, powerful and lethal, but on each occasion he attempted to swallow the lethal drug, he became paralyzed, "thanks to the intervention of an invisible hand which rid my control." Today we would of course easily say that his unconscious had taken control of his hand. After abandoning the idea of poisoning himself, he decided to drown himself in the river, but when he arrived it was at low tidewater, and found himself being observed by fishermen. He then changed his mind and decided to hang himself. He rushed home and strung himself up by a sash and as he lapsed into unconsciousness he heard a voice saying, "tis over," but later awoke to find himself sprawled on the floor, with his neck swollen and badly bruised. The sash had snapped at the crucial instant, his uncle was called and pronounced his nephew unfit for the post, and Cowper was off the hook.

At this moment, perhaps for the first time in his life, Cowper had gained his desire, but was now pledge with religious guilt. Not until then had the element of ungodly rebellion in suicide stricken him. Now he was consumed with an overwhelming sense of God's wrath directed specifically against himself. "Surely I must be uniquely the worst of sinners?" He wondered as he paced up and down in his room, repeating to himself "there never was such an abandoned wretch; so great a sinner." He hardly dared to go out and when he did, he then thought, adding that "the people stood and laughed at me and held me in contempt, the eyes of man I could not bear." He felt deserted, rejected and compared his self to being a monster. He combed theology convinced that he probably committed the unpardonable sin and wrote about "that unique blasphemy against the Holy Ghost, which biblical scholars agreed, put a sinner beyond the bounds of forgiveness and mercy." To Cowper it seems initially to have thought the sin lay in the pharisaical act of ascribing works of providence to mere natural causes, for, on reflection, he recalled that "I falsely attributed my recovery at Southampton to the ozone." Collapsing into hopeless, boundless, self-incriminating despair, he later added. "I was filled with the sense of sin and the expectation of punishment."

He later had an uplifting conversation with his brother and his Evangelical cousin, Martin Madan, eventually feeling even more alienated from God, wild and incoherent, he was taken by his brother John to the lunatic asylum at St Albans, which was ran by Dr. Nathaniel Cotton, a medical doctor of Methodist leanings. In his writings, Cowper recalls he went gladly, and for eight months Cowper languished in Cotton's *collegiums insanorum* under the most profound conviction of sin.

He was a bundle of pollution, ever so ungrateful hourly he expected fatal vengeance and the final destructive thunderbolt. He again attempted suicide, but at this point his brother John was able to offer reassurance, questioning him, "might not this certainty of vengeance itself be a delusion and a facet of insanity?" Insisting, he then wondered, "If this be a delusion, then am the happiest of men." Finally accepting and stating that "once more, God showed His merciful providences." This time humbled from foolish pride into the miseries of madness, Cowper heeded them, and he now had a divine vision of being pavilion under a cupola of radiance and seeing glory all around. He later attempted to convince a doubting Thomas of the asylum and a servant, about the reality of special Providence. They later experienced an exemplary thunderstorm, in which a fiery hand clenching a bolt, arrow of lightning appeared in the sky, hurling down lightning flashes to earth, but sparing them. One day, while he was flicking through the Bible, a book he had long neglected, fate directed him to St Paul's Epistle to the Romans, which spoke of "his Savior whom God has set fort to be a propitiation through faith in his blood, to declare his righteousness for the remission of sins that are past, through the forbearance of God." The scales fell from his eyes. The text convinced him of Christ's atonement and forgiveness. Finally, in a dream, Cowper saw a radiant boy come dancing up to him. Cumulatively these experiences had worked a conversion within and brought an epiphany. The burden of sin was lifted and Cowper felt redeemed by Christ. Thanks to his assurance of grace, he would be saved. His complete sanity returned and he added that his madness had been a divine chastisement, the madhouse, the instrument of his reformation, which became the scene of his second nativity."

In later spiritual conversations his brother wrote of Dr. Cotton "restored him to a state in which he could face the world, because he supplied spiritual solace and succor as well as medicine." Although some say Cowper later confessed that Dr. Cotton's behavior was just as crazy as his own. After a year and a half of being in the sanitorium, Dr. Cotton pronounced him cured and Cowper was free to leave. Taking Cotton's own servant boy with him, he got lodgings in Huntingdon, to be near his brother, who was a fellow at Bennett's College, currently today's Corpus Christi's College. While in Cambridge he became friendly with an Evangelical family, the Reverend Morley Unwin and his wife Mary. He began to board with them and after Reverend Morley's death he remained on terms of intimate spiritual friendship with Mary. They moved together to Olney in 1767, partly to be near the Evangelical John Newton, who became their spiritual guide. He finally found security in submission after so much mutiny, now confident in the Lord, he then wrote. "He has never left me, since he first found me, not for a moment. I know that the Everlasting Arm is underneath me and the Eternal God is my refuge. Oh, blessed state of a believing soul. In the Unwin household, I've found a place of rest prepared for me by God's own hand." Cowper wrote his Olney Hymns and penned his *Memoir* as an act of thanksgiving, thus recording his spiritual conversion.

Although not covered throughout this segment, one of the most enduring and most damaging accounts of bad religious madness that we could all attest by which we're all been drastically affected by the Church throughout history, is discrimination. Be it racism, bigotry and phobias.

CHAPTER III

The History of Medicine

Mankind has evolved successfully over time by adapting ourselves to encounter the hazardous found throughout our environment. We have learnt to use plant, minerals and animal life around us to provide food, clothing and shelter. Nevertheless, disease is one of the enemies, we have been unable to fight on an equal playing field. Parasitic organisms too small to be seen by the naked eye, still bent on invading our organisms, living, infesting and feeding themselves off our prime substance, until they have weakened and finally killed us. Deficiencies in any of our basic needs, such as food or warmth, reduces the body's basic defenses against attack, however, even when these basic necessities are available, disease may arise through ignorance or neglect of basic simple hygiene. Although man, is not completely helpless against the onslaught of disease, nature has its own defense mechanism by which a species gradually adapts itself to its environment by developing immunity to such diseases that threatens our survival. This form of unconscious biological adaptation is a slow process, but man has been able to add conscious and deliberate adaptation by scientific studies, treatments and surgery.

The many techniques of modern medicine could never had been understood nor devised, without 'profound comprehension of the structures and the functions of the human body, nor an in-depth study on the force, which can shorten our normal life span. Perhaps by focusing our study on the history of medicine, we could then realize, how gradual this process has been, although even by today's standards, the growth toward understanding some of the mysteries the earliest physicians faced still remains a mystery. Ignorant of the physical causes, caused by disease, made people of primitive societies look at an illness as being caused by evil spirits, or evil doings, "this still happens in many cultures of today." Some may still even seek cures in worships and sacrifices, in many cases, the functions of the doctor and that of their priest is inseparable. However, during the early days of medicine, progress toward a more practical approach was on the horizon and the lore of the medicine man, became more of a nature based study rather than that of a scientific approach. Plants came to be used in a form of treatment, it medicinal properties, were later extracted. Surgery was on it heels, for it too had its early beginnings. Prehistoric skulls found in many parts of the world, appeared with holes bored in them, shown signs of primitive medical tool usage. *"This process known as trepanning was generally intended to allow the escape of evil spirits, which was thought to be causing the symptoms of mental illness."* Surprisingly, patients did survive these operations, many of the uncovered skulls, were found with the rims of the perforations blunted by the healing process in the bone tissue, thus indicating that these patients did survived for a period of time.

In later years medicine evolved and grew to become even more sophisticated in the great civilizations of the ancient world. In Egypt, there were doctors for different parts of the human body. Studies on influential people in Egypt, shows, degrees of specialized treatment, even more sophisticated and at times taken to an extreme, even by today's standards, e.g. an Egyptian pharaoh, had a different doctor for each of his eyes. By the year 2000 B.C. Egypt already had what could perhaps have been the world's earliest national health system set in place, with doctors, whom where paid by the state and free treatment for the sick, while they were traveling, or injured in wars. Medical papyri from around 1500 B.C. shows that although Egyptians had recognized and treated various diseases affecting many parts of the body, including mental illness, their medicine remained primarily a religious practice and their knowledge of anatomy, was extremely limited. The ancient civilizations of China and India also had well-established systems of medicine, the Indians had little knowledge of anatomy, but their surgeons could remove tonsils and limbs, using a range of instruments, which included scalpels, saws and forceps. The ancient Greeks, who showed that man's power of reasoning could be applied in so many fields of philosophic and scientific inquiry, today are still being considered the fathers of rational medicine. Although first they needed to divorce themselves from religious beliefs and mere speculation. These breakthroughs came with the realization that certain common symptoms, always appeared together and that certain drugs caused relief.

The founder of this new group of scientific medicinal of thinkers was, the ancient Greek physician, Hippocrates, whom is considered to be the father of modern medicine, Hippocrates wrote several volumes by which he scientifically described his findings of a number of diseases and their treatments, based on detail observations. He was also the first to disconnect modern medicine from any particular religious superstition. Hippocrates, who lived on the Aegean Islands off Cosin, during the (5th Century = 460 – 377 B.C.) although he too, was hampered by an inadequate knowledge of anatomy physiology, he believed that a disease was caused primarily by an imbalance among the four basic 'humors' of the body. His method of diagnosis, was primarily based on reason and on careful observation. This became the basis of medical practice for centuries that follow. Hippocrates also placed great emphasis on importance of a doctor's duties toward their patients for future outcomes. This, which is now enshrined in the 'Hippocratic oath', which remains the basis of today's medical standard practice and ethics. Hippocrates, also emphasized on the healing powers of nature, the values of personal hygiene and a correct individual's diet, "One man's meat, is another men's poison." His primary belief, was that the physician's task was to assist nature in the fight against the disease, not by dangerous remedies for minor ills, but rather by observing and waiting for the right moment when medical intervention was most appropriate. However, this new scientific school of medicine founded by Hippocrates, would not survived for long and would swiftly be swept away by early religious treatments based on cultural religious beliefs.

This would later became known, as a system of temple medicine, which was dominated by the cult of Aesculapius 'the god of medicine,' which survived throughout the ancient Greek history. Thousands of people flocked for cures to vast sanctuaries in Athens, Epidaurus and even Cos, Hippocrates's homeland.

The treatment at these sanctuaries, always began with a ritual purification, followed by the use of drugs, hallucinogenic or hypnosis to induce sleep and mind control. These patients were then liked by snakes, at which point temple gods would appear to them to diagnose their sickness. Upon reawakening, the patient would then relate their dreams to temple attendants, who would then later interpret them and suggest a cure. Offerings of afflicted parts of the body were left behind at the temple, presumably in gratitude for successful cures.

Another historic figure in the history of modern medicine, is Galen.

Aelius Galenus = Claudius Galen, circa 130 A.D. He was born in Perganum, modern day Turkey of Greek parents. He studied medicine in Greece, Alexandria and throughout Asia Minor, Galen was the first to recognize and document that our muscles are controlled by our brain. Galen, was originally the chief physician to the gladiators at Perganum, where, he gained vast knowledge and experience with treating and repairing severe wounds and obviously the understanding of the functions of the synchrony between the brain and the muscles.

Galen, was a surgeon, and a philosopher in the Roman Empire, he later served, as the first physician to five different Roman emperors. In his writings, Galen summarized the results of five centuries of medical inquiry. However, he later added findings of his own, the principle one of these being incorporated into his teachings that everything in nature has its functions and injuries, brings about change in these functions. Unfortunately, Galen's usual method of argument by analogy from animals rather than by clinical observation on human patients, led him to make many serious errors, e.g., *'he thought that blood passed directly from one side of the heart to another, thus ignoring the arteries and veins and had no idea that it circulated right around the body.'* Nevertheless, the skill with which he presented his theory caused his errors to go unchallenged in Europe for centuries, until the Renaissance period, more than 1400 years later. With the fall of Rome in the 5th A.D. all medicine and all medical treatment ceased to exist throughout Europe.

Other important historic aspects of modern medicine are the Arabs

Following the fall of the Roman Empire, the Arabs had collected, studied and translated numerous Greek manuscripts on science and medicine, thus not only preserving them for later generations, but also making useful comments and additions.

Rhazes = Abu Bakr Muhammad Zakari al Razi, circa (865 – 925), Persian polymath, alchemist, philosopher, was and important figure in the history of modern medicine, who also wrote on logic, astronomy and grammar. He was the chief physician at the hospital of Baghdad, and was also the first scientist to distinguish between small pox and measles.

Avicenna = Abu Ali Sina, (980 – 1037). Persian polymath, Avicenna has been regarded as the father of early modern medicine. He compiled a *Canon* of medicine, which became compulsory reading for medical students in universities across Europe throughout the 17th century. The interest in medical knowledge and ancient Greek medical schools began to resurface during European medieval times throughout Western Europe in the 10th century. Latin translations of the medical classics were made from the Arabic versions and a school of medicine at Salerno, in Italy. Medical students learnt their lessons in verse form, as an aid to memory, the school specialized mostly in surgery and the diagnosis of ailments, which was conducted from patient's urine. The revival in medical teaching spread from Salerno to other newly founded medieval European universities, e.g. Bologna, Padua, Montpellier, Paris, Oxford, etc. Medicine was still only being studied for its mental discipline, rather than for its healing values and the practical effects of the revival, was strictly limited. Medical research, however, was still discouraged by the widely held beliefs that sickness, was God's punishment for the sin … in the words of the Bible, *"the sins of the fathers, are visited upon his children."*

The First Act Geared Toward Removing the Mentally Ill From Jails

The odyssey of repeated incarceration for severely ill people, was common in the United States throughout the 18th and 19th centuries, although back then many Americans found such practices inhumane and uncivilized. Their sentiments found, organized expression in the Boston Prison Discipline Society (BPDS), which was founded in 1825 by the Reverend Louis Dwight, a Yale graduate and Congregationalist minister. Due to the shocked received by what he saw, when he began taking Bibles to inmates in jails, he established the society to publicly advocate improvement in the prisons and jail conditions in general, and the hospitals that housed the mentally ill prisoners in particular. According to the medical historian, Gerald Grob, due Dwight's insistence that "mentally ill persons belonged in hospitals" aroused a responsive chord, especially since his investigations demonstrated that large numbers of such persons were confined in degrading circumstances. Dwight's arduous campaign, led the Massachusetts legislature to appoint a committee in 1827 to investigate conditions in the state's jails. The committee's investigations report directed to the State General Court, concluded in its documentation that in fact many lunatics and persons suffering from mental illness, were being confined, often in inhumane and degrading conditions. The report showed that in one jail, a man

had been kept for almost ten years that "he had a wreath of rags around his body, and another round his neck. He had no bed, chair or bench, a heap of filthy straw, like the nest of a swine, was in the corner." The report concluded "the poor wretched lunatic, was indulging in some delusive expectations of being soon released from such wretched dwellings." In its report, the committee concluded, "The situation of these wretched beings, calls very loudly for some redress. They seem to have been considered as out of the protection of laws. Less attention is paid to their cleanliness and comfort than to the wild beasts in their cages, which are kept for show."

Among the specific recommendations of the committee, was that all mentally ill inmates of jails and prisons should be transferred to the Massachusetts General Hospital and that confinement of mentally ill persons in the state's jails should be made illegal. Three years later, the Massachusetts

General Court "overwhelmingly approved a bill providing in its budget monies to build a state lunatic hospital for 120 patients"; this opened in 1833 as the State Lunatic Asylum at Worcester. When the hospital opened, "more than half of the 164 patients received during that year came from large work houses, almshouses, and prisons." One-third of these patients had been confined in these institutions for longer than 10 years. Dorothea Dix, the most famous and successful psychiatric reformer in American history, would pick up where Dwight had left off. In 1841, with the American asylum-building movement under way, Dix began a campaign that would focus national attention on the sad plight of the mentally ill in jails and prisons she was directly responsible for the opening of over 30 state psychiatric hospitals.

Historic Overview of Institutional Psychiatric Care In America.

It wasn't until during the late 18th to early 19th centuries that hospitals and asylums assumed the care of the mentally ill. The first hospital to accept and treat mentally ill patients, was the Pennsylvania Hospital, which was founded by the Quakers in 1752. Treatment there was the same as for other patients, clean surroundings, good care and nutrition, fresh air and light … in short, one could perhaps believe that the mentally ill were finally beginning to be seen and treated as human beings.

The word 'asylum' literally means temporary shelter or refuge. One definition found in the 10th edition of Webster's Dictionary describes it as an institution for the care of the destitute or sick and particularly the insane although some strongly believed that during such times, the permissive term represented more of a security or a protection, rather than relative care. If we were to rest on this thought, we would subsequently realize that the mentally ill back then, weren't actually running and seeking out essential treatment, they simply ran, because they were vehemently being persecuted and punished by society. Of course, they just wanted to live … they certainly wanted to save their selves from being burnt at the stake. The first actual mental asylum built in America, opened in 1769 under the guidance of Doctor Benjamin Rush, who became known as 'America's first psychiatrist.' Dr. Rush was an esteemed professor at America's first psychiatric hospital in 1769. This hospital, located in Williamsburg, Virginia was to be the only such institution in the country for over fifty years. As we identified the historical origins surrounding the concept of insanity, three different perspectives come to mind, "the medieval, the enlightened and the modern era." At this point, however, since we covered in detail different aspects of enlightened period, we will exclude such and focus primarily, on the existent differences between the medieval and the modern concepts of insanity.

One of the significant differences between these periods, is that medieval men successfully acknowledged what insanity was, meanwhile, we, throughout this modern era, still do not. That is, medieval lawyers, doctors and theologians were certain of the symptoms and particular significance of insanity; however, many may have defined it according to their specialized interest and diagnosed it in terms of behavioral signs. In recent decades, most legal treatises and psychiatric texts have reflected the meaning of the term 'insane' and the border-between sanity and insanity. Pertaining to us as the modern culture, we do not have profound knowledge and perhaps do not care much about the meaning nor the intellectual concept of insanity, but are rather more concerned about our own personal growth and the level of earning potential. One might easily notice that in many cases, psychiatrists, psychologists, nurses and social workers, lose central focus on those for whom they are to effectively provide professional care for. They later find themselves more interested in rapidly becoming institution directors and, or working their way into mental health commissioner appointed positions. This, in combined essence, is not a bad thing if their heightened target and particular interest, was to actively continue treatment oriented improvement toward patient care.

Secular Perspectives: Chronic Mental Illness, Versus Faith Base Initiatives

The moral, the enlightened and the modern perspectives are the three known general perspectives of mental health. Throughout history, each of these has led us into a very different approach to care. According to historians accounts, the cult of St. Dymphna is based on a legend dating back to 1247 A.D. Petrus Cameracensis first described it in his writings that his story was primarily based on oral accounts that would later take on Christian tradition. He wrote about, Dymphna, a 14 year old girl, who'd consecrated herself to Christ, and took on a vow of chastity. Her mother died shortly thereafter, Damon, whom was her father, and also happened to be a seventh century Irish king, refused to marry any other women unless they were as beautiful as his beloved departed wife. His mental health severely deteriorated and he sunk into severe depression. At his point, counselors demands he needed to remarried, once pressed to remarrying by his counselors, finding himself unable to locate anyone as beautiful as she was, due to their close resemblance, Damon grew strong desires for Dymphna, and wanted to marry his daughter, following the death of his wife. When she resisted his wishes he threatened her life and she had fled the country, with her confessor, Father Gerebernus, several trusted servants and the kings Gester. Together they sat up a hospice for the poor and the infirm in the town where they'd seek refuge. He traced her spending through the usage of her wealth, as some of the coins used, traced and lead them back to Belgium. He then had his agents followed their trace, who'd found her in the town of Geel, Belgium. Damon, ordered his soldiers to kill her confessor, and rest of her trusted servants, then tried to forcing her to return with him back to Ireland, but she refused. A furiously demented, out of control madness, led Damon, to draw upon his sword, thus he struck off his daughter's head. The legend tells us that from the eleventh to the twelfth century, miraculous cures of both mental and physical illness were said to have occurred, right on the spot where St. Dymphna was martyred. This area is located in the town of Geel the spot later became very popular and remained a regularly visited shrine. By the end of the thirteenth century a hospital was built, and by the second half of the fourteenth century, Geel, Belgium widely became known as a place of pilgrimage for mental patients. The town then became so popular that the church and the religious order could no longer care for the large numbers of visitors afflicted with mentally illness still thronged and gathered there, in search of a cure. At such point, the local people began to take them in at first, though only for a brief period of time. During mentally ill pilgrimages to the shrine for still unknown reasons, they extended the length of their stay. Since the seventh century, large numbers of mentally and chronically ill people have boarded with Geel families, yearly increasing in numbers from an estimated 285 patients in 1804 too much over a thousand in 1847, and twice that amount in modern times. Although veneration of the relics of St. Dymphna continues, there has been a gradual shift over the years to a more modern approach to treatment. According to historic documents, parts of her remains has since been transferred and are now kept at the Shrine of St Dymphna, in Massillon, Ohio, right here in the United States.

The Age of Enlightenment.

At the close of the middle ages, there was a sweeping shift in perspective on the horizon, regarding mental illness that took a more enlightened and humanitarian viewpoint. However, early on during the eighteenth century, mental illness was no longer considered to be the result of sin or a devil possession. Instead of viewing the disease as the visitation of God, it was considered more of an unfortunate weakness or undeserved affliction. Of course, this was after the royals and the noble class, realized that they too were not excluded. Hence forth, there was an immediate movement to release the mentally ill who'd still languished in prisons or almshouses, followed by a renewed sense of public responsibility for the care of these individuals. An illustration, which depicts these changes, is the dramatic painting of *1792 Striking of The Chains Off The Chronically Ill*, in Paris insane asylums by *Pinel*. This period, despite its enlightenment mistakenly produced institutions such as *Bedlam*, official name being, the Saint Mary of Bethlehem Hospital or Bethlehem Royal Hospital, in London England. Bedlam was an institution designed to provide benign custodial care for the mentally infirm. However, this proved to be somewhat worse than prison, because on Sundays the general public was encouraged to go to Bedlam and for a few shillings, they could view live show, taunt, and dehumanize the mentally ill as a form of cheap unimaginable way of amusement or entertainment. This period, however, is considered to be the first documented account of reduced stigma; it also provided the first attempt of humane type of treatment. It is believe that this period is also credited with reducing the amount of fear previously associated with mental illness and the mentally ill and therefore, also creating the beginnings of a genuine social, conscience toward the mentally ill. These treatments however, were no more effective, in alleviating the symptoms or altering the course of these illnesses than the preceding era.

The Enlightened period, terminated in the nineteenth century with the emergence of one of the major figures in social reforms for the mentally ill.

At a recent United Church of Christ symposium on justice and equality, I mustered the courage to ask the panel "what was the Church doing to help ease the situation of the mentally ill, today?" A young minister somewhat confused about my question then replied, "well we really don't know what to do, because we don't know how these people may react, we also do not feel comfortable being around them, because we are not equip with sufficient knowledge." I could not help but to remind the panel that the first major impact that brought positive change in mental health treatment occurred due to the Church's indirect involvement almost 150 years ago, and that perhaps it was time for the Church to again become involved.

The name synonymous with social reforms concerning the plight of the mentally ill, is that of Dorothea Lyn Dix (1802-1887). As a Sunday school teacher, Miss Dix, had an opportunity to visit prisons and poorhouses, in which the chronically mentally ill were confined and she was appalled at the conditions, in which these people were forced to exist. Almost single handedly, she mounted a campaign to arouse the public awareness to provide special funds and build better places for the care of the mentally ill. Prior to Dorothea Dix's time, throughout the New England states, as in many other parts of the world, the colonist's shared belief was that all Native American 'Indians,' mentally ill and witches, formed part of Satan's army. They constantly launched campaigns against them, in an attempt to exterminate and wipe them off the face of the earth. This belief also spilled over to the way in which the supposedly righteous, industrious, moral minded, viewed the mentally insane person and likewise they treated them accordingly.

Recorded events, dating back to the mid-sixteen hundreds, shows us that if a local insane woman, could not be cared for and supported by her husband, the town would be obliged in assuming some of the responsibility and financial burden for her care.

These perhaps are the first documented public care records, regarding mental health establishing a precedence for towns to take responsibility for their poor and insane individuals. Perhaps it should best be recognize as the very first welfare act. Approaching the middle part of the 1600, strict laws were passed referring to "paupers," drifters and undoubtedly the insane. These such laws, ordered each town to care for their poor; laws were later enacted to help to provide means to individual towns that abdicated 'renounced' the responsibility to care for indigent strangers. This moved was to secure the first general law concerning the insane in 1699, known as 'the Act for the Relieving of Idiots and Distracted Persons,' it was passed by the General Court of Connecticut. Such Act reads as followed: *It is ordered and enacted by Governor, Council and Representatives in General Court assembled and by the authority of the same that when do so often as it would happen any person who appear to be naturally wanting of understanding, so as to be incapable to provide for him or herself, or by the providence of God shall fall into distraction and become non compos mentis and no relation appears that will undertake the care of providing for them, or that stand in so near a degree, as that by law they may be compelled thereto; in every such case the selectmen or oversees of the poor of the town, or peculiar where such person was born, or is by law an inhabitant. Be and hereby are empowered and end enjoyed to take effectual care and make necessary provisions for the relief, support and safety if such impotent, or distracted person, at the charge of the town or place whereto he or she of right belongs; if the party hath not estate of his or her own the incomes whereof shall be sufficient to defray the same. And the justice of the peace within the same county at their county courts may order and sis pose the estate of such impotent or distracted person to the best improvement and advantage towards his or her support, as also the person to any proper work or service he or she may be capable to be employed in, at the discretion of the selectmen or overseers of the poor.* Of course laws were later reenacted in 1711 and 1715 that would amplify the 1699 law, reiterating the family responsibilities toward the care of their own. Although in many cases, these laws went much further, as far as to punishing with imprisonment, or striking with severe fines, or penalties to those relatives, whom were able to care for their own, but refused and neglected to do such. By 1715, public assistance became available to compensate non-family members who opened their doors and cared for the mentally ill in their own homes. However, this was not the end of the dilemma, but rather just the beginning. Many mentally ill persons without homes, still roamed the street homeless and uncared for. Often times, these persons became a threat to public safety, while others endangered themselves by idling around, or becoming vagabonds. Without a voice in their favor to advocate for them, and during such a time when their behavior immediately became an apparent insult to the industrious minded, this led to the passage of the act of 1727. This act directed for the building of workhouses that were geared not to treat, but to further punish and suppress the rogues, vagabonds, common beggars and other lewd, idle dissolute and disorderly persons. In addition to punishing, this law also restricted movement and freedom and placed mentally ill persons into a qualified form of slavery, free labor, or indentured servitude. This law also restricted and striped their rights, while empowering and giving the rights to any county court, or any two justices of the peace, or any court assistant and justice of the peace to commit the insane to these workhouses.

The following act read as follows:

All rogues, vagabonds and idle persons going about in towns or counties begging, or persons using any subtle craft, juggling, or unlawful games, or plays, or feigning themselves to have knowledge in physiognomy, palmistry, or pretending they can tell destinies, futures, or discover where lost and stolen goods may be found. Common pipers, fiddlers, runaways, stubborn servants, or children, common drunkards, common night walkers, pilferers, wanton lascivious persons either in speech or behavior, common railers or brawlers, such as neglect their calling, misspend what they earn, and do not provide for themselves or the support of their families as also persons under distraction and unfit to go at large, whose friends do not take care for their safe confinement.

This legislation was rather incomprehensive and broad. It also linked the insane with criminals, thus it obviously became the first approach toward institutionalization. The act also indicated and generalized the fact that anyone committed to workhouses, had to work. They were also submitted to routine and regulatory whippings and lashes if their behaviors were found to be uncooperative. They were also shackled and starved, until they cooperated, or otherwise, just left there to die. It took over a half of century before any new laws were changed, in favor of disallowing the justice of the peace and county courts authority to rid themselves of absolute control over the lives and freedoms of the mentally ill individuals.

This law did not only break and remove their chains, while freeing them from the workhouses, but it also authorized all selectmen to commit any dangerous mentally ill person to a more suitable and safe place, thus including jailhouses if needed to. However, the public still remained stuck with the dilemma of how to best care for the harmless mentally ill individual, e.g.

The developmentally disabled, or mentally challenged or retarded cases, etc." Such a dilemma, however, would then lead to creating the customs and practice of holding public auctions twice a year where they then sold these developmentally disable persons to the lowest bidders, who would in turn agree to take charge of these persons care. Nevertheless, those who weren't sold were left homeless and subjected to abuse and to wander as they endured daily hardships.

Despite well established, advocating committees disapproving of the inhumane treatment of people with psychiatric disabilities. And expert teams visiting hospitals throughout the world and gathering clinical and statistical data to prove that patients do recover, it would still take over another decade for these changes to take place throughout the United States and other parts of the world. Moreover, clinical researchers of the time had proven facts that even those patients being kept in cells naked, filthy that were often times fed like animals, responded well to non-abusive treatment. They would later become calm, ate and were able to behave like human beings, once treated and placed in appropriate caring institutions. In 1797, almost a hundred years after the enactment of the 1699 law, the General Assembly finally amended the 1793 act, thus an annulment to the laws, which favored the jailing of the mentally ill persons, was then passed. Though during those four previous years to which they were not only incarcerated, but were also kept inhumanely in cages, manacled and kept in shackles. For it was not until during the 19th century, when the ill treatment geared toward the mentally ill would finally undergo it first serious scrutiny, throughout most of the country. It was also around this same time when the decrease in the treatment of bloodletting, whipping, purges and the continuous beatings with chains would gradually begin to cease from existence. Thus, the first official report was written concerning the welfare and appropriate treatment in regard to the mentally ill.

These committees unanimously agreed that the mentally ill should be treated as unfortunates, rather than as criminals, as objects of compassion and not of punishment. The committee also recommended that restoratives alone can reform them and that punishment, would further aggravate and decrease progress. Such documented reports would, however, go almost unnoticed and perhaps somewhat unchanged until the early part of the 1840's, when Dorothea Dix launched her worldwide and lifelong campaign, as a plighted to improve the treatment for the "insane and mentally ill persons." Though still in mid infancy, however, her focus and progress, was aimed toward its cure and perhaps the eradication of illness, and not just simply the stagnant dependable lifetime incarcerations.

Dorothea Dix, was the undisputed world-renowned social reformer born in Hamden, Maine on April 4, 1802. She devoted her life's work to the welfare of the mentally ill struggles. Through her efforts, special hospitals were built to enhance treatment for mental patients in more than 15 different states and Canada. Throughout her arduous commitment for the treatment of mental illness in America, her plight also came to light throughout Europe and Japan, where psychiatric treatment not only gained notice, but also was redeveloped and enhanced, and hospitals for the mentally ill, were also built. Histories first account toward Miss Dix's social reform spirited journey takes us back to her teenage days, when she opened and ran a school in Worcester, Massachusetts. She later founded and operated a school in Boston, but her health conditions would soon force its closure in 1835. She would later begin teaching Sunday school classes at the East Cambridge Massachusetts's jail. It was there and during such time, where she saw firsthand the thoughtless confinements of mentally ill persons, locked away in cages, in chains, manacled, or thrown into cells with criminals. However, this disturbed her deeply and after touring similar jails throughout Massachusetts and the Northeast, while noting that these conditions only worsened, she wrote a stunning report. In her report, she revealed the shocking conditions found throughout her tour. This report helped to bring about major reforms in the treatment of mental illness and to the system as a whole. Ms. Dix died in Trenton, New Jersey on July 17th 1887.

From Sunday-school teacher to World Renown Social Reformer

In 1841 Dorothea Dix, a young Sunday school teacher, appalled at the conditions found throughout the jails and mental institutions, where the mentally ill was being warehoused, began a forty-year quest and championed the plight of the mentally ill. Through her arduous efforts, she managed to get more than thirty hospitals for indigent patients with mental illnesses built.

To merely recognize, Dorothea Dix's accomplishments and efforts toward the treatment of mentally illness, enumerate them and simply call her a social reformer could easily be considered not much more than an understatement by today's standards. Dorothea, carried out a monumental s crusade for the insane, from Massachusetts, to New York, New Jersey, Tennessee, North Carolina, Mississippi, Alabama, Florida, and beyond our borders into Canada and across the oceans throughout Europe. Her impact on the care and treatment for the mentally ill, here in America and abroad, was remarkable and to this day, it should still be applauded cherished, considered and received more than merely some form of slight attention in historic passing of a footnote. And quite frankly by now the mental health industrial profession should have erected several monuments, commemorating her struggle and perhaps even honor such a remarkable human being, with a national holiday. Her accomplishments and her life long struggle in the name of mental health, still remains unparalleled by any standards.

Miss Dix, was born on a farm several miles outside of Bangor, Maine, her paternal grandfather was Dr. Elijah Dix, a descendant of an honorable family. Although his parents were poor and could not afford to have him attend college, he become an apprentice to a physician in Worcester and later studied pharmacology in Boston. He then went into a partnership with Dr. Sylvester Gardner, in 1770. Dr. Dix, was also very successful in real estate speculation and manufacturing, he owned a fleet of small ships that transported goods back and forth between the West Indies and the United States. He married Dorothy Lynde, the belle of Worcester in 1771 and together they had seven sons and one daughter.

Joseph Dix, Dorothea's father, did not inherit any of his father's ambitions, neither the medicine, nor his business abilities. He lacked both and was considered frail, nervous, and showed disinterest in any kind of successful drive or pursuits. He vaguely managed to study theology at Harvard and for a short time, became a frontier preacher. Later he met and married Mary Bigelow. Mary was almost eighteen years his senior. His parents also found and thought of her as ignorant, uncultured and refused to ever accept her as a member of their family. Unable to support his family on a preacher's salary, he resigned from the ministry shortly thereafter. He later found himself unable to hold a job for any length of time and became an alcoholic. At the young age of twelve, Dorothea, became intolerant of her father's vagaries and constant drunken abusive behavior. She then revolted, ran away from home and went to live with grandmother, Dix in Boston. While in Boston, she enrolled in school, but due to her stubborn and headstrong teenage attitude, she could not get along with her grandmother. Therefore, on several occasions, she was sent to live with her grandmother's sister, Mrs. Duncan and her daughter Sarah, in Worcester, Mass. Mrs. Duncan, Sarah and her husband, Dr. Fiske, were somewhat more understanding and kind to Dorothea. There she found herself happier, by which she responded and flourished. Shortly after her arrival, she developed considerably, intellectually and became a charming, amiable, cooperative young woman. When she was only 14 years old, she sought approval from her aunt to start a school for small children in 1816. Though young, she displayed herself as a strict disciplinarian, an attitude by which her school greatly benefited and prospered. Though her school remained open and flourishing, three years later she opted to return to Boston to attend public school. Of course, by then a much-changed young woman, though unusual for a girl to attend public school in those days, she also took private lessons for which, she then qualified as a teacher shortly thereafter. Dorothea's father Joseph died in 1821 at the age of 43 and later two of her brothers also came to live with her and her grandmother after the death of their father.

Shortly after her father's death, she opened another school for poor children in Boston. In addition to operating and running two schools, she also wrote and published several books in the space of about five years from 1824 to 1829. During this same time period Dorothea, became ill with lung congestion and constant hemorrhaging and had to give up teaching. Due to her suffering mostly during the winter months, in the fall of 1830 she agreed to tutor for a physician's children in exchange for traveling to the United States, Virgin Islands. She remained in St. Croix, Virgin Islands throughout that winter and did not return to Massachusetts until the spring of the following year. Upon her return to Boston, almost immediately she proceeded to open another school, this time it being at her grandmother's house. The school remained open and thrived for almost five years, until she suffered a nervous and physical collapse and was forced to shut it down in 1836. At such point, her physician recommended a sea voyage and a change of climate. She embarked on a trip that would take her to England, but it was short lived, due to the passing of her grandmother in 1837. Although Dorothea returned to America immediately after her grandmother's death, she found herself, being forced to spend winter in Washington D.C. and Virginia, due to her lung condition, before finally returning to Boston in the spring of the following year. However, she emerged three years later in 1841 when a young Harvard divinity student conducting Sunday school classes for the women at the East Cambridge jail approached her. Informing her of the urgency of their need, "I believed a woman would be far more suitable and effective in this position." She marveled at the opportunity to again teach. Armed with a Bible and a hymnbook, she began teaching at the jail that following Sunday.

After the services, she toured the prisons, met and spoke with other prisoners, as well as with the insane, and became rather shocked with her findings. She found that the conditions in which the insane lived in were far beneath human standards, this experience became the stimulus that propelled and launched her career as a social reformer at age of 39.

Throughout the next two years, Miss Dix, would tour, survey and write about her findings in a cohesive report geared toward the inhumane conditions of all poorhouses, jails and workhouses throughout Massachusetts. She would then write her petition in the form of a memorial and delivered it to the Massachusetts Legislature. In it, she cited two facts (that of people and that of places.) Her petition was presented to the Legislature in early 1843 and as expected, it made a considerable commotion among its members. She was immediately denounced by its representatives and the newspapers. The local press accused her of being a slanderous, sensationalist and argued that her report was based solely on lies. Nevertheless, a committee was appointed to investigate her charges and these, however, were all substantiated. The committee recommended that immediate action be taken to improve the conditions within these institutions. Miss Dix, however, would not stand still and throughout the next five years that followed, she covered more than 70,000 miles in travel. Throughout which, she visited almshouses and jails across the country and like in Massachusetts, she traveled to other states, where she would again write memorials and present her findings to the Legislative bodies of each particular states she visited.

Her visit to New Jersey in 1845 spearheaded the building of an asylum in Trenton. Such would become the first hospital for the insane to be built and paid for directly through her efforts, with public funds. She would spend the next three years writing her national memorial that was finally completed in the early summer of 1848 and presented in the form of prayer to the Senate and House of Representatives of the United State Assembly, in the first session of the 30th Congress. In it, she requested a grant of land for the relief and support of the indigent, the curable and incurable insane in the country. She estimated that based on her findings there, existed one insane person per each thousand (1 per 1000) and that such population amounted, to well over twenty two thousand (22,000) nationwide. Incidentally according to estimates at such time the U. S. population, was approximately 22,000,000. Her report also stated that only nineteen of these thirty states currently had public institutions for the mentally ill and that even if all private institutions were added, we would merely accommodate thirty seven hundred 3,700 mentally ill individuals. While stressing that such would leave over eighty-two 82 percent still confined to jails, almshouses, or to just wander about the streets. Her memorial arguably stated to Congress, "I've seen more than nine thousand idiots, epileptics and insane in these United States, destitute of appropriate care and protection. I've seen thousands bound with galling chains, bowed beneath fetters and heavy iron balls, attached to drag-chains, lacerated with ropes, scourged with hot rods and terrified beneath storms of profane, execration and cruel blows; now subject to gibes. And scorn, torturing tricks-now, abandoned to the most loathsome necessities, or subjects to the vilest and most outrageous of violations."

The impressive thirty-two page document is to this day, perhaps the most eloquent appeal ever written on behalf of the mentally ill by anyone, throughout the entire history of mental health. In it, she cited innumerable instances of mutilations, deprivations and horrors, she had personally witnessed in almost every state of the Union and in the District of Columbia. She also documented and introduced statistics that clearly pointed toward incidence of insanity by state and incidence of cure and of improvement, when the insane received proper and adequate moral, spiritual and medical treatment. She maintained that insanity was daily increasing at alarming, epidemic proportions, among the rising population. She also stated that her attributions, was based on a society that proudly endorsed its civil and religious liberties, one that believed in extreme competitions, in which one could aspire to the highest office, or honor, regardless of their humble beginnings. A society, in which, wealth, education and material possessions, as well as scholastic achievement, were still held in a high esteem. In her report, she also argued that "insanity knows no boundaries," as she stood up and reminded Congress that "Statesmen and politicians, as well as merchants, the wealthy, and the poor, were all uniquely susceptible to insanity."

The grant of land she requested from the Senate and House of Representatives, were to allocate for the relief and support of the indigent curable and incurable insane throughout the United States. It consisted of five million acres of land, if such were granted, she planned the building of institutions for the insane throughout the country. Of course, Congress denied her petition. Nonetheless, she continued raising public awareness regarding her crusade on the plight of the mentally ill. However, this time around, she traveled not only throughout America, but also through Japan, England, Italy and the rest of Europe. And before her journey would end, the United States was in the midst of a civil war. Upon her return, she heard about Union soldiers being mobbed and wounded in Washington. She enlisted as a volunteer, shortly after and joined a team of nurses to aid in their care. Although she wasn't a nurse, on June 10th of 1861, she was commissioned as Superintendent of the United States Army Nurses. Her responsibilities, stemmed from organizing and implementing military hospitals, to recruiting and supplying nurses to where they were mostly needed. Her duties and responsibilities also included receiving, controlling and distributing the supplies, donated by wealthy individuals, and associations for the comfort of the soldiers and their families. In this position, she again displayed herself as a born leader by establishing, strict and rigid regulations throughout her department. Therefore by showing concerns regarding the nurse's age, dress code, behavior, attitude and appearance, during and while off duty!

She subsequently abandoned the profession, when the Medical Bureau and the Sanitation Commission was reorganized, thus eliminating the position of the Office of Superintendent of Nurses though she still remained somewhat involved, until the war ended, then she formally resigned in August of 1865. The following year, she was awarded a stand of the United States Colors, which was presented to her on December 3rd 1866 by the Secretary of War, in recognition for her valuable services during the war. After the war ended, she reinitiated the push for reforms in the mental health field and would later re-embark her visits to jails, poorhouses and mental institutions. Upon her arrival to Trenton on October 1st in 1881, she became seriously ill and a private apartment, with beautiful views were fully furnished and set up for her usage. Miss Dix, remained there for the next six years, until her passing on July 18, 1887, at the age of 85. Though she came from modest beginnings and could have dedicated her life to making money and to perhaps dying in a palace somewhere in Europe, she instead chose to humbly end her days in a place that she help built at Trenton Psychiatric Hospital, New Jersey.

This is the same hospital in Trenton, was the same place where forty-two years earlier, she had helped to gather funds and support for its building. Ironically, it was also the first state, public hospital for the insane built in America directly through her efforts, but it would not be the last.

Dorothea L. Dix, the social reformer and strong advocate for the humane treatment of the mentally ill, should be historically credited for stimulating public interest worldwide, regarding the plight of the insane with her well-publicized reports on behalf of the insane during the 1840's. By this time most states throughout the Union were awakened to the realization of her report and they began building institutions to house, treat and care for the mentally ill. Her courage, inspiration and hard-work, is instrumental to many of us, whom still remain committed to the care, growth, progress, recovery and the development of all of our brothers and sisters still suffering with mental illness.

The mentally ill began reappearing in America's jails and prisons in large numbers approximately 90 years after the 1880 census. In 1974 and 1975, following the Glenn Swank and Darryl Winer assessment of 545 inmates in the Denver County Jail reported that "the number of psychotic persons we encountered in the jail was striking, as was the large number of them with a history of psychiatric hospitalization, particularly long-term or multiple hospitalizations." Realizing then that many of the jail inmates with history of long-term psychiatric hospitalizations had previously been in state mental hospitals. They also documented a widespread belief among jail personnel that there had been a large increase in the number of severely mentally disturbed individuals, entering the jails in recent years. Although they had no earlier data available for comparison, concluding that the jail system appears to have inherited responsibility for the mentally ill by default rather than preference.

Throughout the earlier part of 2000, it was estimated the largest mental health facility in the United States of America, was the Los Angeles County Jail, although the number was not fully estimated, to my recollection its alarming numbered neared the thousands.

Historic Facts, About How A Lost Mind Could Find Itself

The First Modern Perspective:

Clifford Whittington Beers, is an individual that could be viewed, as one of the most influential figures in the history of mental health. Clifford Beers, was born in New Haven, Connecticut in 1876 and died in 1943, Clifford Beers shared his experiences with the world and such would help to shine a brighter light upon the treatment of mental illness. In his published autobiography, A Mind That Found Itself, he described the inhumane and ill treatment received as a psychiatric patient during his repeated hospitalizations throughout these public and private institutions. He was the founder of the mental health movement and was convinced that the ill treatment and criminal-like behavior imposed upon the patients by the staff, further influenced in grand part, and help to propel the destructive behaviors of the psychiatric patients. In his writings, he stressed that positive expectations, elicited desirable behavior and that what the mentally ill mostly needed while in the hospital was an ally.

Deprived of any other outlet for his boundless manic energies, during his enforced sojourn in a Connecticut State Asylum at the beginning of the twentieth century, the young Clifford Beers took to rethinking that modern science, might make him more famous than Newton. He had conceived in his mind a refutation of the physics of gravity, asserting that "This is no mere abstract triumph. It could surely have its practical pay-off if it succeeds. In fact, one might be able to defy my conquering imagination, soon tickled me into believing that I could lift myself up by my own bootstrap." Clifford argued and insisted as he followed his newfound delusional venture. Most speculators on the unconscious like, Jung, have had their say on the sexual undercarriage of flying fantasies. Here, however, the fruitful meanings are surely socio-cultural, and lodged in the upper stories of the mind. Not only was Beers taking a flight of fancy from the asylum at which he was imprisoned, he was rather simply alluding to the American dream of individual success, by following successful stories of the time, such as taking off from a log cabin to the White House.

Beers then later wrote. *"I am as good as any man … by my own efforts further, I will rise further. I too can be a high flyer."*

By the time Beers came along, self-help and self-idealistic perfection, had long been living philosophies in the land of the free; the tremendous heroic myths of the New World were by now, secularized optimistic recessions of the protestant ethics of individual salvations. During such times, the lone individual must unexpectedly confront the world through the pioneering spirit of sharp work, dynamism and entitled enterprise, he would decisively win the stupendous success that would promote his inner, spiritual qualities and his dominating inherited character. Self-reliance presupposed a strong self. The potential survival of the fittest, the Social Darwinist creed, had by now been taken over by the great robber-barons, the Carnegies and the Rockefellers, would sift vehemently from weak to egos. This presumptuous arrogant attitude toward life and empirical dogma of daily living, began to appear alarmingly around the 1850s. It seemed, as if many White Americans could not take the tremendous pressure, their nerves became over-stretched and would suffered subsequently go in to a state of weariness, sluggishness, by being overcome by 'lassitude and inertia.' In truth, they couldn't stand up to such high expectations, social pressures and they suffered nervous breakdowns, or as it was simply put back then, 'they cracked up.'

Of course, during such times of the 'Victorian machismo era,' this was only supposed to occur among women, it was to be consistently expected, indeed, they had even defined a specific, racist, misogynist term for it, known as the 'the new women syndrome.' Insisting that women and blacks had falsely tempted to try to emulate the white male counterpart in order to become successful go-getter's in the intellectual pursuits of profound knowledge, the literary scene and public life, which stood against the laws of psychobiology; therefore, they winded up hysterical. Their simple belief back then, was that if women and minorities were to resume their proper place in society they would recover.

Nevertheless, they failed to notice the a particularly large number of all European American men, whom in addition seemed to be caving in, thus not in a position to confer the challenge of the contemporary market, which had long been set into place to primarily focus on shaping their manhood. During these times a new condition was labeled for the consoling and euphemistic term *'neurasthenia,'* which came into dramatic play. Neurasthenia, was viewed as a position on the weakness of the nerves and was later coined as the great *'American disease.'* Intellectual African Americans, would later refer to it as, *'the white man sins upon his offspring.'* The end of the late-nineteenth-century would open the doors for the teachings of psychology and the ministrations of psychiatrists in America. These would later come to play a dominant role in the molding of the American mind, to a degree that is unparalleled to that of any other nation in history. Of course, this wasn't the case for Native Americans or Afro Americans, although some has theorized that these latter cultures were primarily engaged in just trying to barely survive and overcome some of the same obstacles placed upon them by these mad people. Nevertheless, the analysis remains open to a wide range of sociological and scientific debates. Hence, perhaps the 'New World' wasn't free of the contagious diseases of civilization, which, plagued and riddle the Old.' In reality the great democracy had to first democratize psychiatry itself, in other for American to fully develop as a nation. Psychiatry itself, would have to subsequently adapt new techniques to deal with the adjusting achievers into this modern society. Throughout the last century psychiatry in America gradually transformed from a negative to a positive force and eventually discontinued being only for the treatment of mental disease and became a tonic to personal psychic health, a romantic road to self-discovery, and until most recently, a license to just let it all out.

The Americanization of Freud, obviously also help set the stage for European Americans love-affair with psychiatry. American consumers would then bath in the glow of progressivism, trans-Atlantic Freudianism and psychoanalysis became hooked up to success. Freud had portrayed the inevitable and often tragic tension between the individual basic human drives and civilization, with its demands of repression, sublimation and neurosis. The New World formulated a sort of Freud without tears and the ego could forge full speed ahead, with self-realization and social adjustments. But the path had been cleared long before Freud's interwar, which rode upon the crucial creed previously set by the Mental Hygiene Movement, which was evangelized by Clifford Beers. Beers had unknowingly and almost single handedly written weaved psychiatry right into America's fabric, literally stamping it into the American dream. Mr. Beers became the Benjamin Franklin of psychiatry, his writings and talks, provided advice on how to renounce mental illness and embrace mental muscle-power. And like all good preachers, he provided the best personal sinner-turned-saint tales. Clifford Beers could proclaim that what he preached, was indeed true because he had been through it all himself. "My credentials are far better than those of any psychiatrist, insanity is my medical education!" He would insist throughout his lectures "I believe I am one of the few, whom have ever successfully recover from a mental breakdown," he added, "and I did so not in my own interests, but out of altruism, though I have received unexpected personal benefits." He wrote in his spiritual style autobiography, *"A Mind That Found Itself"* (1908). He declared and in it he first established himself as an all-American boy, born to an all American family, descended from the earliest settlers. Born in 1876 of middle-class parents, as a boy he had possessed that mixture of traits, a diffident self-conscious shyness combined enterprising, competitive get-up-and-go type of spirit.

Among his fond schooldays memories, was of being a business manager of the student newspaper, while at Yale University, where he excelled at his classes. From day one as a freshman, he wanted to make contacts, join the fraternities and right away get involved in running things. He rose to the challenge of the 'Yale spirit' and succeeded in all set goals and ambitions. On paper, and perhaps throughout most his young days as a student, while in the classroom, as well as in later on in life, it must be noted that he was always dedicated to as he'd later referred to as, "stamping out the three ills;" 'incompetence, abuse and injustice.' This statement could easily characterize most mental institutions as recent as the first decade of the twentieth century. To this day one cannot justify in good conscience any discussion about the history of mental health and the community without first recognizing, Clifford Beers's, successful mental health movement and its contribution to future great developments in treatment.

The Connecticut Mental Health Association, previously known as the Connecticut Society for Mental Hygiene, was founded a couple of months after *A Mind That Found Itself*, was published. It was the first of its kind in the world. The original founders of this society included, representatives of the courts, the clergy, the field of medicine, faculty from various universities, the association of social work, as well as Clifford Beers himself, a former mental patient, turned advocate, and other several members of his family.

From the beginning its objectives was clearly defined in its institutional mission statement:

1. to work for the conservation of mental health, to willingly help prevent nervous and mental disorders and mental defects.
2. to successfully help raise the standard of care, for those suffering from any mental disorders, or defects.
3. to potentially secure and disseminate any reliable information on these subjects and to work in cooperation with federal, state and local agencies, as well as public and private agencies, whose work is related in any way to that of the society for mental hygiene.

Clifford Beers was appointed Executive Secretary to the society, he devoted the rest of his life to the mental health movement and the extraordinary mission of stated ideal objectives, just as he had promised in earlier statements. Such achievements were, effectively educating the community, spearheading the changing of contemptuous attitudes toward the mentally ill, implementing areas of significant prevention and significant educational improvement of mental diseases and the immediate continuous enhancement of services, and essential treatment for the mentally ill patient. However, his exemplary work and his accomplishments didn't go unnoticed. Washington and other states kept a close eye and Canada and Europe, also took notice of the societies work. The following year on February 2nd 1909, the National Committee for Mental Hygiene, was founded and in 1918, the Canadian National Committee for Mental Hygiene, was also established. Several European countries in addition followed shortly thereafter and by 1930, a delegation representing fifty nations gathered in Washington D.C. to participate in the First International Congress on Mental Health. This led to the establishment of the International Committee for Mental Hygiene. Although twenty-one years had passed since the successful organization first organized, in New Haven, Connecticut, on behalf of the mentally ill. Several

States had also developed similar associations on both regional and state levels.

Twenty years later, in 1950, the National Association for Mental Hygiene joined with two other organizations to form one enterprising entity, The National Mental Health Foundation. Such, which is a benevolent organization developed essentially by conscientious objectors, who'd previously worked in state mental hospitals during WWII. The next branches that developed via Beers original work, was the Psychiatric Foundation, which is the fund raising unit to the American Psychiatric Association, thus emerged the National Association for Mental Health.

In particular aspects, the mental health movement simulates to psychiatry practically in exactly the same ways, in which the civil health movement is to general medicine. One significant difference and that's because the mental health movement to this day, still remains a citizens movement, whereas the latter is now an official, professional organization with the adequate powers and influential authority to establish, effectively enforce and put in to law, numerous public health standards and practices. However, the mental health movement that was officially implemented by Clifford Beers, a former mental patient almost a hundred years previously, has had a tremendous impact. Not only in the progressive development of new and improved services and treatments for the mentally ill, but rather on thorough development in the areas of psychology, psychiatry, psychiatric nursing and social work. In addition, it successively impacts in the areas of educating the public toward mental health awareness, while mobilizing its particular interest and finest efforts in preventive therapeutic and rehabilitative programs. It also still displays its impact upon legislature, where it requests significant assistance and ongoing development for community mental health programs throughout the world. Therefore, one could not justify in good conscience any discussion toward the mentally ill, mental illness and the community, without first officially thankfully recognizing Clifford Beers' mental health movement, its contributions and its progressive development. However, we could legitimately raise the argument that without Mr. Beers, mental health movement being established, the psychiatric profession would've certainly taken another turn, perhaps the wrong one … and we could definitely argue that nonetheless, it wouldn't have been precisely what it is in this day and age. Although time is now long overdue, for another XXI century Beers type to come along and revamp this system! Yet we shouldn't conveniently disregard that one of this movement's significant accomplishments was the passing of the Connecticut Mental Health Act, which vigorously lobbied on behalf of the patient rights. Though today these rights are much taken for granted, the arduous and grueling struggle to obtain such, should never be deliberately forgotten, abused, nor ignored by anyone.

Thanks to the mental health movement, the first outpatient hygiene clinic, opened its doors in New Haven, Connecticut in 1913. Only four years after the act were established and it was sponsored by the Society for Mental Hygiene. The clinic became the first outpatient clinic in the country and it was also the first to effectively provide aftercare treatment for individuals who were recently discharged from state run hospitals. It was staffed with physicians from two state hospitals on alternating basis. Several years later, the clinic was reorganized and a permanent medical director and social worker were employed. The clinic met its definite objective, by first demonstrating the immediate need for the aftercare of patients recently discharged from state hospitals. It also influenced and became the functioning model on which other states would later implement, successfully build and expand their aftercare, outpatient services for the mentally ill throughout America and rest of the world. After a rather turbulent history, characterized by local community problems and political differences, the clinic was reorganized and its name officially changed in 1952. It reemerged as the Clifford W. Beers

Guidance Clinic, Inc. It's stated particular purpose, operating and managing a psychiatric clinic for diagnosis and treatment of adults and children. By this time, patients were being discharged earlier from state hospitals, while the clinic provided community outreach programs and appropriate supervision. The unexpected success of this project led to further collaboration between the Society and the Division of Mental Hygiene. Both groups worked closely together on projects consisting of mental hygiene, education and assisting communities in establishing future child guidance clinics.

Throughout the early thirties during the depression and while most state curtailed their spending, the society intervened, thus preventing cutbacks of any previously established community programs. In addition the Society was also instrumental in its role toward ensuring the passage of the 1945's General Assembly of the Connecticut Mental Health Act. Such act also aided in providing the full operation of state run psychiatric clinics for children, aftercare clinics for state hospital patients and it also secured state grants to general hospitals, by professionally assisting them in creating their psychiatric services. The latter attempt would eventually prove to be far much easier said than done. During the nineteen fifties and sixties, the National Association for Mental Health, increased a nationwide lobbying campaign on behalf of the citizen's, in support of centralized departments for mental health, while advocating for increased community services and the rights of hospitalized and recently discharged individuals, with the Connecticut Association for Mental Health leading the march. The association's member charter, remains to this day, committed to the ideal objectives, academic concepts and models established way back in in 1909, by Mr. Clifford Beers. The significant responsibilities of the Association are not only that as advocates and protectors, but rather as promoters and pioneers in the field of mental health treatment.

Clifford Beers, established and effectively unquestionably started the mental health movement, perhaps out of pure particular concern and the after documenting, and publishing his personal experiences in his book "A Mind That Found Itself" He would later be honored by the Connecticut Society of Mental Hygiene in 1933, on its 25th anniversary.

It was exactly twenty-five years since the publishing of his autobiography, A Mind That Found Itself. In addition he also received tributes consisting of hundreds of rewarding letters, many awards and countless honorary degrees in appreciation for his valuable part in founding the movement. He was also the recipient of the National Institute of Science's Gold Medal Award, in official recognition for his services to humanity. The American Psychiatric Association in addition elected him as an honorary member and Yale University conferred on him an honorary masters of Arts Degree. Clifford Beers also traveled extensively abroad that same year, mainly to obtain several awards granted to him by several members of the European community, one being his trip to France, where he was presented with The Cross of The Knights of The Legion of Honor, King Albert also received him in Brussels.

Just like Dorothea Dix, who came aboard the railways of difficult struggle upon her plight for the mentally ill practically a hundred years before him, he too further pointed and shined the light bright on the plight for the humane treatment of the mentally ill. Not only did he put the spotlight on the negative practices and abuses in psychiatric hospitals worldwide, in the early nineteen century, but he also brought honor and successfully helped earn the respect to all current, former, presently and forthcoming mental patients toward better treatment. More significantly, he gave them hope. He in addition brought honor and notoriety to his home state of Connecticut, with the publishing of his book, A Mind That Found Itself. "When reading or simply seeing anything relating to Clifford Beers and all of his accomplishments, I cannot help, but to chuckle and shake my head in wonders, as to perhaps how those staff members whom had imposed abuse upon him must have felt after he published that book?" points to ponder!

Although perhaps time is now long overdue for another XXI century Beers type to come along and revamp this entire system into a new one that best functions!

Several years back, prior to conducting this research, I was not merrily impressed, but rather highly inspired, by just basically reading highlights of his extraordinary life for a school term paper. Although, as I delved deeper, I just couldn't help, but to become more in depth in this research, to share and tell the world about this amazing human being of a man, his satisfying mission that benefit the world, his contributions and academic accomplishments.

Long before even thinking about writing this book, I was forced to intervene in defense of a patient, as I overheard a colleague, a fellow staff member, making fun of a patient on the psychiatric unit, where I worked overtime during his shift. I immediately thought of Clifford Beers and wondered to myself, as I collectively assumed in my mind, what would the abusive staff said, if this man was to overcome his illness, effectively get discharged and became his next-door neighbor? What would they apparently say … though more importantly, what would they do and how would they subsequently treat him? Of course, my being me and not wanting to change from the individual I am, and since I was the lead on the unit, I thought it my duty and my responsibility, so I later approached the staff member and I did question the relevant issue, as I raised the hypothetical supposition? Though at first they declined to specifically comment, but later insisted mumbling "Oh, well, he'll never get out of here." I still cannot help from wondering how good those clients, whom actually knew Clifford Beers must have felt, to realize that one of their own; one of their peers, had effectively made it out and did essentially recover enough to write a frigging book! That one of their friends, were out there getting positive headlines, was appearing on the covers of magazines, front pages world-wide newspaper, earning prestigious awards, etc. "not long ago, a once fellow inmate, now a real talk of the town!" Although to this day, about one hundred and ten years ago, since the publishing of "A Mind That Found It Self" and with all the computers and technological advances in medicine the medical and psychiatric communities we have yet to see another Clifford Beers emerge. Though we're long overdue for another.

Clifford Whitttingham Beers, was born, raised and educated in New Haven, Connecticut, he was a graduate of Yale University; class of 1897. Beers' oldest brother had been diagnosed with epilepsy, reason for which he became somewhat obsessed, with the idea that he too had contracted the disease. Such fears and the constant episodes of anxiety, clearly reflected in his college performance. He also suffered from prolonged periods of depression. This also interfered, often prevented his verbal participation during classes. After graduating from Yale, he became obsessed with making money and quickly accumulating wealth. He firmly believed that such wealth would've brought him influence, status and power. During and right after college, he spent a year or so working as a clerk, in the Tax Collectors office in New Haven. However, shortly after graduating, he'd gotten a job in New York and went to work for an Insurance firm. While working in New York, he experienced symptoms of acute and emotional distress, followed by episodes of hysterical attacks and became convinced that he too, had now contracted epilepsy. Around mid 1900, he resigned from his job in New York and returned home to his family in New Haven.

Besides the fact of his increased anxiety, he'd also turned to severely depression about the fear of his being an epileptic. By now he was fully convinced that he'd rather die than to live the daily sufferings of such a condition, and opted to jump out of the fourth floor window of his parents' home. Beers had sustained fractures on both ankles and was hospitalized for a short period; certainly becoming convinced that all his delusions had vanished, as he hit the ground during the fall. However, while hospitalized, he'd developed other types of delusions and hallucinations. This time consisting of a more paranoid persecutory hallucination and thought that since he'd committed a crime, when he attempted suicide, the police was now chasing after, and trying to persecute him. Beers, became increasingly suspicious, misinterpreting the activities within the hospital and outside of his barred, secured windows. After being discharged from the general hospital he returned home with a nurse in attendance. Despite all the efforts, his behavior showed no improvement and he was readmitted shortly after to a private psychiatric asylum in southern Connecticut on August eleventh of that same year.

Beers remained there for seven months; depressed, delusional, paranoid and at times mute. In his book Beers noted that "he was at first specialled or 1 to 1 by day and night attendants. Later the day attendant special observation was discontinued, although the night attendant slept in his room, for several weeks."

Canvas muffs were applied at night to his hands, with the straps locked around his wrist. Beers wrote about "good and bad" nurses and the attendants, he also wrote about the mercenary physicians. Although still depressed, he left this institution and for a three-month period lived in the home of an attendant who'd befriended him. However, his condition did not improve and throughout the earlier part of 1900, he was admitted to a private, non-profit psychiatric the then Hartford Retreat at Stamford Hall, currently the Institute Of Living or IOL, in Hartford, Connecticut. During his first fourteen months in this institution the attendants were kind and helpful and although still depressed, his physical conditions improved. Beers then became elated and overactive, their kindness then turned to abusive terror, which caused for his retaliation and often turned into staff provocation, by which staff responded in an aggressive manner. Finally, after an acute episode of acting out, he was placed in a camisole, restraint straitjacket and locked seclusion, or as described in his writings, as "in a small barred room, which was mostly unfurnished except for a bed that was screwed to the floor."

In his autobiography, Beers described his long stay in this cold cell, the brutality of the attendants, and the vindictive behavior of the physicians. He was finally transferred to the then named Connecticut Hospital for the Insane in Middletown, currently the Connecticut Valley Hospital (CVH) and admitted to its "'best" ward on November 8, 1902. Upon his admission to the State hospital, Beers was restless and talkative, constantly expressed delusions and ideas of grandeur. He wrote constantly, he was untidy, but for the first two weeks he was somewhat, cooperative. Until his anxiety grew and one day he decided to barricade himself into a room and taunted the attendants to show him the 'worst conditions' that existed within the hospital. He was placed in a camisole and thrown in a cold, locked seclusion room, where he remained for almost a month. He was noisy, demanding destructive, and frequently provoked by attendants who retaliated by inflicting verbal and physical abuse upon him.

In his book Beers stated, "I have observed that the only patients whom were not likely to be subjected to abuse, were the very ones least in need of care and treatment. The violent, noisy, and troublesome patients was abused because he was violent, noisy, and troublesome and was in need of care. The patients, either too weak, physically or mentally to attend to his own wants, was frequently abused because of that very helplessness, which made it necessary for the attendants to wait upon him."

Beers also wrote, "usually a restless or troublesome patient, placed in the violent ward was assaulted on the very first day; in fact, these fellows nearly all of them ignorant and untrained, I seemed to believe that 'violent cases' could not be handled in any other way."

While he continued taking notes during his stay, some of the documentation found later in which he stated "(one attendant said to me,)" "They are getting pretty damned strict around here these days, discharging a man simply for choking out a patient."

Beers spent almost four months on a 'violent' ward at the Connecticut State Hospital. During that period he frequently intervened on behalf of other patients and became a zealous advocate and protector of their rights. After being transferred to a quiet ward, he resumed his incessant writing, drawing and talking; he was elated and often made unreasonable demands on the staff. On March 12, 1903 Beers wrote a letter to the Governor of the State of Connecticut describing the conditions and abuses at private and State mental hospitals and smuggled it out of the hospital. Although the State hospital, was not investigated, once he informed the medical staff of the strategy he used to mail this letter, several attendants accused by him of abusing patients were proven guilty of brutality and summarily dismissed. Although in it he vividly described detailing vagaries and common treatment practices, found within the mental health system during those times. The attempt of exposure and reforms written by a mental patient from the inside walls of a state hospital, had very little to no impact during those days. Such perhaps would not be the same case today. Quite frankly, there wouldn't be a need for a letter to reach the Governor's office. This is mostly due to the fact that each hospital now has a patient's advocate department, with an office specifically dedicated to handling and investigating their complaints. Although, in part some, patients may engage in abusing the system and will, at times, engaged in venting their frustrations by turning in innocent staff members, based on social pathology, retaliation upon the system, displacement, etc. Equally, we find overzealous advocates whom, at times, tend to feed into and encourage such behaviors or complaints do outrageous and bizarre in nature. Therefore investigations are highly imperative.

Throughout the months that followed, Clifford Beers' behavior and mood progressively improved and by 1903, following more than seven months of hospitalization, he was given ground privileges and in September 1903 he was discharged improved. These, experiences in three different psychiatric hospitals in Connecticut, made a tremendous impact on Clifford Beers and awakened in him a fervent desire to effect reforms on behalf of the mentally ill. He returned to his position in New York and concentrated on becoming successful. In the autumn of 1904, while physically ill, he read 'Les Miserables.' This impressive book, reinforced his desire to write a book that would arouse public sympathy and interest for the mentally ill. Early in 1905, following his brother's advice, he voluntarily readmitted himself to the Hartford Retreat (The Institute of Living). He was elated and excited and spent most of his time writing. After a short hospitalization, he was discharged. Beers was still concerned about the plight of the insane and determined to write about his experiences as a patient so that the public would be informed about the shameful conditions predominating throughout these mental institutions.

He discussed his plans for the book, with several illustrious people and subsequently sent a copy of the manuscript to Professor, William James, an eminent psychologist at Harvard University. Dr. James, after reading the manuscript, encouraged him to publish it and added. *"You were doubtless a pretty intolerable character, when the maniacal condition came on, and you were bossing the universe. No ordinary tact, but rather a genius for diplomacy must have been needed for avoiding rows with you; but you certainly were wrongly treated nevertheless, and the spiteful Assistant M.D. at the hospital deserves to have his name published. Your report is full of instructiveness for doctors and attendants alike. "At its* publication the book created quite an outrage. The furor created, among the press, was enough of an uproar, to further promote A Mind That Found Itself in 1908.

Many questions were raised in regards to the authenticity concerning some of Beers' statements. The Hartford Post conducted and printed the interview with Mr. Joseph E. of Hartford, also a former mental patient. Mr. E., confirmed all of Beers claims and stated, "The Connecticut State Hospital for the insane is a hellhole." While corroborating with Beers' statements of abuse and brutality, he added that "The attendants by the way, said Mr. E., are big, burly backwoods men from Vermont and Maine, who are chosen for their bull strength and size rather than for any efficiency on their part. All they have to do is mix medicine and some bandaging which anyone can learn in no time."

Beers used his unfortunate experiences as a mental patient in a constructive way; he succeeded in funding the mental health movement. A catalyst to all other organizations concerning mental health, and it still lives on to this day under the banner of the *National Institute of Mental Health*. Such, which remains instrumental in effecting reforms in the care of the mentally ill and remains alive, well and ongoing. However, despite all its efforts and accomplishments, it has fallen short on its main targeted goal, which is that of revolutionizing the way in which current medical practices cares for these patients. Ironically, Beers ended his own life by committing suicide, while in a mental hospital in 1943. *The fact that he is so widely known for his amazing recovery from these episodes of mental illness and that so little is known about the circumstances of his death during an exacerbation of his illness, is an example again of the stigma and obscurity that still surrounds mental illness.*

Don't Look Down, On Your Brother if You Are Not Going To Pick Him Up

The Turning of Backs Syndrome Remains Alive and Well

"Mental illness is still not acceptable in our society … it is not acceptable, because we keep turning our backs to the facts. We buy the myths and forget that we're talking about each other."

These very same words were once spoken by the former First Lady, Mrs. Rosalyn Carter in her address, when she took the helm as Chairperson to President Jimmy Carter's Commission on Mental Health. Those were the very first word used at the opening of her speech, as she embarked on her mission to make the plight of mental health a priority, during her husband's administration. Mrs. Carter chose this not as a political platform, but rather to awaken the public sense and to heightened awareness, regarding this national epidemic. She made these statements to highlight one of the most important and most difficult aspects the nation encountered when her husband took office. Although there were established laws, rights, rules, and many, many other problems, she realized that what the mentally ill patients needed most, was a voice and they found it in Mrs. Carter. Mrs. Carter vowed for the continuance of the fight for a more effective and a more humane way of treatment, toward those afflicted with chronic mental disorders. The "turning of backs" statement she mentioned, was to merely put a face before the public and therefore await their response toward those suffering with mental illness. It emphasized the indifference on the long-held stigma that had ridden throughout many generations and lasted through the centuries. However, one must characterize this attitude in two variations, a) the lay population, which is understandable and at best even justifiable and b) the trained mental health professional. This last group, however, is increasingly more difficult to understand, when a "turning of backs" occurs, as it often does among those who'd been trained to deliver mental health services. It appears, as if somewhere along the way they'd lost their vision toward the reality of their profession.

There have been ample discussions and vast documentation in recent years regarding witnessed cases of some mental health professionals, and their attitude of hostility and their indifference toward the mentally and chronically ill individuals. This observation, was made several years ago, as a professional caregiver issued a speech, during which, he carelessly described individual mental health patients, diagnosed with schizophrenia, as "strangers in our midst." Often times, we have seen, or have experienced the indifference displayed by some of our own colleagues in the mental health field, especially from those who have repeatedly represented themselves as professionals in the field. Often times, we drooped, dragged, and waddled in the unwillingness to advocate and address these patient's needs. Instead, we point toward those found missing among the bureaucracies, while we blame other professionals, whose main concern at times is that of the institutional structure. While we should instead be looking toward the growing concern for those patients who are socially disabled and are soon to be discharged into these unsteady environments; much like those being poorly run and operated by the private sector, we again slightly "turn our backs" or simply tune out. Although some strongly believed the private, nonprofit sector to be the new system of care, regarding the future of mental health, we still do not quite see, where the politicians promised monies would indeed be saved, when these large institutions still remain open as revolving doors. This however, is due in part, because the private nonprofit agencies' salaries, benefits and other incentives, are in fact very low and very unsteady. They offer their mental health employees little, to no job securities and are rather unrealistic to the fact that this type of work, is rather voluminous and stressful. Therefore, the turnover rate of their employees is also, rather constant. Most of these changes, are continuously being done without any involvement, implementation, or even an in depth study of this impact and how this might further affect the lives of their patients who are already struggling with their illness.

Indeed, we already know that the individual diagnosed with schizophrenia experiences negative social responses as a first public reaction to the massive social disability and by experience, we know these factors that could cause them to de-compensate. Is it perhaps these social disadvantages affecting this patient group, while out in the community? Is it the lack of opportunities due to a complex variety of reasons to develop social or vocational skills? The third question should then be, is the low self-esteem of the chronically ill a main factor?

Once we have addressed all of these factors and the problems they create, we easily note that these are not so easily resolved and they should not be attributed to a single cause. Therefore, after analyzing all of the data, we then realized that "doing away with institutions and state run programs would not do away with mental illness." What is our backup plan, if and when these private nonprofit programs failed? When these individuals are still in need of treatment and where would we shuffle them off to … where will they then go? Whom is going to be around to rehabilitate them, when the money is long gone? So, in trying to sum all of this up, it only adds up to one thing. "Although laws have changed and mentally ill patients now have rights and sufficient laws to protect them somewhat, politicians and health care professionals, engage in abusing them by way of cutbacks, politically geared, entrepreneurial favors and mal-adjusted changes that are primarily tailored around campaign financing and projected votes." So, perhaps we do need to get the Church involved, perhaps the Church should definitely become involved and therefore, help curved this political imbalance that is long prevalent throughout the system.

As a secular group, we did put up a good fight for our Community Based Initiative (CBI) program and the success of these clients, whom were being cared for and treated in these programs. Nonetheless state officials, walked right in and destroyed every therapeutic accomplishment that both patients and staff had worked so hard to build for the past seven years. "As aforementioned, these programs were a work in progress, tailored toward long term achievement and future success. All of the CBI's were well on the way of becoming perhaps a national model in treatment, one of the most productive tools ever implemented in the history and treatment of mental illness." A former client who'd de-compensated around the time of the closings of these programs, and was later sent back to a state hospital later commented "they weren't broken and they didn't need fixing." Days later, another was overheard as he wondered out aloud "and they have the nerve to lock me up and called me crazy?" I thought they were right!

Clinical Depression Among the Royals, Aesthetic Reasoning Perhaps

Queen Victoria (1819-1901)

While growing up as a boy, I spend many precious times around my grandmother's home, I remember noticing she always had a large portrait of Queen Victoria hanging over her front door. She took it down once a week, dusted it off, and carefully put it back in its place. Noting to my younger sister that she probably took better care of it than she did her own family pictures. As I grew up, I often wonder about the portrait. I believed I was about 8 years old, when I finally asked "whose picture was it?" Of course my grandmother being a diehard *"Britishian,"* born in Grand Cayman. BWI. She had relocated to live on the mainland, Honduras, refused to ever speak a word in Spanish, but maintain, bragged and daily boasted her British origins. She would only tell me that it was the portrait of "Her Majesty, Queen Victoria and that she had unexpectedly died broken-hearted." As I compiled the raw data for this research and ventured eagerly in to the behaviors and the critical fundamental functioning of the individual's mind, "as to the why we behave in ways that we do?" Of course my grandmother's beloved portrait of Queen Victoria, kept coming back to mind, thus propelling me to venture further in, as I researched the varied reasons for her depressing dress-code.

Victoria was the beloved daughter of Edward, the Duke of Kent and Princess Victoria of Saxe-Coburg. She was born in Kensington Palace in London on May 24th 1819. Edward died when Victoria was about eight months old, upon, which her mother enacted a strict regimen that shunned the courts of Victoria's uncles, George IV and William IV. In 1837 Queen Victoria, took the throne after the death of her uncle William IV. Due to her secluded childhood, she displayed a personalities marked by strong prejudices and a willful stubbornness. Barely eighteen, she refused any further influence from her domineering mother and ruled in her own right. Popular respect for the Crown, was at a low point at her coronation, but the modest and straightforward young Queen, won the hearts and minds of her subjects. She expressly wished to be informed of political matters, although she had no direct input in policy decisions.

The Reform Act of 1832 had determine the applicable standard of legislative authority residing in the House of Lords, with executive authority resting within a cabinet formed by members of the House of Commons; the monarch, was essentially removed from the loop. She respected and worked well with Lord Melbourne (Prime Minister in the early years of her reign) and England grew both socially and economically. On February 10th, 1840, only three years after taking the throne, Victoria took her first vow and married her cousin, Prince Albert of Saxe-Coburg-Gotha. Their historical relationship, was one of great love and shared admiration. Together they birthed nine children - four sons and five daughters: Victoria, Bertie, Alice, Alfred, Helena, Louise, Arthur, Leopold, and Beatrice.

Almost immediately, Prince Albert replaced Melbourne, as the dominant male influence in Victoria's life. She was thoroughly devoted to him, and completely submitted to his will. Victoria did nothing without her husband's approval. Albert assisted in her royal duties. He successfully introduced a strict decorum in court and made a point of straitlaced behavior. Albert in addition gave a more conservative tinge to Victoria's politics. If Victoria was to insistently occasionally interject, her opinions and effectively made her views felt strong in the cabinet, it was only because of Albert's teachings of hard work. The general public, however, was not enamored with the German prince; he was rightly excluded from embracing any official political position, was never granted a title of peerage and was named Prince Consort, only after seventeen years of marriage. His vested interests in art, physical science, and industry enthusiastically encouraged him to organize the Crystal Palace Exhibition in 1851, an immensely profitable industrial convention. He used the creative revenue, some £186,000, to purchase lands in Kensington for the establishment of several cultural and industrial museums.

Reflecting back into her childhood, Victoria was consistently prone to self-pity and sadness. On December 14th 1861, Albert died from typhoid fever at Windsor Castle. Victoria remained in self-imposed withdrawal, depression and seclusion for ten years. This somewhat genuine, but rather obsessive mourning, kept her occupied for the rest of her life and played an important role in the resultant evolution of what would become the Victorian mentality. Her popularity was at its lowest by 1870, but it constantly increased thereafter until her death. In 1876, her good friend and Britain's Prime Minister, Benjamin Disraeli, crowned her Empress of India. In 1887 Victoria's Golden Jubilee, was a Grand National celebration of her 50th year as Queen. The Golden Jubilee brought her out of her shell, and she once again embraced public life. She toured English possessions and even visited France (the first English monarch to do so since the coronation of Henry VI in 1431). Victoria's long reign witnessed a conventional evolution in English politics and the collective expansion of the British Empire, as well as political and social reforms on the continent. France had known two dynasties and embraced Republicanism; Spain had seen three monarchs and both Italy and Germany had united their separate principalities into national coalitions. Even in her dotage, she readily maintained a youthful energy and optimism, which infected the English population as a whole. The national pride connected with the name her name Victoria, the term Victorian England, for example, stemmed from the Queen's ethics and personal tastes, which generally reflected those of the middle class. Thus the first documented and unrecognized case of characterized depression would become vogue, though if not utterly a diagnosis thus rather for aesthetic purpose perhaps accepted.

The Evolution of Clinical Psychiatric Treatment

Freud's story, is like most other people's stories, it evolves with others. In his case it ties in with two other chief players, his mentor and friend, Dr. Ernest Bruke and Bruke's patient, better known, as Anna O. Anna O. had been Bruke's patient from 1880 through 1882. The twenty-one year old Anna, had spent most of her time nursing her ailing father, however, somewhere along the way, she developed a bad cough, which at the time proved to have no physical basis. After the cough, she also developed some speech difficulties and later became mute, shortly thereafter; she could no longer speak her native German, but rather spoke only English.

Following the death of her father, Anna began refusing food and developed a rather unusual set of problems. She lost the feelings in both hands and developed paralysis shortly thereafter, she exhibited involuntary spasms in her feet. Ana O, also developed visual hallucinations and tunnel vision symptoms. However, when examined by specialists, they found no specific physical causes for any of these problems. Despite all of these issues going on in her life, she also experienced fairy-tale fantasies, dramatic mood swings, and several rather bizarre suicide ideations, followed by several serious suicide attempts. When Dr. Bruke, diagnosed her, documented in his findings that she was suffering from what was then known as hysteria, or conversion disorder, as it would be called later. This meant that she suffered from symptoms, which appeared to be physical, but were rather psychological in nature. During the evenings, Anna would sink into "states of clouds," as she called them, or what Bruke then called "spontaneous hypnosis." Bruke found that during these trance-like states, Anna could explain her daytime fantasies and other experiences. He then realized that she would soon began to feel better right after giving such explanations and sharing her experiences. Anna O, recognized and named these episodes "the chimney sweeping and the talking cure."

Although often times during chimney sweeping episodes, she would recall emotional events that gave meaning to some particular symptoms. The first example came soon after she had refused to drink for a while. She recalled seeing a woman drinking from a glass that a dog had just drank from, while recalling this, she experienced strong feelings of disgust and then had a drink of water. Clearly speaking, her symptoms and avoidance to water, disappeared almost immediately after she remembered its root event and experienced the strong emotions appropriated to the event. Bruke later called this catharsis, which comes from the Greek word 'cleansing, or purging.' It would take almost eleven years, before Bruke and Sigmund Freud, whom was then Bruke's assistant to record, write and document anything regarding hysteria. Nevertheless, when they did, however, in it they described their theory. In such, which they stated that every episode of hysteria, is the direct result of a traumatic experience, one that cannot be integrated into the person's understanding of the world. They also explained that emotions appropriate to such trauma, are not expressed in any direct fashion, but neither does it simply evaporate. Both Bruke and Freud, agreed that these emotions, expressed themselves in behaviors that in a rather weak, vague and unusual way tend to offer response to the trauma. And that these symptoms were in other words meaningful. They then described that when the patient, can be made aware of the meanings of his or her symptoms through hypnosis, then the unexpressed emotions are released and would no longer have a need to express themselves as symptoms. They compared it to lancing a boil or draining an infectious wound, 'catharsis, or purging;' by these means, Anna, was able to rid herself of symptom after symptom. However, it should also be noted that Ana, needed Dr. Bruke to help her accomplish such. Therefore, when hypnotized, she needed to feel his hands upon her for reassurance, prior to the beginning of her talking. Sadly, problems then began to emerge shortly thereafter.

According to Freud statement, Bruke had realized that Anna, was falling in love with him and that he in turn, was also falling in love with her. Anna O, also began to experience delusions and began telling everyone that Bruke had impregnated her and that she now carried his child. "Had it been in a different era, people would in fact imagined that she wanted it rather badly that her mind had told her body it was true, and that she'd therefore, developed a hysterical pregnancy. Nevertheless, these were during such time of strict Victorian mores,." Dr. Bruke, was a married man, living during the Victorian era. He therefore, opted to abruptly end their sessions together and immediately lost all interest of any further research on hysteria. Nevertheless, Freud would later add that Bruke, refused to acknowledge publicly his secret sexual desires for Anna, which lay at the bottom of all hysterical neuroses. Anna spent quite a long time in a sanatorium. She would later go on to become a well-respected humanitarian activist, credited with becoming one of Germany's first social reformer and social worker under her birth name, Bertha Pappenheim. She died in 1936, at the age of 77 she is remembered not only for her own accomplishments later in life, rather as the inspiration for being the most influential, theoretical personality in psychiatric history.

How Germany Exterminated Their First Social Reformer.

The History of Anna O, is perhaps the first major Jewish contribution to the Field of Mental Bertha Pappenheim was Born 1859 in Vienna, Austria and died in 1936, in Isselburg, Germany. She was a social worker, author and leader of the German, feminist movement. She devoted most of her life to improving the social and economic position of Jewish women and children in Germany. She successfully enlisted a nationwide international support for her causes, as a founder and leader of the 'Juedischer Frauenbund.' She was the third daughter of four children born to a wealthy Viennese Orthodox family. Bertha Pappenheim, envied the attention and opportunities given to her younger brother Wilhelm and lamented her traditional upbringing and being treated only as 'a girl.' Bertha Pappenheim attended and graduated from a Catholic school in Vienna, with fluency in French, Italian, and English languages. Although her intellectual potential was stifled, while she dutifully awaited marriage and the leisured womanhood that was expected of her during such times by society and family members. She engaged in occasional charity work. She would later encourage and persuade idled women of privilege to embrace charity and social justice campaigns. After nursing her dying father, Pappenheim suffered debilitating psychological problems, then classified as severe hysteria. Distinguished psychoanalyst Ernest Bruke, who treated Pappenheim in Vienna from 1880-1882, documented her case, and made it known to Sigmund Freud, who referred to her in his writings as Anna O. Her symptoms, paralysis, hallucinations, inability to eat and drink, and suicidal tendencies, were relieved through hypnosis and explication of her memories, therapy, which Pappenheim referred to as 'chimney sweeping' and 'talking cure.' Prior to meeting Freud, she had eventually been trained by Bruke to treat herself. Pappenheim, would later by hailed journalists and commentators, as being the 'true discoverer of the cathartic method.' Pappenheim suffered several relapses and occasionally entered into sanitariums, following her treatment by Bruke, until her relocation to Frankfurt in 1889.

With the help of concerned relatives, Pappenheim, cultured her growing interest in social justice and once in Frankfurt, she became attracted to German feminism. Above all, she was influenced by the work of activists like Helen Lange. In 1890, under the fictitious name of Paul Berthold, she uttered concerns for children and the poor in a book of short stories entitled, *In the Second Hand Shop*. Pappenheim, devoted herself to incorporating her newfound passion for feminism, with her concerns for social justice and her identity as a Jew. These newly developed interests, were the groundwork and the theme of her 1899 play, *Women's Rights* that prompted her to publish the German translation of Mary Wollstonecraft's A *Vindication of the Rights of Women*. After a series of jobs as a soup kitchen volunteer, a nursery school administrator and headmistress of a Frankfort orphanage, Pappenheim, published two pamphlets in 1910 that connected the poor to the educational opportunities and the real life poverty, prevalent among Jewish girls. The first of these being: *'The Jewish problem in Galicia'* and *'The Condition of the Jewish Population in Galicia.'* In 1902, Pappenheim, also founded the Care for Women Society *Weibliche Fuersorge,* which was designed to place orphans in foster homes, educate mothers in childcare and provide vocational counseling and employment opportunities for women. As a representative of the Care for Women Society, Pappenheim traveled throughout the Middle East, Europe, and Russia. She became greatly concerned with prostitution and issues surrounding white slavery. These were later publicized, in one of her widely recognized publications, *The Sisyphus Work*. Bertha Pappenheim also saw the need for a larger, nationwide organization devoted to Jewish social issues and women's concerns, independent of and rival to the then comparable institutions being established by Jewish men. Along with several other activists, Pappenheim created the *Juedischer Frauenbund* in 1904, and served as its president for over twenty years after its inception. *The Frauenbund* campaigned against the white slave trade, especially in Eastern Europe and worked to enhance legal protection for women worldwide. Pappenheim characterized this aspect of her work as *Sisyphean* or endless uphill task, because the progress she made in awareness rising, often brought about strong resistance from Jewish communities, whom denied the extent of such social problems within their own ranks. Ironically, Pappenheim later had to witness the Nazis use her own reports of white slavery, among the Jewish circles as anti-Semitic propaganda. The Frauenbund also worked to establish women's equality with men, in other secular community matters. Pappenheim encouraged women to penetrate the ranks of the highly regulated Germeinde, (German Jewish community). Career training, a third emphasis of the Frauenbund, was to encouraged and foster means to financial independence and personal fulfillment for women. Despite all, training was narrow and only provided opportunities in those fields traditionally associated with women, such as housekeeping, nursing and social work. Pappenheim ensured that knowledge of Jewish traditions, concerning holiday and family observances, was the central element to such training. In addition to the editing and the publication of the *Frauenbund's* periodicals, Pappenheim translated into modern German the Memoirs of Gluekl von Hameln, a distant relative in 1910. In 1913 and 1916, Pappenheim then published a play, *Tragic Moments* and several short stories, sharing the themes of the status of women in Judaism, anti-Semitism, and assimilationism. Pappenheim criticized Zionism harshly in her writings, considering it divisive to families and neglectful of women's issues. After leaving the presidency of the Frauenbund, due to her declining health, Pappenheim translated the *Maaseh Buch,* a collection of traditional Jewish narratives, the *Ze'enah u-Re'enah,* a 16th century women's bible, the *Five Megillot,* and the *Haftarot.* Toward the end of her life, Pappenheim patriotically spoke out against emigration of Jews from Germany, despite rising anti-Jewish legislation. She died shortly after an extensive 'torture,' as she was being interviewed by the Gestapo in 1936. The interview was in regards to several anti, Hitler's remarks made by one of her former stewards. Her death, was commemorated with only a small funeral, she herself had written her own obituary prior. In 1904, she founded the *Juedischer Frauenbund,* its importance, benefited Jews throughout the world. Therefore, Jews worldwide, men and women, are very much in debt of gratitude to her, as a thanks for this social achievement. However, they would instead continue to withhold such.

Our guess was perhaps due to the stigma attached to her previous battle with mental illness, they were unable to overcome such … or perhaps because she simply told the truth.

Hypnosis

Hypnosis is an extraordinary phenomena, to this day no complete satisfactory definition, has yet been developed to describe it. As a matter of fact, debates still rage over the findings of its origins and the exact nature of its components. The British Medical Association and the American Medical Association, have tentatively defined it in part as a temporary condition of altered attention, in the subject that may be induced by another person, but there is still much about hypnosis to be understood. Although the condition resembles normal sleep, scientists have found that the brain wave patterns of the hypnotized subjects, much resemble the patterns of deep relaxation. However, rather than just a psychic or mystical phenomenon, hypnosis is now generally viewed as a form of conscientious, approachable and highly alert awareness, in which all external or unimportant events are omitted and disregarded. When hypnosis first came to scientific attention, it was then called 'animal magnetism' or 'mesmerism,' after Franz Mesmer of Vienna, who first used it in the late 18th century and had claimed it to heal certain nervous ailments. His belief was that some sort of magnetism was transferred from him to his patients and in tern it redistributed their body fluids. Although mesmerism, was criticized for many years by medical practitioners, whom simply discounted hypnosis, whom quickly associating its outcome, with theatrics and stage performances, fraud and superstition. Nevertheless, it became widely used as anesthetics by physicians, who began using mesmerism throughout the 19th century, during surgery before the discovery of anesthetics. They found that a deeply hypnotized patient would lie perfectly still, appearing unaffected by pain. Hypnosis later was used even during operations as serious and as painful as amputations.

Around 1840 a doctor named James Braid coined the term hypnosis, which means 'a nervous sleep.' The new name was more acceptable than mesmerism, with its implications of fraud, and it soon supplanted the previous term. In the mid to late 19th century, several physicians, including Jean-Martin Charcot and Sigmund Freud, became interested in the usage of hypnosis during their practice of medicine. Today hypnosis is still widely accepted and successfully used by medical practitioners as surgeons, dentists, and psychotherapists. Physicians may use it to relieve anxiety or as an anesthetic. Psychotherapists use it to relax the patient, to reduce resistance to therapy, to facilitate memory, and even to treat some conditions. Hypnosis, is also used in specialized therapies, such as those that help a person to stop smoking, eat less, or fight specific fears, such as fear of flying. It is unclear, however, if such procedures have any positive long-term effects. Hypnosis, has also been used during police interviews to enhance the memory of witnesses. Regardless of the application, hypnosis should be left to those whom are properly trained. When used by novices and untrained persons it could have undesirable and even dangerous effects.

CHAPTER IV

The Uniquely Interesting Life and History of the Mental Health Worker

> *The Evolution of Treaters: From Keepers to Custodians to Attendants to Doctors to Psychiatrist to Psychologist to Sociologist to Clinicians to Social Workers to Psych Nurses to Psychiatric Aids to Psych Techs to Mental Health Workers to Mental Health Assistants to Case Managers.*

The first state institution built exclusively for the mentally ill, was known as *the Hospital for Idiots and Lunatics,* renamed years later, as the Eastern State Hospital. It was located in Williamsburg, Virginia and opened in 1773. However, it was forced to suspend services during the Revolutionary War, due to lack of funds and was instead used to hose the troops until 1783, when it was again reopened as an institute for the insane. This time being administered by non-medical personnel, known as keepers, until around 1841, when the State Assembly discontinued the position and passed an Act specifying that the institution were to be directed by a hospital superintendent, whom had to be a physician. At such time, its name was also changed to Eastern Lunatic Asylum. Dr. John Galt II, 1819-1862, a graduate of the University of Pennsylvania, became its first medical superintendent. Dr. Galt, is also best known, as one of the original thirteen founders of the Association of Medical superintendents, known today as the American Psychiatric Association (APA).

Dr. Galt, is also best remembered throughout history, for being one of the first physicians in the field, to recognize the value of fresh air, recreation, musical, occupational and industrial therapy. He also encouraged games and carriage rides for patients, as well as a well-stocked library, regular classes of music instructions and a choir. During his tenure at the hospital, he ensured that there was a carpenter shop, a shoe-making shop and a crafts shop, making leather goods, brooms and of course a sewing room. His administration lasted a little over twenty-one years, until May 6, 1862. His life was cut short when the hospital came under a threat of attack during the Civil War, and he was ousted by the Union Army. It is uncertain whether he committed suicide via an overdose of laudanum, which was often dispensed patients, as a neuroleptic substitute. Although it is believed his death was rather accidental, some researchers have also documented that Dr. Galt, also suffered from bout of depression. The hospital then entered into a somewhat of a stormy period that lasted more than three years, during the Union Army's occupation. Although during these times Army medical officers, continued providing care exclusively for the mentally ill; white and black civilians and military, Northern, and Southerners alike, administered it.

After the Union Army withdrew, the institution was again operated by the State of Virginia and in 1894, it became the Eastern State Hospital. During this period, there were still very few institutions devoted exclusively to the care of the insane, before 1800. The few that were in existence, functioned more like jails rather than hospitals. The main purpose of these institutions, were to keep the inmates in custody for their safety, as well as the protection of the attendants and the public. That was their objective and that is what was achieved, usually by any necessary means. The caretakers in these institutions charged with providing care for the insane during the late seventeen hundreds and throughout most of the eighteenth hundreds, were the attendants. They were generally uncultured, uneducated, of poor character, with unstable personalities, intemperate undisciplined, untrained and oftentimes even illiterates. They were society's rejects whom often displaced their hostility on the mentally ill, which involuntarily became the victims of their brutality. Male attendants, were assigned to wards for men; and female attendants, were assigned to wards for women. Generally speaking, it is believe that the female inmates, fared somewhat better than their male counterpart. Usually, two equally untrained supervisors were also employed; one, a male, which was assigned to cover the building and grounds occupied by male patients and their male attendants; the other a female, usually called the 'Matron,' she was assigned to those occupied by the female patients and their attendants. The attendants worked long hours, had little time off, they were paid poorly and generally lived on the wards.

Before 1850, each had a 24 hour responsibility for about fifty patients. Since they were no night attendants, the inmates were not only locked up, but were often times also restrained, or even chained to their beds, so that the attendants could get some sleep. A few years later, a watchman was employed to make rounds during the night hours.

The long hours, low wages massive responsibilities and poor living conditions only contributed to further inflame the already hostile environment. There was no appreciation for the job, rather a deep seeded belief that the disturbed agitated behavior of the patients, was rather reinforced or even precipitated by these external factors. During these times, the attendants relied heavily on seclusion, restraint and medication (chloroform, ether, paraldehyde, chloral hydrate, bromide and compound alcohol) to control and keep them quiet. The inmates, were confined to their beds for long intervals. Urine and feces incontinence, was also a noted serious problem. Atropine, belladonna and periodic catheterizations, as well as enemas at bedtime, were often administered to reduce the situation, which was seen back then rather as a problem. In general, these measures were merely used to help decrease the attendant's workload, rather than as a form of clinical treatment. Log books found in hospital archives throughout the United States, dating as far back, as early eighteen hundreds, clearly indicate the various documented medication, list used by these institutions. Among those listed, each ward kept a bottle of whiskey and a strong bottle of sleeping medicine of bromides and chloral which attendants dealt out at their discretion. Though not documented in the log books, but one could assumed that the attendants, both males and females, helped themselves quite largely from the ward's whiskey bottle, which was then refilled at their discretion, or when desired.

Around 1884, the first journals cautioning institution administrators against the abuse of power toward the mentally ill emerge, when George L. Harrison published *Legislation On Insanity,* throughout which, he wrote, petitioned and persistently argued for a more humane treatment toward the insane. In such written petitions he stated, "There is a need for constant watchfulness against the negligence, recklessness, the self-will, the cruelties and the abuse of their immediate power." "It's all about their little brief authority."

Harrison, cautioned and raised claims against some of the subordinate attendants of these institutions. Harrison also voiced concerns surrounding the facts in which, the hospitalized insane were isolated from the community against their free will and stated that "the social experiences of the inmates of almost all hospitals for the insane, are designed by nature to induce insanity, where it does not exist, to intensify it where it does exist, and to drag down to irremediable madness, unhappy victims of such companionship, as they are consigned to in these institutions." Though sad the reflection upon the treatment of the mentally ill, throughout these publications, Harrison's comments toward the behavior of the attendants and the attitudes of the public during the late 19th century, was right on target. Beers witnessed these treatments only 14 years later and confirmed this type of behavior in 1908, when he published his autobiography *A Mind That Found Itself.* Despite the fact that Board of Trustees of hospitals for the insane throughout the country, had already began publishing revised work rules for the 'Government of Persons Employed' at these institutions, dating back as early as 1887, it still did not seem to matter. One such published piece of work, was found in the Connecticut Valley Hospital's library dating back to the year 1887. Almost twenty years after the Connecticut Hospital for Insane now the *Connecticut Valley Hospital,* such, being the first public institution, built exclusively for the treatment and care of the mentally ill in Middletown, Connecticut.

Been considered myself rather fortunate and more blessed for the opportunity given, for the richness to have served my fellowman for seven in a half years at such a fine historic institution, such as Connecticut Valley Hospital.

These listed rules at CVH, clearly reflect the emphasis during such times, about the hospital expectation of a good employee, the strict discipline and the long arduous hours imposed upon the attendants. Considering the fact that they were generally known and were labeled, as a group of uncultured, uneducated of poor character, with unstable personalities, ill temper undisciplined, untrained, illiterates. Still hospital administration, imposed upon them and expected them to work long grueling hours and that they provided somewhat of a humane care and treatment, to an already overcrowded patient population. In order to make a sound historical judgment, one must keep in mind that during these times, there still weren't any specific types of psychotropic or neuroleptics available in the forms of medications, therapy, nor even rational treatment by which to treat the mentally ill. The attendants, were perhaps given a simple basic list of rules to follow, these, which were rather implemented or enforced, as they worked side by side, with un-medicated chronically, mentally ill individuals. However, still to this day, administrative personnel in certain hospitals, tend to treat mental health workers, nurses and direct care givers as such. I still recall an article published in the late 1980's, in which a member of the Connecticut Legislature, had addressed a group of psychiatric aids and direct caregivers as 'goons.' Insults and comments of this nature, discredits and simply makes it a bit more difficult for those whom provide care to mentally ill individuals by lawmakers, should never be made nor furthermore tolerated. Thus far it simply encourages displacement and it is rather offensive.

Copies of documents published in late 1800's relates specifically to hospital scheduled regulations. A daily routine for day attendants was as follows:
Rising: bell at 5, 5:30 or 6 A.M. according to the season of the year.
Breakfast: bell. ½ hour after rising bell.
Physician's rounds: 9 A.M., and after supper.
Dinner: 12 N.
Supper: 5:45 P.M.
Out-of-door exercise: four hours daily in summer, in winter according to the weather. Bedtime: 7:30 P.M.
Before breakfast every patient should be washed, dressed and hair combed.
The beds will be opened for airing and soiled bedding removed.
After breakfast, beds will be made up neatly, floors swept, furniture and walls dusted and everything put in order by 9 A.M.

(Attendants should be prepared to inform the medical officer on his rounds of all circumstances in their patients requiring attention, such as loss of appetite, constipation, suicidal tendency, etc.) These rules mainly elaborated upon the duties and responsibilities of the attendants and reflected the moralistic philosophy and the custodial care in existence at that time: Taken also into consideration, was the cleanliness of the patients, their safety and comfort, diversional activities, the application of restraints and seclusion; outdoor exercise; the locking of doors; and so forth. Little to no attention, was focused on the rigid schedules of the attendants, whom were forced to work long hours, due to the fact that many of these hospitals, strived to remain self-sufficient and independents of their community. This in addition, managed to further isolate the patients from their families and their own communities. Several of these hospitals also ran and operated their own factories, producing everything from shoes, to clothing, to mattress's, bed linen, to smoking and chewing tobacco, etc. Such which was used to help clothe the patients. Many of these hospitals also maintained their own farms and raised livestock, which fed the hundreds of employees and over a thousand inmates. It is now also known that often times, these hospitals also supplied and sold their produce and meats to the surrounding towns. Nevertheless, patients continued to be locked in their rooms at nightfall. The rule though they weren't any significant reasoning concerning this practice, it required that: *"After taking every precaution for the security and comfort of each patient, each attendant, is to bid their patient's good night and lock them in their rooms."* Some of the night attendants were assigned to watch epileptic, suicidal or other special patients; others made hourly ward round, charged with the responsibility of assuring themselves "that the patients were secure that the outside doors were fastened by the night locks that neither water, gas, nor steam was escaping … that no fire had been started and that at least five minutes was being spent on each ward while doing rounds." Filthy patients, were as far removed as possible, thus preventing them from becoming offensive to others, or were simply ignored until the following day. In addition to reporting about changes in the condition of patients, the attendants were also responsible for reporting employees, who came in late. *This practice is still vividly carried out throughout the much-antiquated state hospitals systems, and is very much encouraged by some supervisors, bent on further stressing out nurses, mental health workers and other direct caregivers. Equally and fairly, some mental health workers and nurses also inconsiderate toward their peers and often chooses not to release them on time.* They also reported on lights burning after 10 P.M. and any irregular behavior on the part of the employees. Depending on the size of the institution, availability of attendants, administration and need, usually one, or more attendants, was also assigned to visit the barns and out buildings at regular intervals every night, to guard against fire and intruders and especially to give necessary attention to live stock. Apart from nine hours off duty, presumably to sleep, the night attendants spent about fifteen hours on duty.

The day attendants in these hospitals, also worked long hours, seven days a week and if their supervisor granted permission, they were free one afternoon. These permissions, were carefully monitored and they extended from after the midday meal to suppertime, about five hours, or one evening to 10 P.M. and alternate Sunday mornings from 10 A.M. to 12:45 P.M. This however, was usually to attend church services. All hospital employees, were expected to comply with hospital guidelines according to these directives and to devote themselves entirely to its interests, faithfully to regard its rules and to cheerfully contribute all of their talents to the advantage of the institution. *"Apparently these institutions were designed to literally suck their employees dry as they served, as a trickledown effect of displacement. e.g., The Trustees displayed upon the administration, the medical staff, in turn displayed upon the attendants, who then dumped it back on the inmates, whom would become a bit more psychotic than when they were first admitted."*

Judging from the extent and specificity of these rules, the Trustees were authorized to establish policy and were also responsible for the daily administration of the hospital and the discipline of the employees. The medical superintendent apparently functioned more as a physician than an administrator. This practice however, still is in effect among Doctors, Nurses and Social workers. The fact that nursing schools, diploma programs in general hospitals throughout the country, were long established and had been producing nurses since the last quarter of the 19th century, had little to no impact in the care of the mentally ill. Graduates of these early nursing schools, apparently shunned both state and private mental institutions. They all shared the negative misconceptions and negative attitudes expressed by the general public, toward the mentally ill. They ignored the plight of the mentally ill, did not perceive them as being sick and could not be induced to work in psychiatric hospitals. Mental hospitals, particularly state mental hospitals and all those who worked them, alike their patients, were being constantly criticized. The overcrowding, the unsanitary conditions, the isolation, as well as its allegedly disreputable employees, only served to further reinforce their fears toward the mental patient ... the fear of being hurt and of even becoming mentally ill themselves. Such myth still remains alive and well among many lay persons, mainly those, whom have had no type of contact with a person suffering from some form of mental illness. *Even during the Great Depression, nurses had not risen above such deep-rooted stigma, nor fear, mainly due to deep-rooted prejudices. Unemployed nurses, ignored opportunities for employment at state hospitals, which desperately needed their services and skills. These attitudes persisted at least through the 1930's and 40's.*

During the late nineteenth century, the care of the inmate, remained the responsibility of the states, based primarily on the malady, which entitled them to the most thoughtful sympathy. The recovery of the patient often depended on the character of the nursing, seclusion, chemical, mechanical, and manual restraints. Apparently, the trustees were aware that these protective practices, were being abused. The following is from one of their documented explanations printed in a late 19th century newspaper. In it, they expressed their concern by stating that:

A patient, for whom a physician has prescribed restraint by mechanical means, requires more attention than others, because of being less able to wait on themselves. Mechanical restraint must never be applied except as or-by a physician. Neither may a patient be secluded for any considered length of time without the physician's order. The patient is to be secluded, be locked in a bedroom - not in a closet nor bathroom.

Throughout the darkened days, the segregation of patients and staff by way of sexual gender, persisted. Patients were deprived of their liberties and kept behind locked doors, subject to the authority of the attendants and the rules and regulations of each institution. Custodial practices prevailed. Patients, were dehumanized and isolated from sustained contact with friends and relatives. The attendants during such times, had no status, little self-esteem and fared little better than many of the patients themselves. The instability and transience of this group, proved further evidenced by the following regulation. With reference to protection from the peculiar embarrassments, incidental to sudden withdrawal from service on the part of the ward attendants, *no persons are engaged in this department of labor, unless willing to contract agreeing to forfeit one month's wages if they leave without a month's notice.* The early attendants were literally laborers, who worked long hours for very low wages. Documented records have noted that as late as the mid 1900's, it was not at all uncommon for the psychiatric nursing personnel attendants to be working fourteen-hour day shifts, or a ten-hour a day for six and a half days a week.

At the beginning of the twentieth century, few graduate nurses were employed in public mental institutions. Often, showing very little distinction if any, between the nurses and attendants, their functions, titles, fringe benefits nor wages. From the onset women, although well trained, were paid less than men with comparable background.

Documents collected from a New York State Institution's Archive, shows that in addition to a room and meals: female attendants received monthly wages ranging from $16.00 to $22.50; whereas male attendants received from $22.00 to $30.00; female nurses, $31.25 as compared to the $31.25 to $37.50 paid monthly *the male nurses. These nurses were generally trained in mental, hospital nursing programs that ranged in length from two to three years. It also shows were newly employed female nurses received only $3.00 more than the male attendants and their maximum wage exceeded that of male attendants by only $1.25.*

It was also noted that female patients reportedly received better care, one could assume that the female nurses received better supervision during their training, than the male nurses and that they functioned at a higher level. However, the male nurses were paid a beginning wage comparable to that of the maximum wage paid to female nurses.

More than half a dozen pages of recruitment leaflets for nurses and attendants in state institutions dating back to the late 1800's and early 1900's was uncovered during this research that help to provide clearer explanation and more of an in depth detail, regarding hospital practices on hiring and their specific requirements:

Previous experience is not required of applicants for the position of nurse or attendant in the State service, but those certified from other institutions, or having had valuable experience, continue at salaries above the minimum. Appointees new to the work are assigned to duty with an experienced attendant who understands all the duties of his position and could instruct the newcomers. Supervisors also to look after the interests of the newly appointed, who would be given every opportunity to learn the work. The service requires men and women of good habits, who are sufficiently matured to take up their duties intelligently, but who are not too old to do their work efficiently, or to be ambitious to advance. The age limit for applicants for the position of Nurse or Attendant at this hospitals for the insane, varies somewhat, but is practically placed at 18 to 35 for women, and 21 to 35 or 40 for men, when entering on the work. Salaries cannot be definitely stated for all departments, but at the hospitals for the insane at entrance from $16 to $20 per month for females and from $20 to $25 for males, with maintenance or its equivalent. There is assurance of promotion for continued efficient service up to $30 and $35 per month. Graduate Nurses and those with experience at other institutions, are taken on at salaries above the minimum entrance wage, with the same promotion opportunities. While employed, the entire time of Attendants and Nurses is at the service of the state, they are certain of lodging, meals and laundry, in addition to their regular salary, they'll enjoy homelike surroundings. Recreation hours are provided for them and there is much outdoor exercise, with time of at stated periods.

The large majority of persons afflicted with mental or nervous insanity are not violent or dangerous, but should be treated as unfortunate sick people in need of kindness and help. Firmness is necessary at all times, but with ordinary self-control on the part of the Attendant, and with the cooperation of one's fellow Attendants on the wards ... the work will then proceed comfortably and smoothly. Certainly the occupation has a noble purpose, and the men and women who take up this work are helping others while making a very comfortable living for themselves. During Colonial times nursing the sick was mainly a task, left to be performed by mothers, wives, or neighboring women and it was usually done in the patient's own home. These women nursed literary in the dark and against great odds, without any real knowledge on any specific diseases, what caused them, or even how and what treatments to provide. They mostly depended on familiar medicinal herbs, peels, barks, fish oils, garlic, fowl fats and household remedies handed down by their ancestors. Trying to care for the sick during the long, cold winters were especially difficult. One must keep in mind that during such times, central heating, electricity and modern lavatories were nonexistent these women had to be resourceful and creative in meeting every simple and daily physical needs when, concentrating on maintaining basic lives.

The first Medical hospital was built in 1731, in Philadelphia. Nevertheless, it functioned more in the form of a salad-care system. As a combination of a hospital for the sick, the insane, orphans and prisoners; it also serve, as an almshouse, a workhouse for the poor, a home for the aged and to the mentally infirm. During such times, the sick were in the hands of servants, paupers and criminals. Several other hospitals were established later during the eighteenth century.

However, nurses were from the lowest social classes. Generally they were unable to read, write and were mostly hardhearted drunkards. Valid reason perhaps, as to why mainly the very poor, the indigent or those without friends nor relatives visited hospital back then. The frequency of infection, the unsanitary conditions, the poor character of the employees and the high mortality rate, help brought about the negative attitudes toward hospitals. During those days, people also found it disgraceful and disrespectful, not to take care of their sick or loved ones at home. Throughout great part of the Revolutionary War, medical and nursing care, left much to be desired. There existed very little organization and discipline, was almost excluded from the medical vocabularies. Hospitals for the sick and wounded soldiers were usually makeshifts tents, mostly overcrowded and very unsanitary. Field transport of the wounded, was primitive and often compounded their injuries. Soldiers often suffered and died though mainly not just from combat wounds, but from fevers and infections, which helped to contribute in the decimation of the armed forces. Nevertheless, during those times, untrained men, mostly performed nursing … they were then called *orderlies*.

In 1777, George Washington, while trying effortlessly to improve conditions among his wounded soldiers, ordered that women be employed to nurse the sick. However, these women functioned more as cooks, while trying very much to limit their contact with the sick, thus reducing their duties to merely serving the soldiers their meals. Hence, whatever nursing was performed upon the soldiers, was left up to their wives and other camp followers. Throughout most of the first half of the 19th century, treatment of the sick was still mostly done in their own home and nursing still would remain the responsibility of the women. *Specific remedies for common afflictions were transmitted* verbally from mothers to daughters,' colonial cookbooks of these times included a section on elementary, first-aid and the care of the sick. These books, were also given as wedding gifts, while young brides regarded them as vital resources for their kitchen and home. Their contents also included, basic rules that reflected their superstitious beliefs and the lack of knowledge about diseases during such period. e. g., keep windows closed at night; avoid night air like the plague; don't live near a cemetery, do not take warm baths, then step right out into the cold air, etc. These books also contained certain health concepts that are still being recommended today, such as avoid overeating and start each day with a nutritious meal!

The first medical school, with planned instructions and some guidelines for admission, had been opened since 1765 in Philadelphia, yet no uniform laws, regulating medical practice was in existence throughout most of the country. By 1840, only about one third of the practicing physicians had graduated from a medical school, while the majority had received their medical training as apprentices to physicians. The quality and nature of this training varied considerably to the individual's mentor or medical practitioner … the time ranged from several months, to three years. This medical training, was based solely on learning by doing and observing. The results depended appreciably upon the intuitive and experiential skills of the practicing physician as well, as his personal and intellectual qualities.

During the Civil War many soldiers died from neglect, dysentery and smallpox. This was the beginning toward raising awareness of our need for trained nurses. Nevertheless, the deep-rooted prejudice toward employing women as nurses in hospitals, persisted. During the Civil War era, there were only 68 hospitals in the country, but by the year 1872, the number had increased to 178, a tremendous growth in less than a decade. The Civil War had brought about a phenomenal impact in the development of new medicine and progress in the field of medicine and neurology. Although accomplishing great strides in medicine; nevertheless, psychiatry and nursing, would remain still in the prehistoric dark-aged. Almost eighteen years after Dorothea Lynde Dix's birth in America, and twenty years before her 'worldwide' crusade on her plight for the insane, Florence Nightingale 1820-1910 would born in, Florence, Italy.

The difference between these two remarkable women, is that same which, would make their lives that much more similar and rather interesting to the world. Florence was born to a well to do, cultured English couple. Dorothea's father was a frail, nervous, disinterested drunk, who'd chosen not to work. Her mother was considered, ignorant, lazy and uncouth by her in laws. However, by the time of Florence's birth, Miss Dix had already opened and successfully operated a school for children and by the closing of the 19th century, these two remarkable women, would have made contributions to humanity that would prolonged throughout history. Such contributions, wouldn't only serve their respective countries, but rather the world as a whole, these still yet to be equaled by any other two individuals, either male or female. Accomplishing all, despite the social limitations surrounding them. The "narrow-minded discrimination and prejudicial, dependent status, women faced during the early 19th Century." Dorothea and Florence, dared to depart from roles and customs and did things that reflected their religious philosophies, their intellectual powers, their convictions, their social consciousness and their concerns for the sick and the helpless, the neglected and the oppressed.

Their unconquerable spirits, surpassed their physical frailties; their courage and perseverance permitted them to accomplish the greatest historical reforms for the care and treatment of the physically and mentally disable. The difference between Dorothea and Florence's childhood, was that one was reared in a wealthy, cultured, stimulating and stable environment and the other barely stood a chance in life. Florence's family, spent the winters in London and France and the rest of the time at Embley Park, Hampshire, England. Florence's paternal grandfather, was a Member of Parliament and a religious zealot and her father had tremendous influence, on her early development. Her father, contrary to the existing public attitude, believed in education for girls. Hence not only that provided a governess for Florence and her older sister, in addition, he personally participated in their education. In contrast to Florence's, Dorothea spent her early childhood running from her father's vagaries and verbal abusive language to her grandmother's home in Boston, or to her aunt's in Worcester. Dorothea had nothing in common with either of her parents, but found it easier to model after her aunt, in whom she also found discipline and with whom she clearly identified. Meanwhile Florence, identified with her father, but had little in common with her mother and sister whom, were mostly satisfied with Victorian society, enjoyed privileges, inherited, in their social class. Although Florence was customarily presented at court, she found such social life foreign, grim and unfitting to her independent nature. She was usually disinterested in developing any relationships with the men of her class, who appeared interested in her. Florence displayed, an early appeal to nursing, but her father refused to let her engage in the field, which, of course during such times was primarily consistent with disreputable, uneducated individuals of low moral character. Inspired by her grandfather's religious philosophy, she turned to the church and began working with the poor and the deprived, to which she would devote most of her time, energy and care.

At age 31, Miss Nightingale would travel to Kaiserwerth on the Rhine; there she spent three months at the Institution for Deaconesses. She became so impressed with this institution, which in less than twenty years had grown from a two-hospital bed to 100 beds, plus an orphanage, an asylum, a school for infants, a penitentiary with twelve inmates and a school for training teachers. She worked very hard and found no task too menial or disagreeable and quickly learned a great deal. By 1854, she was now 35 years old and had learnt rather well, how to successfully manipulate family contacts, within political figures and gain access. Through such contacts, she was able to get permission to take thirty-eight lay and religious female nurses to Scutari, to help care for the sick and wounded soldiers during the Crimean War. The simple thought of having these women, replacing untrained orderlies, while caring for the sick was deplorable and offensive to the army's medical officers. They fervently voiced their objections and vehemently resisted. Nevertheless, Florence and her small group of pioneers would persevere. She was sickened and disgusted by the condition in which she found the sick and wounded. Most of the sick and wounded men, were still fully clad in their filthy, bloody uniforms. The mortality rate, nearly approached the fifty percent mark, Florence and her army of nurses worked tirelessly to combat cockroaches, rats, bedbugs, diseases, filth and mud. She remained intolerant to army rules and regulations; and placed her priorities on saving the lives of the soldiers. This group of dedicated women, confronted tremendous and difficult obstacles, but in the end they would prevail. Although many of these women, had given up their privilege lives of ease and luxury, in exchange for these hardship and deprivations, endured, they soon learned to cope. It would take them over six months, for their efforts to succeed. Not only did the sanitary conditions improve, and the soldiers were now clean, comfortable and well fed, but the mortality rate had declined from almost fifty percent to less than two percent. Miss Nightingale had proven her genius for organization, administration, though more importantly for getting things done. She would later convinced the army that she could definitely bring order out of chaos ... she gained the respect of the medical officers and the War Department. Florence and her team of nurses, were showered with the love and admiration to the soldiers from the people of England. During the Crimean War, she proved by her experiences that nursing of the sick and wounded could be done successfully; and that trained nurses are an asset, which provides a valuable contribution to humanity. Though one might find it somewhat sick and at best hard to justify, nevertheless, wars were the truthful cause for the success of modern day nursing. Such was the positive result of the outcome of Crimean War and the tireless efforts of Florence Nightingale and her crew.

Two years later, upon her return to England in 1856, Miss Nightingale would exhaust every political and social contact, in order to implement reforms that would improve the lives and health of all English people. Long before documented findings or scientific knowledge of any bacteriological diseases, she advocated for cleanliness throughout hospitals and recommended the isolation of patients with contagious infections. She lobbied arduously for the comfort of sick people, while instructing that patients have access to well-trained nurses. During this period, she wrote and published her book, *Notes On Nursing* that to this day remains an inspiration to all those who read it.

The untiring roll she played throughout the years brought her effort to fruition, when the Army Medical School was founded at Fort Pitt, Chatham, in the fall of 1860. The opening of this school, also brought fort the beginning of new reforms, which included a rigorous military hygiene practice into its curriculum. Subsequently, the school was later moved to London where it became one of the leading medical schools at that same university. Florence Nightingale, truly believed in self-discipline and self-evaluation, though more importantly, she believed in a healthy body and soul. Based on those beliefs and her arduous efforts that same year the *Nightingale School for Nurses* was established in London in 1860. The school is best known for being the first in the world to teach the nursing profession. At first, it was affiliated with St. Thomas Hospital, however, this later became a challenge for Florence, due to the large number of overgrown egos among the medical staff, opposing the nurses. Doctors at this hospital, considered nurses to be not much more than confidential, obedient servants, responsible for keeping their patients clean, or as trained waitresses ready to obey doctor's orders.

However, not only did Florence Nightingale, advocated for their training to be a formal one-year professional nursing education, but she also insisted that the individual guidance; be taught both, the 'how and the why in nursing;' and that they be treated as a physician colleague, not as their maids. In addition that they may be provided with ample opportunities to learn and study. She stressed about how the importance of relationships and the treatment of the person and not only the disease be treated.

Florence Nightingale's enthusiasm did not stop there with the sick. She was as passionate in successfully formulating and developing a more adequate environment of significant growth for her nursing students as she was in implementing appropriate care and effective treatment for the sick. In addition, she single handedly revolutionized many ideas toward the proper functioning of general hospitals and in her *Notes On Hospitals,* published in 1863; she made a significant impact on their structure, vital construction and on their sanitary conditions. This impacted not only hospitals in her native England, but rather caused a ripple effect in the design, building, running, environmental maintenance and operation of hospitals throughout the modern world. She was in addition very independent and of course, very outspoken. In one of her many statements, she made a distinctive affirmation that to this day still guarantees a genuine respect for all nurses throughout the world. She later noted that: *"A Nurse Should Do Nothing else, but Nursing. If You Want A Charm-woman, then you should hire one … Nursing is a specialty."*

Although in today's healthcare system, many would argue otherwise. Given the fact that nurses lose central focus on what their profession actually means? One could not blame them for looking toward securing their future by climbing the political ladder, similarly to the doctors, the social workers and other healthcare professionals. In fairness to all nurses, whom have become nurses, due to their love for the distinguished profession … in today's climate, nurses still struggle in hospitals throughout the world, while trying to adhere to the Florence Nightingale's creed and put forth her philosophy. The reason for this, being that the technical expertise of trained nursing personnel is utilized less each-day in direct-care service, thus rather expended to non-nursing duties, which could easily be done by other disciplines. And in my defense to those nurses and other healthcare professionals who may aspire to key political positions geared toward nursing and medical policies, we unquestionably see the immediate need for such and therefore, we should support their effort. Because often times, we need trained and competent personnel within the psychiatric healthcare field, within those key political positions, who could best serve as advocates for the mentally ill. *Only those who have been on the frontline of psychiatric care, knows what functions could best provide valuable growth and could best benefit patient needs, regardless of the cost, thus rather measuring the effectiveness.*

Mental health work is a specialty, psychiatric nursing is a calling and each patient, client and consumer in the system, is an individual with unique categories and specific set of everyday changing needs. Therefore a lawyer, a businessperson, the clergy and a career politician could only assume and speculate what they have read about the individual. It is the mental health worker, the nurse, the case managers, perhaps a collaborative effort of entire team of healthcare professionals, the only ones whom have witnessed, listened, and understands what best suits a patient's need in order to make a full and complete recommendation. Although often taken for granted, in reality we carry a heavy burden upon our shoulders and for these reasons, we should persistently remain morally and ethically upright. *We should therefore have the outmost respect for each other, regardless of whether an individual is a doctor, a nurse, a mental health worker, a case manager, a social worker, an orderly, or a nurse's aid.* We are advocates, we are blessed we are of a benevolent nature; for health care is a selective calling and not just a job. And even if we managed to climb to the top of our careers and are unanimously chosen to serve in key governmental or administrative positions, we must insist in staying morally, ethically and spiritually upright. Moreover, we should never forget whom we were selected to serve. In recent years however, like Mr. Clifford Beers, there have been a number of mentally ill individuals whom have recovered and are now working in the field. Some has carried on to become psychiatrists, others as trained nurses, psychologists, advocates and volunteer members for grass-root organizations, together, all advocating for patient rights and a more humane treatment for individuals with mental illness.

The pride Miss Nightingale instilled in those nurses over a hundred and fifty years ago, have been handed down throughout the generations in the profession of nursing. Therefore one could not help notice that although the profession has since expanded from GN, to LPN, to RN, to APRN, etc. And some nurses would later go on to further their education and obtain PhD's, yet they still use and fundamentally recognize the letter 'N' at the end of their formal title when legally signing their names. Of course, since the 1870's, the arrogant attitudes of physicians toward the Nightingale School of Nursing have progressively changed. Doctors have since learnt to respect and to appreciate the significant importance of the role nurses play on their teams, although *it wasn't that long ago, when nurses and the nursing staff, were widely expected to stand up and practically salute the doctors, as they appear on the psychiatric wards.*

In the 1 870s, the caliber of academic and moral standards for admission to the Florence Nightingale School of Nursing began to drop below expectations. Florence Nightingale, became active virtually immediately in administering supervision to the esteemed institution, therefore restoring its standards for enrollment. In 1875, she implemented several reforms, stating that formal educational training at the institute is *"A home, a place for moral, religious and practical training ... A place for the shaping and educational training of character, habits and intelligence, as well as for acquiring profound knowledge."*

Considering that both Dorothea Dix and Florence Nightingale's childhood were immensely different, their venture did not differ in their pursuit of ideals, nor in their attributable representation and optimistic dedication toward their fundamental convictions. They were both, perhaps, the two most exceptionally successful women, in the field of environmental scientific health and care, and in many distinct endeavors. Both were writers, teachers, organizers, statisticians, recognized leaders, disciplinarians, advocates to the poor, the sick, and the oppressed. They were social reformers and crusaders, and they were doers, not just talkers. They were both able to get things done against all odds. They were in addition, the two very first women to collectively and proactively serve in official, governmental capacities during wartime. And likewise both of them, were also the two first women to be honored by their respective governments for their services in the health care field during the Crimean and the Civil Wars. Surely, their benevolent spirit and their vocational service to humanity, must have prolonged their longevity. They both also lived to see their efforts on behalf of humanity come to fruition. Miss Dix lived to the age of 85, and Miss Nightingale, to see her 90th birthday. Their sacrificial breakaway from 'Victorian era,' social tradition roles, did not only served humanity in the health field for approximately two centuries, but their extraordinary achievements, additionally paved the way and successfully help to secure the respect, admiration and the freedom that all women throughout the world continue to benefit from today.

Perspectives on Psychiatric Hospitals, Under the Colony System

Our view toward the modern period, is an indication as to where most states engaged in the construction of large, centralized park-like psychiatric hospitals, although during this time most medical and nursing schools wanted nothing to do with mental health, nor with having any of these institutions in their back yard. The majority of these hospitals were built in remote areas, at a far distance away from society, far removed from any neighboring metropolis. Though out in the country, they were primarily located on enormous, manicured grounds, aesthetically simulating, Victorian parks; reason for which, it is believe they were then nicknamed 'pauper's palaces.' Perhaps the original idea for such designs was done with a benevolent cause in mind, it was believed that the mentally ill, would benefit from pleasant and tranquil surroundings; arguably, it was the main reason for placing these hospitals out in the country.

Unfortunately, the size of these institutions defeated their purpose and these large institutions, would later become the epitome for mass brutal and dehumanizing treatment. Such was caused mainly by the difficulty in staffing such large institutions, a continuous problem that placed the care of most patients in the hands of undereducated and underpaid individuals, often without the supervision of professional staff. Historically, there were even recorded instances, when shortages became so drastic that patients, were then given uniforms and placed in charge of large groups of their fellow patients, or inmates; (noted points in history was during the Great Depression and WWII). This system became known as the "colony system," it was doomed and clearly showed signs of failure from its early beginnings. It should also be noted that during such times, no 'Blacks' African Americans, were allowed to work in the mental health field, as direct care provider. In the state of Connecticut's Department of Mental Health, African Americans were only allowed to work as janitors, laundry department and perhaps in dietary.

I was fortunate enough to have had the wonderful opportunity to work side by side, with the first African American person to ever work directly with psychiatric patients, as a mental health worker, at the Connecticut Valley Hospital, in the state of Connecticut. The Gentlemen name, is Mr. Ronald Poindexter. During conversation, Ron reminded me that he was transferred from the dietary department in the mid to late 1960's. During our conversation, I recall him telling me that "it was as if I carried the entire race upon my shoulders. I was supposed to represent the whole race. And I was warned by every other black man throughout the hospital. Do not to mess this up. This is not about you, it is rather about everyone of us. Because if you make it, we'll all make it. So I had to succeed, I had no other choice, but to succeed, in other to keep the doors open for the hiring of more black people to these positions."

Early on, the system was involved in purchasing large farmlands, on which these large hospitals were built. Although, the original intention, was to simulate normal village life within the confines of an institution, they were gaudy, rambling, Victorian exteriors and were often referred to as 'pauper's palace.' Their structures, were cheaply built and very little attention was paid to utility or the internal design, however, the second half of the nineteenth century brought an era of competition among these hospitals. Hospital administrations, commissioners and local politicians, soon began to grossly inflate their findings according to treatment and research, therefore, boasting toward rapid rates of cure. This period of time, was characterized by falsified, inaccurate and inflated statistics as each hospital attempted to outdo the other in its claims of treatment successes. During this period, several states did not yet have hospitals for the mentally ill and those that did, were having difficulties keeping up with the demand for admission. Some of these buildings, were erected so hastily that states paid no attention to detail, quality, or structure, their objective, were merely to accommodate the rising demand for the exaggerated care being promoted..

As the sham of cure-rate became rapidly overexposed and these Mental Asylums architectural, fiscal, medical and psychological inequities became evident, the public view became pessimistic, about the early claims of curability, being issued by proponents of these hospitals.

Even so, there were still too few hospitals to accommodate the growing indigent population of mentally ill individuals, which by now were overflowing in the almshouses and jails. Some of the primary architects of many of these buildings included *H.H. Richardson, George Kessler, Gordon W. Lloyd, Stephen Vaughn Shipman* (who also designed several state capitol buildings) *Elijah E. Myers, Ward P. Delano, Isaac Perry, John Notman, Frederick Law Olmsted* (landscapes and grounds), *A.J. Davis, H.W.S. Cleveland, Edward O. Fallis, Warren Dunnell, Charles C Rittenhouse, Richard Karl August Kletting, John A. Fox,* and others. *Thomas Story Kirkbride,* although not an architect, he devised the basic floor plan many of these architects used in the design of their main asylum buildings. *Many of which, carried his name during such era, are still known today as the famous Kirkbride style.*

First Renowned American Psychiatrist

Although rarely mentioned in passing, Dr. Benjamin Rush has for long been recognized, as America and the world's first psychiatrist by his peers. In 1769 Dr. Rush became the first professor at the first American psychiatric hospital. This hospital, located in Williamsburg, Virginia, was to be the only such institution to care for the mentally ill in the country for over fifty years. Dr. Rush graduated from Princeton University at the age of fifteen. In his twenties, he studied medicine at the University of Edinburgh. Right after graduation he began to practice medicine, realizing shortly thereafter that his primary interest was geared toward the treatment of the mentally ill. He divided the mentally ill into two groups, those who suffered general intellectual 'derangement' and those whose problems seemed only partial. Dr. Rush completely disapproved of the usage of restraint of any kind for long periods of time. He outlawed the use of whips, chains and straitjackets and developed his own methods for keeping control. Although looking back at some of the methods for which he advocated, one might think he was quite harsh. But in those days, his methods were considered exceedingly humane compared to what else was out there.

First Humane Methods of Treatment: Dr. Benjamin Rush is credited for inventing the *'Tranquilizing Chair.'* This therapeutic tool, is considered to be the first humane method of treatment known. The chair is preserved and could be seen when visiting the *National Library of Medicine* in Bethesda, MD. *The Tranquilizing Chair* was a device, whose projected goal was to heal by lowering the pulse and relaxing the muscles. This contraption was designed to hold the head, body, arms and legs immobile for long periods of time and helped enable the patient to settle down. Dr. Rush is also known for revolutionizing *'The Gyrator.'*

Comparable to what its name suggests, the *Gyrator* was a contraption similar to a spoke on a wheel. The patient would be strapped to the board, head outward and the wheel would then be rotated at high speed, sending the blood racing to the patient's head, supposedly relieving their congested brain. Dr. Rush, also believed deeply, and depended highly on the usage of the *'Circulating Swing.'* This swing worked similar to the gyrator, with the patient bound in place and in a sitting position. As we look back today, we could clearly see how obviously primitive were these types of treatments, however, changes in treatment were on the horizon. The Quakers would build the second American asylum near Philadelphia and called it *The American Friends 'Asylum.* This asylum and several others, that soon followed, would embrace the teachings of the Englishman William Tuke. Tuke's emphasis consisted mostly in providing moral treatment for his patients. No chains were used and violent patients, were separated from the others. By the mid 1800's, many institutions, were making the effort to truly help their residents, yet by today's standards, their efforts were still rather crude. Real changes began to take place with the arrival of the twentieth century, during and after World War 1.

Following World War I, it was discovered shortly thereafter that a large a numbers of soldiers, were returning home incapacitated due to emotional problems. Rapidly, it then became apparent that not just a few, but many of the soldiers, suffered from abnormal behavior. Scientific researchers and mental health treaters, then reasoned that if a direct trauma such as a 'war' could cause widespread symptoms, then it would be reasonable to assume that lesser trauma, occurring daily, frequently and for a prolonged period of time, could perhaps produce these same effects.

The Dawning of the Psychopathic Hospitals

Convincing general hospitals to recognize the mentally ill as patients and to treat them with dignity, kindness or perhaps to even see them as humans, was not as easy as easy task as we might think of it today. Nearing the end of the 19th century, mental illnesses, was finally beginning to gain some understanding and a gradual recognition, of being in the realm of medicine in origin. Although as to the classification type and symptoms that which still proceeded. At the beginning of the 20th century, the public's interest in social reform and their acceptance of social responsibility, began to show an increase, although the stereotype, prejudices, stigma, fear and hatred toward public facilities for the mentally ill, still persisted. Nevertheless, there was an activist movement, already set in gear toward recognizing the need for better services for the mental patient, hence the term 'psychopathic' evolved. It was the term used to describe institutions providing diagnostic evaluations and short term, intensive treatment services, it also engaged in training and research. The first psychopathic ward in a general hospital, was established around 1902 in Albany, New York. Several years later, various state Governors petitioned their General Assemblies, supported provisions and statutes, enabling the enactment of laws and special Acts that created special commissions to investigate.

The purpose for such commissions, was to investigate the need for each individual state to have a psychopathic hospital, while at the same time it questioning, why there wasn't one yet in place? These comprehensive reports and investigations, produced thousands of pages of data, consisting on everything from the existing private and public facilities for diagnosis and treatment of the mentally ill; to the physicians, their educational background and the extent of their psychiatric knowledge. More importantly, they also contained data on general hospital attitudes, toward providing psychiatric care for the mentally ill. One of the commission's chief recommendations, was that "every state in the union should have a psychopathic hospital in operation."

Although the year was now 1922, none of the twenty-eight general hospitals in Connecticut were treating psychiatric patients, nor had there yet been established any psychopathic hospitals throughout many of the states. Years later, a new commission was formed. Its recommendation was that a state psychopathic hospital be established in Connecticut. Yale University agreed to donate the land if the state provided the building, the nursing staff and building maintenance. The university, would provide the medical staff and New Haven General Hospital provided the clinical resources. Out of this state-corporate-university concept came, the development of the Connecticut Mental Health Center, (CMHC) in New Haven, Connecticut. A survey was then put into place to further monitor progress. The majority of these general hospitals, including the New Haven General, did not knowingly admit patients with mental illness back then. They instead argued that their facilities were not adequately set up to provide diagnosis and treatment services for these people. In the 1940's and 50's, medication to help the severely mentally ill, were now being discovered. Great hope been placed upon these drugs, though it would soon be discovered that these new scientific breakthrough did not really provide complete cure to the illnesses, thus often, rather a temporary relief. Although, in certain specific cases, they were quite successful at ameliorating some of these symptoms to the individuals. Many of these medicines, especially the antipsychotic medications still currently being used to this day. Followed by insulin therapy and ECT, both which came around the quarter part of the 20th century. During such times, circa 1933 insulin therapy was discovered and rapidly put into use, followed by ECT in 1939. It would be noted almost immediately that ECT went a long way in helping those patients suffering with depression. ECT therapy is still being used to this day, although it is done in a more refined and very humane mode, compared to how it was previously administered. Several serendipitous discoveries in the following years, nearly revolutionized the treatment of the mentally ill. New medications were discovered to help in most cases of severe mental conditions, and researches for new ones are constantly being funded.

World Renowned Psychologist and Neuroscientist

If you were ever asked to rank by name someone whom do you believed made the greatest contribution to the field of mental health throughout the 19th and 20th century, whose name would you mention? Although some theologians would dispute this claim in reality and to some degree they also have a valid point. Some theologians consider 'psychiatry to be the illegitimate child of psychology,' due in part to the vast number of grand-claims made throughout the years by an almost defunct system that fast continuously failed to reach a scientific significance. According to a statement made at a symposium of "progress on psychiatry" back in 1955 by a then eminent member of the American Psychiatric Association, stated that "psychotherapy today, is in a state of disarray, almost exactly as it was 200 years ago." The following year psychiatrist Percival Bailey, also stated "the great revolution in psychiatry has solved few problems. One wonders how long the hoary errors of Freud, will continue to plague psychiatry?" also adding that "the success of the Freudian revolution seemed complete. Only one thing went wrong. The patients did not get any better." Other critiques throughout the years have included that "psychotherapy has not yet been proven any more effective than general medical counseling, in treating neurosis or psychosis. In general, therapy works best with people who are young, well born, well-educated and not seriously ill." Another long- time one of Freud's strongest critiques, Dr. Thomas Szasz is quoted in his book *The Ethics of Psychoanalysis,* as he strongly argues these views. *The adherents of this exaggerated faith used it as a shield of illusion, concealing some ugly realities."* In it he arguably questioned, "thus when must we be given the papers, indicating that the alcoholic, the rapist or vandal must be given 'psychiatric care?" We are assured that the problem is being effectively dealt with and we dismiss it from our minds. I contend that we have no right to this easy absolution from responsibility." While some modern day Christian leaders challenges and takes this notion a bit further by asking themselves and questioning others of these facts ... *there seems to be a little question, then that much rethinking is called for?"* Others also point to the fact and state that *"Christians ought to be foremost among those engaged in such rethinking."*

Other theologians have since confronted the 'Freudian ethics,' and have asserted that the only achievement Freudianism should be given credit for, is for the leading role he plays in the present day collapse of responsibility in the American society! They have also pointed toward Freud's contribution to fundamentalism and presuppositionism, as the decline of a new view in morality. That he adopted such from his French instructor, Charcot and popularized it under the medical model. However, it could be seen openly that back, then and even today that (*he simply gave the illness a human face.*) Prior to such, mentally ill individuals, were seen as malingerers, rather than as patients or even as human beings. Other critiques have challenges Freud's ethics in psychoanalysis by challenging psychology itself. Within the pages of, "Psychiatry and Responsibility," 1962, we find a direct quote, stating that "psychiatry have been trying to dull if not actually extract the teeth out of the law, and this is on the distinctively Freudian assumption that it is entirely natural for the criminal to act as he does and quite unreasonable for society to make him stand trial for being his antisocial self."

So, regardless of whether we disagree with much of his learning's and much of his teachings, we must agree to disagree with the answer to the question:

If you were ever asked to rank by name, someone whom you believed to have made the greatest contribution to the field of mental health throughout the 19th and 20th century? Just say the name, Sigmund Freud, first. "Simply put, Freud is to psychology, what Einstein is to physics ... he is its great leading light!"

Sigmund Freud was born on May 6, 1856, in the small town of Freiberg, Moravia.

His father was a wool merchant, with a keen mind and a good sense of humor. His mother a lively and much younger woman, was 20 years younger than Freud's father and was merely 21 years old, when she gave birth to her first son, Sigmund. Freud, had two older half-brothers and six younger siblings. When Sigmund was five years old, the family moved to Vienna, where he lived throughout most of his childhood and adult life. He was a brilliant child, always remaining at the head of his class. The same year Freud visited Vienna and later relocated to live there with his parents, was the same year, Charles Darwin had published his book The Origins of Species. Such was destined to revolutionize man's conception of man. Prior to Darwin's writings, man mainly differed from the animal kingdom by virtue of us having a soul. The following year after Darwin's publishing, Gustav Fechner, would become the founder of the science of psychology, by demonstrating that the mind could be studied scientifically, and measured quantitatively. Psychology, would go on to take its place within the hierarchy among the natural science, and Darwin and Fechner, would have a tremendous impact on the young Freud. This would latter shape and develop Freud's intellectuality. Sigmund went on to medical school, which was then one of the few viable options for bright Jewish boys during such in Vienna. There, he studied medicine and later became involved in research, under the direction of a physiology professor by the name Ernest Burke. Burke, believed in what was then a popular, radical notion, known as reductionism, which actually means that no other forces than the common physical-chemical ones, are active within the organism. Freud spent many years trying to reduce personality to neurology, but he would soon give up on these studies. Freud proved himself, very good at conducting research, concentrating mostly on neurophysiology and in the process; he invented special cell-staining techniques.

During such time, just a limited number of positions were available for a young Jewish scientist. He could not afford to support a wife, six children and other family members, who depended on his earnings. Although there were several others ahead of him, his mentor, Dr. Burke, assisted in obtaining him a grant to further his studies abroad.

Freud began studying at first with the great French psychiatrist, Charcot in Paris and later with Burke's rival, Bernheim in Nancy. Both of these men, were engaged in investigating the usage of hypnosis and the study of hysterics. However, after spending a short time as a resident in neurology and as a director of a children's ward in Berlin, he returned to Vienna and married his fiancée of many years, Martha Bernays. Almost immediately upon his return, he sat up a practice in neuropsychiatry, with the help of his mentor and friend Dr. Ernest Burke. Unfortunately, at this point, his books and lectures simultaneous would bring him, a combination of both fame and ostracism from within the medical community's mainstream. However, from Freud drew a large number of bright sympathizers, who later became the main core for the growth of the psychoanalytic movement. Unfortunately, Freud raveled in his fondness for rejecting those who did not fully agree with him, several separated and broke ties with him on a friendly basis, others did not and simply moved on to find other competitive schools of thought.

Freud, later emigrated to England right before World War I, as Vienna was in the midst of becoming an increasingly dangerous place for Jews, especially for Jews as famous as himself. Shortly after moving to England, Freud died from a cancer of the mouth and jaw, he had suffered with such for more than 20 years of his life.

Freud, Sigmund 1856 -1939

Freud was born in Freiberg, now Príbor, which was then part of the Czech Republic, on May 6, 1856. He was educated at Vienna University. His family uprooted and moved from Freigberg to Leipzig, when he was merely five years old while, the anti-Semitic riots that raged throughout Freiberg shortly thereafter, the family settled in Vienna, where Freud would remain throughout most of his life. Although his childhood dream had been a career in law, he decided to become a medical student, prior to entering Vienna's University at the age of 17 in 1873. The German poet Goethe's, scientific investigations, would further inspire Freud's highly driven passion and desire to study the natural science. Such inspirations, drove his desire to solve some of the most challenging problems confronting contemporary scientists. In his third year at the university, Freud began conducting research work on the central nervous system, in the physiological laboratory under the direction of the German physician, Ernst Wilhelm Von Bruke. The neurological research, was so engrossing that Freud neglected the prescribed courses and as a result, remained in medical school three years longer than it would have normally required him to qualify as a physician. In 1881, after completing a year of compulsory military service, he received his medical degree.

Unwilling to give up his experimental work, he remained at the university as a demonstrator, in the physiological laboratory, until in 1883. At Bruke's influence and encouragement, he would reluctantly abandon theoretical research and go on to gain practical experience in the field. Fortunately for humanities sake, he was forced to practice medicine. One could assume that if he'd remained a scientist, with ever having patient contact to further arise, his stimulus, dynamism to psychology, would have remained rather illogical to this day. Freud spent the following three years at the General Hospital of Vienna, successively devoting himself to psychiatry, dermatology and nervous diseases.

In 1885, following his appointment as a lecturer in neuropathology, at Vienna University, he left his post at the hospital. Later that same year, he was awarded a government grant, thus enabling him to spend 19 weeks in Paris, as a student under the French neurologist, Jean Charcot. Charcot, was then director of the clinic at the mental hospital, the Salpatrire, which was then treating nervous disorders via the usage of hypnotic suggestion. Freud's studies under the guidance of Charcot, was centered largely on hysteria. This influenced him greatly in channeling his interests toward psychopathology. In 1886 Freud, established a private practice in Vienna, specializing in nervous disease. Due to his strong support of Charcot's, unorthodox views on hysteria and hypnotherapy, he encountered an almost violent opposition from the Viennese medical profession. The resentment he incurred, would seriously delay any acceptance of his subsequent findings on the origin of neurosis. Freud's first published work, "on Aphasia" appeared in 1891; it was a study of the neurological disorder of which, the ability to pronounce words or to name common objects is lost, as a result of organic brain disease. His final work in neurology, an article, *Infantile Cerebral Paralysis,* was written in 1897 for an encyclopedia, only at the insistence of the editor. During this time Freud, was occupied largely with the psychological rather than the physiological explanations of mental illnesses. His subsequent writings, were devoted entirely to that field, which he would later name, psychoanalysis in 1896. Freud's new orientation was, heralded by his collaborative work on hysteria, with the Viennese physician, Ernest Bruke. The work was presented in 1893, in a preliminary paper and two years later in an expanded form under the title, *Studies on Hysteria.* His work, the symptoms of hysteria, was then recognized, as manifestations of un-discharged emotional energies, associated with forgotten, psychic traumas.

This therapeutic procedure, involved the use of a hypnotic state, in which the patient was led to recall and reenact the traumatic experience, thus discharging by catharsis the emotions causing their symptoms. The publication of this work, which marked the beginning of the psychoanalytic theory, was formulated on the basis of clinical observations.

During the period from 1895 to 1900 Freud, developed many of the concepts, which he would later incorporate as a psychoanalytic practice and doctrine. Soon after publishing his studies on hysteria, he abandoned the use of hypnosis, as a cathartic procedure and substituted it, with the investigation of the patient's spontaneous flow of thought, which he then called free association, to reveal the unconscious mental processes, at the root of the neurotic disturbance. In his clinical observations, Freud found evidence for the mental mechanisms of repression and resistance. He described repression, as a device operating unconsciously to make the memory of painful or threatening events inaccessible to the conscious mind. Resistance, is defined as the unconscious defense against awareness of repressed experiences, in order to avoid the resulting anxiety. He traced the operation of the unconscious processes, by using the free associations of the patient to guide him in the interpretation of dreams and slips of speech. It was the concept of Dream analysis that led to his discoveries of the infantile sexuality and the so-called, 'Oedipus complex.'

This constitutes an erotic attachment of the child and parent of the opposite sex, with the displaying of hostile feelings toward the other parent. In these years, he also developed the theory of transference, the process by which emotional attitudes, established originally toward parental figures in childhood, are transferred later in life on to others. The end of this period was marked by the appearance of Freud's most important work, *The Interpretation of Dreams,* in 1899.

Through this body of work, Freud analyzed many of his own dreams, recorded in a three year period of self-analysis, which he had started early on in 1897. Throughout this body of work, he would give further details about all the fundamental concepts underlying, the psychoanalytic technique and doctrine. In 1902 Freud was appointed full professor at Vienna University. However, this honor wasn't granted not in recognition of his contributions, but rather based on the result of the efforts of a highly influential patient, he'd previously treated. The medical world still regarded his work with hostility. His next writings for years to follow, *"The Psychopathology of Everyday Life,* published in 1904 and his three others, including the Contributions to the Sexual Theory, published in 1905, only managed to further increase their bitterness toward him. As a result, he continued to work virtually alone. Freud, appeared more at peace during such times, was when by which he coined the phrase "splendid isolation." However, by 1906, a small number of pupils and followers had again began to gather around him, including the Austrian psychiatrists, William Stekel and Alfred Adler, the Austrian psychologist, Otto Rank, the American psychiatrist Abraham Brill, the Swiss psychiatrists, Eugene Bleuler and the other Switzerland born, Carl Jung. Other very notable associates whom would later join this circle in 1908, was the Hungarian psychiatrists, Sándor Ferenczi and the British psychiatrist Ernest Jones.

Neuroscientist Seeks International Acceptances ... Like A Rock Star.

In 1909 Freud would receive his first world academic recognition, after being invited to speak at the twentieth anniversary celebration of Clark University, in Worcester, Massachusetts. Doctor Stanley Hall, the president of Clark University, himself a distinguished psychologist, had recognized the importance of Freud's valuable contribution to humanity. Following Freud's monumental speech, Doctor Hall, immediately embarked on promoting Freud's views in America and throughout the rest of the world. An increase in recognition of the psychoanalytic movement, made possible the formation of a worldwide organization, called the International Psychoanalytic Association, in 1910. The movement spread, gaining new supporters throughout Europe and the United States. During such times, Freud became resentful, and was rather troubled by the disagreements that arose among members of his original circle. Most disturbing, was the turncoat attitudes among members of the group, such as Adler and Jung, each of whom by now had developed their own respective theoretical basis for disagreement, differing from Freud's emphasis on the sexual origin of neurosis. Freud, dealt with such setbacks by further developing his basic concepts and by elaborating his own views to the world, through a large number of publications and countless lectures. Freud, would later receive more recognition following WWI, and his name would become known to millions throughout the world. The term psychoanalysis, would soon began to appear in daily conversations among his peers and laypeople alike and its influence, being felt throughout daily lives, theaters, literature, art, religion, social customs, morals, ethics, education, and the social science. Life and education as it was then known, suddenly began changing. People dragging out of the Victorian age, could now say and used cool phrases, such as "being psychoanalyzed" and put in used new words, such as the subconscious, repressed urges, inhibitions, complexes and fixations within their daily conversations.

Following the onset of WWI, Freud devoted little time to clinical observation and focused his concentration mainly on the application of his theories to the interpretation of religion, mythology, art, and literature. In 1923 he contracted cancer of the jaw and mouth, for which, he underwent constant, painful treatment and a number of surgical procedures. Regardless of his physical sufferings, he remained focus on his literary activities. For the next 2 years, he continued writing challenged mostly by the cultural and philosophical problems of the time. In 1938, when Germany occupied Austria, Freud being a Jew, was persuaded by friends to flee to England, with his family, where he would die a year later in London on September 23, 1939.

Freud, fashioned an entire new approach to the understanding of human personality by his demonstration of the existence and force of the unconscious. In addition, he founded a new medical discipline and formulated basic therapeutic procedures in which, his modified forms are still being widely applied in today's treatment of neuroses and psychoses. He never felt, as if he matched full expectations, or attained full recognition during his lifetime, neither did he felt his work was ever completed. He was always searching for new evidence among his patients and colleagues, while continuously revising and expanding his theorists. Today, Freud is acknowledged, as being one of the greatest creative minds of modern times. Although many of his critics still challenged this statement today, in reality, who was Sigmund Freud? Freud, was a physician by profession, whom engaged in treating the sick by methods, he himself had created. Today he would be recognized as a psychiatrist. Psychiatry is a form of medicine used to treat mental diseases, or abnormalities. Freud was one of the founders of the school of modern psychiatry. Although he admitted to earning his living by practicing medicine, it wasn't by choice. (He later stated.) *"I became a doctor through being compelled to deviate from my original purpose."*

His original purpose was that of understanding some of nature's riddles, thus contributing in part to their solutions. In reality Freud was a physician, a psychiatrist, a psychoanalyst, a scientist, a psychologist and a philosopher. Philosophy actually means to have a love of knowledge. "And we know that there's no one in their right mind, who'd try disputing the fact that Sigmund Freud, didn't have a love for knowledge?" Similar to other great icons, such as Leonardo Da'vinci, Shakespeare, etc. He illuminated and breathed life into everything he touched. He was not merely just a very wise man, in fact only one word, could best be used to describe this man, "genius!"

Although Freud did not invented the idea of 'the conscious mind, versus the unconscious mind,' but he was certainly responsible for making it popular. The conscious mind, is what you are aware of, at any particular moment, your present perceptions, memories, thoughts, fantasies, feelings, what have you done and whom you are. Working closely with the conscious mind is what Freud called the preconscious. This is what many of us might call today, 'available memory.' That which is anything that can easily be made conscious. The memories you are not at the moment thinking about, but can readily bring to mind. Now, no one has a problem with conceptualizing these two layers of mind. However, Freud suggested that these were the smallest parts. The largest part by far is the unconscious; this part includes all of those things that are not easily available to awareness, including many things that have their origins there. These include our drives, or instincts and things that we have put there, because we cannot bear to look at them, like the memories and emotions associated with trauma. According to Freud, the unconscious, is the source of our motivations, whether it be simple desires for food or sex, neurotic compulsions, or the motives of an artist or that of a scientist. And yet, we are often driven to deny or resist becoming conscious of these motives, nevertheless, they are often available to us though sometimes only in disguised forms.

Freudian, psychological reality, begins with a world full of objects. Among them, is a very special object known as the organism. The organism is viewed, as special in that it acts to survive and reproduce, and it is guided, toward those ends by its own needs, such as hunger, thirst, the avoidance of pain, and sex. A very important part of the organism, is the nervous system, which is one of its characteristics sensitive to the organism's needs. At birth that nervous system is little more than that of any other animal, it is then considered an "it" or id. The nervous system, as id, translates the organism's needs, into motivational forces, which in the German language, is called "Triebe." This is translated as instincts, or drives.

Freud also called them, wishes. This translation from a need to a wish, is known as the primary process. These three major systems, are commonly known as the id, the ego and the superego. In the minds of healthy individuals, they form a collaborative, unified and harmonious orchestra. They are well synchronized and work in unison, thus enabling us to establish efficiently, by satisfying daily transactions within our lives. These transactions, are imperative to the fulfillment and the accomplishment of our basic needs and desires. However, when any of these three systems of personality are at odds with the other, the individual's functioning abilities and efficiency, is vastly reduced and they tend to appear dissatisfied with themselves and the rest of the world. And it is then that we as individuals are considered by society, to be estranged, disturbed, maladjusted, and warped.

The Id ... The id's sole purpose, is to provide rapid discharges of massive excitement, energy, or tension, which is released within the organism by internal or external stimulation. Freud called this "the pleasure principle." The id, actually works in keeping up with the pleasure principle, which can be understood, as a demand to take care of the immediate needs. Any doubts? Just picture in your mind a hungry infant, screaming until it begins losing its breath and starts to turn blue?

In a true sense, it doesn't really know what it wants, it just knows that it wants and it wants, right now! Its mother, father, grandparent, or babysitter, picks it up, walks with it, feeds it, or simply places a rubber nipple of some sort into its mouth and it immediately quiets down.

According to Freudian studies, the infant is pure, or nearly pure id. "The id is nothing, if not the psychic representative of biology." Unfortunately, a wish for food, such as the image of a thick, delicious, juicy broil salmon steak, might be enough to satisfy the id, but it wouldn't be nearly enough to satisfy the organism. The need only gets stronger and the tribes or the desires would just keep on nagging you. At this point, we become aware and noticed that when some needs go unsatisfied, such as the need for food, the demand grows stronger, requesting your outmost attention, until there comes a point where we cannot think of anything else to offer it. This is the wish or drive, breaking into consciousness. Luckily for the organism, there is that small portion of the mind discussed before the conscious that is hooked up to the world through the senses. Around this little bit of consciousness during the first year of a child's life, some of the "it" becomes "I," some of the id becomes ego. The ego relates the organism to reality by means of its consciousness and it searches for objects to satisfy the wishes that the id creates to represent the organism's needs. This problem-solving activity is called the secondary process.

Approach to the Theoretical Models

Needless to say a scientific, medical perspective on chronic illness is not always the answer, though it still is possible to take a variety of theoretical perspectives that might lead to a redefining definition of the illness. Not only changing the viewpoint of the illness, but also a different definition of patient populations, are considered chronically ill. Differences in defining illness and patient populations, naturally enough could also lead to a very diverse set of treatment needs that are desirable and which are agreeable. We must now study the historic precedent and justification of these conceivable methods, used for defining and treating the chronically ill. There are five essential methods, in which chronic illness could still be viewed. A) the theoretically, is a method, which obviously takes a medical approach form; B) the epidemiological approach, which is concerned with incidence and prevalence of the disease; and C) the sociological approach, which places its focus on the ills of society and the nature of the institutional structure. However, there is also the intrapsychic approach, where just like the sociological, it tends to lean toward the social perspective, though its focus is placed on the individual, rather than the group and at some point, swerves enough to dismiss chronic illness, as a myth. Each of these perspectives holds its own set of theories, its own focus and takes its own unique form of intervention. Theoretical approaches that places focus on the nature of the problem, should be carefully examined.

Although this study, concentrates primarily on the body's ailing, by targeting pronounced interest in the central nervous system and the brain, it places focus on the organic piece, rather than on the functional phenomena, such as the ego or the psyche. It is often highly criticized for its chief role of humanizing mental illness, as a legitimate medical illness, due to its major investment within physical interventions. Some sociologists, researchers and other critics, have viewed it, as "science in the form of research and medical technology, as a panacea that has been for the last 95 years or so, the mainstream of psychiatry and has resulted in psychiatry's establishment as an accepted medical specialty." Others argued that "it has promoted the training of the nurse, the mental health worker, the rehab worker and the social workers, as intricate parts of treatment, while also helping to solidify the treatment team." The reality though, thus has created a nursing subspecialty that firmly places the care of the chronically mentally ill into a care system. Although the chronically ill, is still being treated in hospitals, group homes, or hospital-like community mental health centers, its long-term goal, is to reduce the psychopharmacological field, with its related host of blessings miracles and tribulations. At its worst, it has dabbled in a wide range of failed cure-all's, such as psychosurgery, insulin shock therapy, ECT, etc.

The medical model, has generated our most effective intervener in chronic illness-medication; however, it has locked up a health care system, already overwhelmed with multitudes and organizational funding. At best, it has recently begun to show some progress with a wide list of recently approved, newly released modern day psychotropic medications. These medications have arrived as a blessing for many of those patients previously hospitalized for long periods of time. Today, many are now being allowed to live for extended periods of time in communities with less supervision. Gradually, many are also able to assimilate into society. Of course, it helps to have available resources in place. Psychologist and sociologist involved in research concerning these illnesses, as analysis of these present medical models in psychiatry, often ignore the importance of documenting the progress attained by these patients for reasons, often overlooked by patients themselves. This practice then, easily takes a political pattern of care, which sometimes is deemed necessary to attract more funding via statistical routes. Generally speaking, the patient progress, is ignored and the political purpose is served under that banner of 'jobs versus votes.' The patient is once again hospitalized, the stigma, is again hidden and the threat to society is again removed.

When there is a threat to life, or when the acutely disordered organism, is being returned to equilibrium, the need for quick, precise reaction, brings with it the need for an overt, hierarchal structure with a clear chain of command.

In other words, the medical model is the acute illness model. If this is considered to be true, then we could easily say that the care of the chronically, ill is currently locked within a system that is clearly geared to the acutely ill individual. Experts in the field, has also placed blame on this 'medical model' by stating that "since the disease comes from within and without any serious illnesses, it ought to be cured from without –by another, then the sick persons when feeling helpless and turns to the physician . The physicians alike the disease, which invaded the patient, then solves the problem from without. Thus again helplessness, hopelessness and irresponsibility are the natural results of the medical model. Because if a person's problems of disease and sickness rather than problems of behavior, he has no hope, unless there is medicine or therapy, which can be applied to his case. Since there is no medical cure for people in such trouble, they move from despair to deeper despair.

This model has generated much research and much literature throughout the years. It is primarily concerned, with incidence and prevalence of the disease. It places its focus on the accumulation of data and the establishment of a data base interest, which is in the demographics of affected individuals, their causative factors and the onset of the illnesses, as well as patterns of transmission and ease within each population. It is related to the medical model in view of a chronic psychiatric disorder, as an illness, in which it then helps to assume a medical definition of such. However, it is not directly concerned with intervention itself, rather it plays the complex role of information resource for clinicians.

Such collected data, directs us to the number of previous hospital admissions, which is at times, the single and best predictor of relapse within the outpatient population.

One of its greatest contributions, has been to provide us with an invaluable estimate of the scope of the problem that we face when caring for the chronically ill. In addition, it provides us with a readymade conscience, pointing out the true impact, or the lack of an impact in the health care system. We could then feel safe to admit that in both, the incidence and the prevalence of chronic illness, until in recent years, have remained relatively at the same base level since the turn of the century. Quite clearly, what it has accomplished to show us, is that we do not yet cure patients, but we rather simply move them around for pure administrative and political reasons and by doing this, they're either more or less visible to the general public. "It all depends on which way the political pendulum swings." This model's worst effect, have been to obscure the real problems of chronic illness-the levels of functioning, symptom control and quality life-in a mass of numbers and an overgrown maze of imaginary tables. A clear example of this, would be the closing of the Norwich State Hospital and the Fairfield Hills State Hospital in Connecticut. These two hospitals were closed in the 1995 and the reason given by politicians to the patients, their families and hospital employees, was that they would instead place the money into community-based programs. "That this would help give patients more independence and help them get reestablish in their own communities more effectively." They also told healthcare employees that they would maintain their jobs, gain promotions and in some cases even work side by side with these same patients, within these community programs. The idea appeared rather sound and promising on paper, a great in theoretical concept, however, in reality it was pretty much baseless and lacked common sense.

Some patients did rather well and even gained astonishing progress with these changes, so did the employees, who busted their humps and worked side by side, assisting them accomplish these goals, nevertheless, they were in small numbers. Though in the end, large numbers of chronically ill patients, were severely affected. Following a seven year research, many remained semi ignored, still struggling to adjust to group homes and shelter living conditions, others spent countless hours in and out of emergency rooms. Moreover, they also dealt with group home shortages, due to an oversight or inability to proactively estimate and prepare for sufficient available occupancy for this newly released population. Safety and liability was also largely ignored, as was the lack of well-trained staff and a concise data system of patient's past history. Despite of all of this, almost six years after closing these two major hospitals, the state finally came to the baseless realization, determined via politics that the Community Base Initiative programs, CBI's, which was operated by well-trained, state employees, was now too expensive to maintain, than previously estimated and decided to close and privatize these valuable programs, rather than to expand.

With the only two remaining state hospitals currently finding themselves caught in the midst of an administrative battle, (but appearing genuinely concerned about overcrowding, nevertheless, despite their political skirmish's), the only one who's lives had been disrupted and yanked around from place to place for the last seven years, was that of the patients.

One must pause to realize that we were a part of a bargaining unit, so all hospital employees kept their jobs, quite frankly some even received promotions out of the deal, just as state officials had been previously warned. They'd also been warned of how such severe impact wouldn't just disrupt these patient's lives, but would rather affect the system of care for years, going forward. Members of our 1199, New England Health Care Union staff, also shared their research and warned state officials, surrounding outcomes found within drastic and abrupt closings, throughout the nation. Nevertheless, perhaps propel via the governors political ambitions, they refused any listening even to the people whom worked side by side with the patients. Clearly underestimated their sufferings, their being taken advantage of, if these moves were to fail. In short term, this is a classic case of "the epidemiological models gone wrong." The chronically ill individuals are human beings with an illness; mental health is an illness that needs treatment. Your average person on the street or even fresh out of college does not understand it, mental health profession takes time, it involves trust building in treatment. Simply put, patients cannot take care of themselves. Data merely amounts to what is imputed into a system and viewed via a computer terminal, it is not scientific and more importantly, it does not specifically deal with direct care.

The Sociological Models

This model places its focus on society's ills and on the nature of the institutional structures that have been created, to deal with the chronically ill. It comes to us, primarily, as a social science base. In contrast of focusing solely on one individual, it studies the ills of each group. Prevention, planning and structures are its main concern. Social engineering, focuses on any of these changes, be it institutional or social. The theoretical concepts for this particular model, is a deviant society and an environmental community. It has told us much about the process of socializing into the patient role, about loss of power and about roles and development. Clearly enough, it has pointed out to us the many ways in which mental illness, specially chronic mental illness, is often wrongly viewed, as deviance rather than illness. That many of our best interventions, are merely forms of socially controlling deviant behavior. In past years, sociological essays have arguably created a viewpoint, which lends itself to the notion that society always reaches out, searches, finds and picks a behavior form, in which it defines the normality of boundaries.

Once such claims are made and sustained, we could clearly admit that mental illness only became repugnant and utterly disgusting, in our sight after leprosy died out during medieval Europe, then mental disorders came to light! With it being initially shunned, then balked at, criticized, dreaded and ultimately considered a disease. This perception sets its views and at times sees chronic illness as a social class and circumstances of economic modus vivendi. Sociologists and some mental health professionals have suggested previously that, unknowingly, individuals with meager financial resources, low social status and no money, clearly do not have the means to take vacations like a middle and upper class persons, so they must often resort to a mental hospital. Although this belief have been highly debated.

We have observed that often times, patients refused to leave the hospitals, some have been known to have injured themselves, or even create chaos, in order to manipulate and lengthen their stay. Sarcastically speaking, such behavioral syndrome, though hushed, but known among treaters throughout the business of mental health as *"job security."*

Historically, this behavior has furnished research material for literary works such as, *Methods of Madness, The Mental Hospital as a Last Resort,* and many other literary research documentation. These, which view chronic re-institutionalization, as an avenue in which to pause from the pressures of community daily living and it gives creed to the perception that helps to characterize chronic illness, as a learned social behavior. It also lends itself to the notion that if social and occupational adjustments were better attended to, *"the chronic lower socioeconomic class patient, would be more accessible to treatment,"* in all areas of pathology, social as well as psychological. What it overlooks is the specifics, the real symptoms of the psychodynamics of their disorders and the fact that individuals from a wide range of social and environmental backgrounds seem to develop similar problems. It also fails to acknowledge that known forms of social engineering, have not been able to build inroads into the problems of chronic psychiatric illness. It manages to sensitize us toward the broad issues of social reform and brought us community psychiatric resources to pull it off successfully. Nevertheless, some hardliners would still argue that individuals experiencing chronic re-instiutionalization, simply use these hospitals, as a social enjoyment that they enjoyed being there, because they regain some control, once they get to know all of the rules. That they're guaranteed three meals, a cot, clean clothes, a nurse, and a dozen servant's maids and of course they regain all of their rights, which usually have been trampled upon by members of their inner circle, while on the outside.

However, even if such is suspected, one should never judge and should always be ready to treat each and every patient as an individual, and with the outmost respect. We should rather try to educate these people on how to use all of their natural resources, while out in their communities, how to find, or build new ones. My belief is that at times the hospitalized mental patient, unrealistically views the mental health professionals, to be living a problem-free life in a problem-free world, with little or no difficulties. Though, as caregivers, many of us tend to gain invaluable power through this method of thinking… meaning, "we feed our egos, with such an unrealistic thinking." However, as mental health professionals, we should continue to steer them in the right direction. Of course this should be done without engaging in our own private affairs, but rather by pointing out to them that *"life is difficult and that the sooner one realizes that life is difficult, it is difficult no more, rather it simply becomes life."* Furthermore, we must insist that we all experience stressors, but that one must assist in building healthier environments for themselves that, set goals in which to gain access. Of course this conversation could only be accomplished, with patients whom are coherent and able to comprehend. Put into practice, it should be done in small steps and with a goal oriented outcome. Patients must also be taught how to deal with stressors and real life anxiety factors. I once questioned a colleague "wouldn't that sufficient clues, if an individual believes that a psychiatric ward in a hospital is the best place in the world?"

The Intrapsychic Models

This model also comes from a social perspective, but it is concerned with the individual, rather than the group. It places its concern toward the ills of the mind. Its primary goal is to alter the patient's interpersonal environmental factors, via individual or psychotherapy groups, in which we could explore and structure their mind or psyche. This model's primary goal is concerned with whether the source and problems are considered functional rather than organic. It studies the internal experiences of each individual during the process of first growing up and how they have lived as an adult. This process is seen as sources of difficulty in their own right, thus without underlying organic pathology.

This viewpoint leads the way to another perspective on intervention, since treatment could now finally be viewed from the psychological or interpersonal perspective. Of course, compassion, social interaction and pleasant environments had been previously analyzed as therapeutic however these interventions were performed in the same manner in which we have beneficially treated the medically ill individuals, such as those suffering with AIDS, or cancer. In years back, these interpersonal environmental adjustments, would have been considered, either as helpful attachments to conventional forms of medical interventions, or as useful calming measures, when medical treatment was inaccessible.

Before Freud's time, it was virtually impossible to imagine the sources of illness, as coming from the intrapsychic and interpersonal aspects or experiences; 'except in those cases, where one was thought of as demonic possessed.' Although even today, there is a tendency to believe that environment must be interactive, with some inherent genetic predisposition to disorder for a psychiatric illness to be produced. This is especially true in the case of chronic psychiatric illness.

It is difficult for many medically trained clinicians, not to be seduced by a perspective that looks for an underlying structural weakness, as causative. Freud also enabled us, to put mental illness on a continuum with normal behavior, to view chronic illness as not so different in kind, but in a degree from what we all experience. This perspective, allows us to put chronic illness, within the territorial reach of human experiences, rather than outside the walls of it, while enabling us to view and treat the mental patient as one of us, rather than if they were less than humans. This psychodynamic perspective, is deeply concentrated on the interpersonal or intrapsychic causes of mental illness. It analyzes structures of the mind, such as the self or the ego. It strives for illnesses insight and behavior modification, on the basis of understanding. Many psychoanalytic psychiatrists, starting with Freud or ego psychologists, such as Eriksson, fall into this category. They view chronic illness, not only as a social label or a learned set of social behavior, but also as a set of learned behavior in the service of certain, very real psychological needs. These needs, must be met in more productive ways before new data can be accomplished. Although undeniably so, the passive clinging and demanding attitudes of many of the chronically ill toward clinicians, could be viewed as ego defenses in the service of health, rather than as simply hostile, aggressive acts. Such behavior, could be seen as a healthy alternative to psychotic disintegration; certainly, the chronic illness itself, can be viewed as a cry for help, rather than a withdrawal into the illness. It has been suggested that if acute psychoses, can be seen as a growth struggle, psychoses may be viewed, as an unsuccessful struggle toward continuing development. This perspective adds many helpful insights into the origins and the nature of chronic illness; it heightens the appreciation for the significant past experiences, and allows for a positive developmental view of the illness itself.

It also allows us to have a broader perspective on life as a whole, one that enables us to view the patient's life as a whole, and each patient, as an individual, rather than primarily as a member of a group or simply belonging to a group of individuals.

It overlooks, however, the very real place of social and environmental pressures, beyond the individual's immediate family or experience. It has also failed to demonstrate any effectiveness, in the eradication or alleviation of chronic psychiatric illness, despite the very long-range effort of a multitude of dedicated clinicians, trying to prove otherwise. At best, this model has given us a broader perspective on disorder and the complete view to the whole person, including his unique personal history.

This model, has also promoted a genuine concern for the individual, rather than a fragmented social concern for the group, it has also served to help attain a sound, theoretical justification to kindness and a mandated to humane therapeutic treatment, rather than a simple ethical overview. At its worst, it has failed to appreciate the very real impact of social and environmental pressures on the family and the individual.

Viewing Mental Illness as a Myth …
Understanding the Patient Rights Model

This model is really the antithesis of the preceding ones. It is perhaps the most extreme of the perspectives on chronic psychiatric illness and one that attempts to refute the existence of the phenomenon altogether. Supporters of this view, have suggested that it is the conventional and that it is the sane individuals who are rather mislead. They've strongly argued and stated that it is the ill who is sane and whom also possesses a true creative insight, into the nature of this world of ours. This is the logical extension of the long prevailing notion and belief that somehow, some of the chronically mentally ill individuals, are indeed superior in intelligence or imagination, than those leading more conventional and rational lives. The artist, the playwright, the poet, the composer and the painter, have all been roles played by a number of chronically ill individuals. At times, a performance is seen as brilliant and at other times dull, but there is tolerance and even admiration for this type of deviant behavior. Proponents, alike, Dr. Thomas Szasz and others have argued vehemently and raised claims toward advocating for the dismissal of mental illness, especially chronic illness, as it is commonly understood. Szasz became the number one champion of the chronically ill patients' civil rights, while arguing persuasively that any kind of long-term treatment, is nothing more than an involuntary hospitalization and incarceration. Hence in defense of his arguments, he also points out that "even the criminals, guilty of committing serious crimes, have the right to an appeal and their length of imprisonment clearly stated. But that the mental ill patient, traditionally have been without recourse and are often times imprisoned for a lifetime, relatively for harmless behaviors." In reality, this perspective have made real contributions to our understanding of the current and potential abuses throughout the system of mental health services in the United States and throughout the world. This particular model, have encouraged, and ultimately demanded a humanitarian and enlightened approach to the treatment of mental disorders.

It has also pointed out the lack of tolerance for relatively minor forms of deviances and the injustice of many forms of treatment. Nevertheless, this model perspective, has overlooked the fact that the problems patients face, are not imaginary, but that they are rather very real. Patients face daily difficulties that are painful and debilitating and these could not easily become alleviated, simply by having compassion, nor a greater social tolerance. It has also minimized the role that the chronically ill patient themselves play, in creating negative attitudes toward their plight. It is clearly a nonscientific-based model and one whose concern, is more of a pure morality issue, and a humanity base. In many aspects, this concept, focuses more on the ills of the spirit; nevertheless, it has alerted us to the fact that patient needs assertive and stronger advocates within the present health care system.

However, it also reminds us that there are political and legal forces at work, shaping the chronic illness's experience, and that we, as a society have a limited tolerance for this form of deviant behavior. It has attempted to show us where we as professionals have unknowingly punished patients, under the guise of treatment and where we have assumed control over the lives of individuals, whom otherwise, might be capable of existing perfectly well without our help, although, perhaps, not according to our values and our standards. Its chief proponents, are indeed famous in both the professional and the lay circles, Laing and Szasz, are champions of its causes. Szasz, states that *"mental illness is no more than a symbolic phrase geared to resemble a medical diagnosis and he takes a defensive stance by arguing that mental illness is nothing more than a stigmatizing label applied to persons whose behavior annoys or offends others."* In Mary Barnes novel, *Two Accounts of A Journey Through Madness*, several years ago, proponents strongly suggested that attempting to explain this peculiar perspective on illness by arguing that *"the worst form of mental illness, is something called schizophrenia and that the definition of this illness, could never be matched with the reality of the people whom were supposed to manifest it."* They see schizophrenia as a career, rather than an illness and that this career always involves at least two professionals, a patient and a psychiatrist. However, more often than not, it is launched with the aid and encouragement of the patient's immediate family.

Furthermore, they have argued that "the experiences occurring in these persons labeled schizophrenics, whom are then subsumed under the term 'psychotic,' are not at all unintelligible, nor crazy and that those, they simply occur at a different order of reality, akin to a waking dream." That "the social invalidation of such experiences is gained by calling them 'sick' or 'mad,' is no more than a basic interpersonal maneuver of people throughout Western cultures, in which dreams and dreamlike states, are not considered a valid vehicle for conveying reality no matter how much truth they may express." It is therefore strongly believed that this model, has alerted us to the many real and potential flaws and abuses found throughout our mental health care system. However, it has managed to deceive a great number of people with a romantic notion that the mentally ill persons, are to be rather envied than treated. In reality, it tends to minimize the very real symptomatic suffering of the chronically ill persons. "Wishing that chronic schizophrenia was not real, is quite a beautiful dream nevertheless; just wishing it, will not make such dream come true." Perhaps it is the same shared belief of a dream that stems to emanate off the desks of some hospital administrators offices, with the overly enjoyed daily mandatory and forced overtime. Such practice, should not only be considered an abuse upon the system and its employees, but more so an abuse upon the patient's, whom is expecting to receive a one hundred percent service, safety and good quality of treatment of care..

In reality by mandating someone to work more than the stipulated amount of hours required throughout their shift, in a mental institution, is merely setting up that person to become hostile and rather abusive toward the most vulnerable. Such, could only be seen as slavery, or at least as modern indentured servitude, regardless of it being a negotiated and forcible paid overtime. It is unsafe and unhealthy for both, hospital staff and patient.

The Integrated Models

If chronic mental illness could not be viewed from a medical, epidemical, sociological, or from an intrapsychic model and if it cannot be seen as a myth, how should it then be viewed, assessed or examined? It is essential for us to have an integrated approach that includes all of these perspectives, not limited to any single one. It becomes more critical for clinicians to develop a coordinated perspective one; one that isolates the unique and essential components of the chronic illness experience.

Components are critical in the diagnosis, treatment and proof of chronic illness. It is in some sense easier to say what psychiatric illness is, rather than to actually define it directly. It is neither a diagnosis nor even a specific diagnostic category. Any category of mental illness then may become chronic. This is an important point, since the term chronic psychiatric illness, is frequently understood to mean chronic schizophrenia. Although there are many cases of chronic schizophrenia and many other types of mental illness, which must be considered, while planning these services for the mentally ill as a group. Affective disorders, neurotic difficulties, personality disorders, as well as organic conditions, can be considered as potentially chronic illnesses. We must also keep in mind that chronic psychiatric illness, is not unique to a particular age group. There is a tendency to identify it as synonymous with geriatric problems, by no means are all older persons afflicted with mental disorders; in fact this problem is far from being exclusively the domain for adults of any age.

Due to the fact that children, adolescents, young adults, as well as older persons can and do develop a wide variety of forms of chronic mental illnesses. The fact that chronic illness is neither age, nor clearly developmentally linked, is one of the most difficult five perspectives affecting its prevention and diagnosis. In addition, chronic psychiatric illness is not of a social class related phenomenon.

Although there is a tendency to think of chronic illness as a disease of the poor, when in reality the poor have no monopoly on the chronic illness market. Throughout the middle part of the 1980s, I had the honor and privilege of working at the Institute of Living when it was totally a private facility. Individuals and their families had to have money in order to be admitted to such an exclusive facility. During such times, they only catered to, and treated the very wealthy and the 'super rich.' There are many other excellent private psychiatric facilities, providing long term care to those whom both, need it and can afford it. These treatment centers provides us with ample evidence that money cannot and does not buy a mental health. If chronic illness is not a specific diagnosis, not age related, not a socioeconomic related disorder, then what is it? It is possible to look at the properties of the chronic illness experiences, crossing a life age, diagnosis, sex, and social classes. It is even possible to find common areas of difficulty that crosses the boundaries between the various forms of psychotherapeutic interventions. It is clear that the major problem of chronic psychiatric illness, is one of perspectives, on finding a perspective that 'works' and that includes consideration of important properties of this phenomenon. Once a patient's difficulties have been categorized as 'mental illness' of whatever variety, the illness can be considered chronic, if four properties are found to be present.

These four special properties, clearly differentiate chronic disorders from acute or transient situational disorders. These four are present when an illness is … severe, permanent, stigmatized, and contagious.

When there is always a sense that something is seriously wrong, regardless of the specific symptom pattern. When it is agreed by all involved that the afflicted individual, can no longer live with the problem as it exists and it is further agreed that professional intervention is therefore necessary. When the illness, may be characterized by recent episodes of severe disability. When there may be varying degrees of actual impairment in functioning. When there is usually a sense of varying degrees of emotional stress for, the patient a family member or significant other. When the total burden of the illness, appears intolerable even with intervention … When the recognition of the enormity of the burden of the illness to patient and others, is a prominent feature of chronic illness. When this burden is generally caused by the degree of social and occupation impairment, created by the patient's symptoms. Since many of these symptoms, are not completely controlled by either medication or psychotherapy, frequently massive alterations in the lifestyles of the patient and his family must occur.

Although disorders may alter or inhibit patient's ability to solve problems in their everyday living. Difficulty either thought or affect may hinder the patient's significant role relationships. The patient may then be totally incapable of engaging in usual occupational role or may never had acquired one in the first place, then problem is never viewed as benign. There is a feeling that symptoms will persist and that this is not just an acute episode that will rapidly be resolved. Although some symptoms may be relatively, mild such as disturbances in mood, sleep, appetite, or sexual functioning, the total number of symptoms, may add up to a more serious picture of disability and if persistent, it may be additionally threatening to life, therefore creating both a social and a psychological problem. Difficulties are always apparent in conventional adult roles, such as occupational or social interaction, there may also be an increased risk of death by suicide, but beyond the threat of either, active or passive, many patients might put themselves at risk for a variety of problems, through neglect of their physical wellbeing. The severity of impairment, may then indicate a need for more groups, one to one counseling, or a form of institutional care. Even when hospitalization is not indicated, there may be a need for continued supervision of physical needs such as clothing, food, hygiene, etc. Additional problems such as confusion or wandering, could easily make the patient become an easy prey for a variety of antisocial or criminal acts. The lack of proper nutrition, proper hygiene and appropriate self, care, should also be factored in.

Although less frequent the appearance and persistence of bizarre symptoms, such as inappropriate speech or violent behaviors, often make community treatment impossible. This goes beyond the mere unavailability of sufficient numbers of sheltered unavailability living situations for such chronically impaired individuals. There then becomes the very real question about the feasibility of maintaining many individuals outside of total care institutions, due to the severity of the psychiatric difficulty they may be experiencing … considerations of risk to self or others is then critical. Throughout this segment, I will attempt to list by names and definition the different types of mental illness that uninterruptedly continues to plague and disrupt so many lives. In my attempt, I'll also try to show how families struggle daily, when a member is afflicted with such. At the top of this, list is schizophrenia, of course. Why schizophrenia… because it is one of the most disrupting and debilitating of the mental illness categories.

Schizophrenia

Perhaps you've noticed that schizophrenia, has been mentioned more, throughout this body of work, than any other of the various mental diseases? According to the specifics guidelines found in Diagnostic Statistical Manuals (DSM's) criteria, indicates that in order to diagnose someone with schizophrenia, a person must have been suffering from this illness for at least six months and exhibiting at least two of the following five symptoms: *Delusions, hallucinations, disorganized behavior, disorganized thought and speech and negative symptoms.* In addition, they should not exhibit significant manic, nor depressive symptoms and of course both substance abuse and other medical conditions must have also been ruled out. The reason for this is because Etoh and other substances, whether be it an intoxication, or withdrawal, can also cause psychotic symptoms much like those exhibited with schizophrenia. Certain medical and neurological conditions can also produce psychotic symptoms that might not meet the criteria for diagnosis.

Schizophrenia … *Schizophrenia and other psychotic disorders: Types of psychotic disorders:*

Schizophrenia, Schizophreniform, Schizoaffective, Delusions, Brief Psychotic, Shared psychotic, Psychotic disorder due to a general medical condition, prescribed medications, which could also lead to substance induced psychotic disorder, and various other types of psychotic disorder. According to the *DSM,* it should take Schizophrenia +6 months, 1 month in active phase and show 2 or more of the following symptoms: *Delusions, hallucinations, disorganized speech, grossly disorganized or catatonic behavior, negative symptoms before making such diagnosis.*

Subtypes of Schizophrenia: Paranoid type disorganized type, catatonic type, undifferentiated type, residual type. The positive related symptoms of schizophrenia, are the following:

Delusions, hallucinations, disorganized speech, grossly disorganized or catatonic behavior, negative symptoms.

The Negative Symptoms of Schizophrenia:

The emotional expression is flat, or affective flattening, thoughts and speech are reduced *alogia,* decreased ability to initiate goal directed behavior *avolitional.*

Schizophreniform, is much the same as schizophrenia, except the symptoms are from 1 less than 6 months.

Schizoafective Disorder is same as Schizophrenia symptoms, plus a major depressive manic or mixed episode of delusional disorders, with one or more non-bizarre delusions, lasting about 1 month = +1. No criteria for schizophrenia. Types of delusions are: *erotomanic,* grandiose, jealousy, persecutory, somatic mixed. A brief psychotic disorder, could be categorized as a sudden onset that usually last from 1 day to a month. One of the following is exhibited, hallucinations, delusions, disorganized speech, disorganized behavior, or catatonic behavior.

Shared Psychotic Disorder, or *Folie a deux,* is categorized as a delusion, which develops in an individual in the context of a close relationship with another, whom has an already established delusion. The delusion is similar to the person with the established delusion.

Psychotic Disorder, Due to a general medical condition, hallucinations, delusions, due to a direct, physiological condition, does not only occur during delirium.

Are also interconnected connected with hallucinations and delusions that are directly connected to the specific effects of a substance, medication, drug abuse and toxins?

Manic Episodes: The person must exhibit the following behaviors for at least one week: Displaying signs of being elated, ecstatic, or in a state of seventh heaven. Sometimes, they might also appear irritable, talkative, grandiose, grandeur, hyperactive, distractible, and or exhibiting bad judgment, which could indeed lead the individual into grave social, or work impairment

Mixed Episodes: In this case the patient would have fulfilled symptomatic criteria for both the manic and major depressive episodes, but has lasted as briefly as a week.

Hippomanic Episode. This is much like the manic episode, though it is brief, much less severe and is usually treated in outpatient clinics.

A Mood Disorder: Is generally categorized by a pattern of illness, which is due to an abnormal mood. Although most patient's experiencing mood disorders, have experienced depression at some point. However, some display highs and others display lows. Nevertheless, not all mood disorders are diagnosed on the basis of mood episodes. A patient must first fit into the following categories in order to be diagnosed as such:

Depressive Disorders:

Major Depressive Disorders: These individuals must have exhibited no manic, or hippomanic episodes, but have exhibited one or more major depressive episodes. These episodes could be either recurrent, or a single episode.

Dysthymic disorder: This type of depression, is not severe enough to be considered a major depressive episode, though it lasts much longer than major depression and has no high phases.

Unspecified Depressive Disorders: This category is studied when an individual displays depressive symptoms and does not quite meet the criteria for a depressive diagnosis in which depression is a featured.

Bipolar Disorders: About 30% of individuals with mood disorders, also experience manic, or hippomanic episodes and about 95% of these individuals, will also experience depression. However, the severity and duration of the individual's highs and lows would help to determine the specific bipolar disorder.

Bipolar 1 Disorder Type: There must be at least one manic episode however most bipolar 1 patients would also have experienced a major depressive episode.

Bipolar2 Disorder: This diagnosis requires at least one hippomanic episode and at least one major depressive episode.

Cyclothymic Disorder: Individuals prior to being diagnosed with cyclothymiacs disorder must have repeated mood swings, but none severe enough to be considered a major depression, or manic episode.

"Mood disorders, however, could also easily be mistaken by a medical condition."

Be aware that highs and lows in an individual's mood could be caused by a variety of physical illness. Substance abuse, could also mask the substance induced mood disorders. Alcohol and other substances can cause the high, low trademarks of the mood disorders, but those that do not meet the criteria for any of the fore-mentioned criteria for a diagnosis. Other causes for mood disorders could be personality disorder's dysphoric mood, which is mentioned in the criteria for Borderline Personality Disorder, though it is a depressed mood, accompanied by avoidant, dependent and histrionic personality disorder. Depression could also be found, in many other mental disorders, included, but not limited to schizophrenia, eating disorders, and somatization disorders, sexual, gender and identity disorders. Mood symptoms could also be noted in individuals suffering from anxiety disorders, panic disorders, obsessive-compulsive disorders, phobic disorders and posttraumatic stress disorders.

The Severe Personality Disorders

Via the abnormal 5 axes in the Diagnostic Statistical Manual (DSM), is the way in which the whole persons are primarily address during a diagnosis. In the DSM IV, clinical disorders are listed on 3 separate axes, as described below. Axis 1, refers broadly to the principal disorder that needs immediate attention; i.e, a major depressive episodes, an exacerbation of schizophrenia or a flare up of panic disorder. Axis 2, lists any personality disorders that maybe shaping the current response to the axis I problem. Axis 2 also indicates any developmental disorders, i,e, learning disability, etc. that may be the predisposing factor toward the Axis 1. Example, someone with severe learning disability, mental retardation or paranoid personality disorders, maybe quickly to succumb into a clinical depressive state, when faced with a life stressing situation. Axis 3, list any medical or neurological problems that may be relevant to the individual's current or past psychiatric challenges. Example, someone with severe asthma, who's also dealing with psychiatric problems, may believe that they're suffering from an anxiety or panic attack due to upper respiratory symptoms. Axis IV, serves to effectively code the major psychological stressors of the individual. Axis 5, codes the level of functioning the patient displays at the time of assessment. This code may also serve to indicate, a highest level of functioning, the client may have achieved throughout the past year. Example, 0 – 100 scale, with 0 being the lowest and 100, being almost perfect … although none of us would score that high, quite frankly!

Throughout the years, researchers have found medications being sometimes helpful in the treatment of severe personality disorders. This they've studied and documented extensively, the reasons for such being, because biological factors, such as changes in temperatures could likely play an important role in the emotional and cognitive coping styles that ultimately shapes a personality. They've also realized that some of the underlying dimensions that influence personalities, such as aggression and emotional sensitivity to separation, are partly biologically inherited and could have a basis in physiology and therefore may be amenable to biological interventions, such as medication. It has also been noted that individuals who develop severe personality disorders, experience extreme or stereotyped responses to common situations, partly because of certain biological vulnerabilities. These biological vulnerabilities, may be shared with other individuals, who develop more acute disorders by showing similar symptoms. Expert-proponents of these studies have also suggested and have proposed that the symptoms of some severe personality disorders overlap substantially with Axis I disorders and even with some neurological conditions, such as Tourette's syndrome.

Some severe personality disorders, could therefore be part of the "spectrums of disorders that reflect common biological vulnerabilities." According to these conceptualizations, research also indicates that severe personality disorders, may well be the manifestation of "sub-thresholds," anxiety disorders, depressive disorders, impulse control disorders, and so on and so forth. And in current debates they've argued that if such reasoning is correct, medications that are effective in managing the symptoms of acute disorders within the spectrum, may also be effective in managing similar chronic symptoms experienced in that "range."

Although clinical facts have showed us that biological interventions such as medication may be of help to individuals with severe personality disorders, we should not invalidate or even challenge the balancing view that other developmental experiences may produce.

These could be as simple as learning the nature of the individual's cognitive processes, which could be of critical importance in the development of each individual's personality disorders, manifestation, and treatment of severe personality disorder. The cause of a severe personality disorder, should not necessarily determine how best to treat it with medications. The choice of

Medications at this point in time, is perhaps very much symptom-based. Therefore, strong recommendations has since been put in place for the clinician's consideration regarding treating individuals with severe personality disorder with medications.

Thus they've been reminded that they should have a clear qualitative and quantitative idea, about the target symptoms to be addressed. It is also important to keep in mind that unfortunately some of the most severe personality disorders, such as Schizoid, Histrionic Narcissistic, Dependent and Obsessive-Compulsive Personality Disorder, do not respond particularly well to treatment with medication, even though their (Possibly) related Axis I disorders, do respond. It may be that we have overlooked some important factor in our classification of those particular severe personality disorders, because although superficially, they seem similar to some Axis I disorders, they do not respond to medications that would be expected to treat those Axis I disorders. These interviews, if done in a systematic manner, would best focus toward bringing out or extracting personality patterns and therefore a severe personality disorder. Behaviors earlier on in life are very important pieces of information, due in part, because a severe personality disorder, would have been formed in an individual since their period of adolescence. "The current opioid crisis and overuse of prescription drug epidemic, currently wreaking havoc throughout our nation, upon our young addicts and non addicts, might be a clear example to these studies that for far too long remained widely ignored."

These studies also, recommended that an in depth and careful clinical interview would in fact, allow interviewers to differentiate between most Axis I disorders that could have been superimposed upon the personality structure and the severe personality disorders. Experts in the field, also believed that all treatments of the Axis I disorders, should be in conjunction with the treatment of the severe personality disorder. The clinical interview of a truthful person, a good historian, whom would clarify whether or not some intervening medical condition or treatment, or abuse of drugs or alcohol, may be affecting these behaviors. If the history is not reliable of course third-party corroboration could be essential. Cultural and family history, could also help to reveal the biological vulnerability of certain conditions. Medical history, including past or current illnesses or medications, are also important, because these may be causing the current symptoms. In the case of impulsivity or aggression, a medical evaluation, becomes rather imperative. These would help to rule-out seizures or other brain disorders, degenerative disorder, etc.

In some situations, a person's very religious family background could affect such. They may have had a very religious relative, probated to the hospital out of concern for the person's safety, while practicing religious rituals. Was the patient behaving appropriately within that cultural context? At times, we're overwhelmed by clerics, who might argue that this individual's religious practices were completely correct, which could perhaps be true. Researchers has also recommended that in certain cases, it would sometimes be rather helpful to stop being distracted by culturally based practices and come to the realization that one could make serious mistakes, due to their own valued judgment. Expert peers and colleagues currently in the field, would agree once again that clinicians should instead decide to place their focus toward the nature of the individual's interpersonal relationship. The main ingredient used, when making a personality disorder diagnosis. In conclusion, we might find that there was a severe personality disorder present within this individual, however it might have not responded to pharmacological treatment.

Finally, although Posttraumatic Stress Disorder may predispose some persons to develop Borderline Personality Disorder, often times we're impressed by the remission of "personality symptoms," when the Axis I disorder has been treated.

As we reflect on the approach and studies of various psychotherapists clinical experiences, we would ascertain that some of their most difficult, differential and severe personality disorders, have occurred, when they have been taken from the persons who had both, a severe personality disorder and some other related psychiatric or medical conditions. Throughout these measures one could learn to avoid premature closure and when to uncover the chief condition that is mostly afflicting that individual. Medical students and physicians, are often relieved when they make a mental health diagnosis and refer a challenging patient over to a mental health professional. One should also keep in mind that there is nothing about having a mental illness or personality disorder that prevents an individual from getting a heart disease, diabetes, multiple sclerosis, or breast cancer, etc. As a matter of fact, studies have shown that people with mental illness, are at far greater risk of contracting complicated medical conditions than the average sane individuals. This is due in part by a long list of possibilities, included thus not limited to medications side effects, lack of appropriate diet, lack of sleep, substance use, poor socialization social skills, isolation. All which is further compound with being sedentary due to the high dosage of medications inability to follow such diet, due to voices depression, etc. We sometimes have had difficulty differentiating Bipolar Affective Disorder (cyclothymiacs) from Borderline Personality Disorder, because affective liability is present fortunately, the medication management is somewhat similar.

Recurrent substance abuse is in addition a challenge, because it may be present in a severe personality disordered individual, whom might be self-medicating. Clinician's whom I've, interviewed, assured me that they've consistently asked such a reliable person what drugs have they taken that have seemed to ably help them feel better?" Several have established that sometimes they can perform biological underpinning of an individual's personality disorder by finding and helping them on the streets where they resided. When the individual realizes that a clinician is not inquiring or investigating about their drug use to later criticize, nor criminalize them, they are far more forthcoming with the information. Another challenge for clinicians, have been determining whether a severe personality disorder, was present in an individual who was receiving medication such as steroids. These particular individuals are essentially those with a kidney transplant, ulcerative colitis, multiple sclerosis, and so forth. Therefore, they highly recommend, we explore all conditions affecting the brain, which could eventually change the apparent 'personality.' I recall reading about a particular group of clinicians, whom overlooked a frontal mass on a man, who presented personality changes. We must always keep an open mind and fundamentally realize that personality disorders simply don't appear and subsequently disappear. The mentally, developmentally challenged person, who is acting out in some way, may or may not have a severe personality disorder. A useful rule of thumb for many therapists throughout the years, highly recommended by the reliable experts, has been to question if the mentally developmentally challenged person's behavior is appropriate for their age of cognitive development, superimposed challenges that puberty may have caused, or is it not? Physicians, APRN's, clinicians, nurses and most of all psychiatric general personnel, have evidently found that medication management in someone with a severe personality disorder is difficult, when the person is medically ill, especially with renal or hepatic failure, or if the metabolism has been altered by other medications. Therefore, before prescribing a mood stabilizer for such individuals, it is not unusual for doctors to try and favorably choose one that is metabolized by an organ system that is reasonably intact. Reason for which, it is believe that lithium pretty much became a drug of choice, back in the 1980's. Throughout the years for the individuals with liver failure, lithium is excreted primarily via the kidney, it is therefore flushed out of their bodies via the urinary tract. Sodium valproate, therefore, in a person suffering with kidney failure is subsequently metabolized in the liver. While compiling my investigation data and questioned several nurses, APRN's and physicians, they all came to an agreement of it being rather fundamental that they basically know, or have a detailed medical history of exactly what medicines the individual is taking, including the doses. In addition to stressing the beforehand importance, and thorough understanding of any abnormal laboratory studies. *In general conclusion, medication dosages may be needed to be increase at times of physical emotional stress and decreased if toxicity, side effects becomes significantly enough to outweigh the benefits.* The difficulties inherent when establishing a therapeutic alliance with someone who has a severe personality disorder and someone whom therefore has significant problems with interpersonal relationships, may make medication compliance problematic. Nevertheless, all whom I have interrogated clearly revealed similar concerns regarding the more impulsive or acting-out individuals and equally they were naturally worried about overdoses. Therefore, it is imperative to operationally define, qualitatively and quantitatively each target symptom for each psychotropic taken. To define the examples of potential target symptoms including impulsiveness and compulsiveness, and not to ignore affective instability, rage, anger, depression, low self-worth, or high responsiveness or low responsiveness, or aggression toward self or others.

All investigative research throughout, has continuously advised clinicians to update toward, precise monitoring methods and significantly document, regarding the levels of anxiety, as well as slower habituation to new stimuli. These, which may be manifested in fear of separation or social phobia, abnormalities in perceptual or cognitive organization, such as transient psychotic episodes, ideas of reference, or paranoid projections and the use of primitive defenses such as; *periods of dissociation, splitting, denial, lack of a conscience, rigid conscience, idealization, or devaluation of self.*

Most of the clinicians and health care professionals, I interviewed, practically have unanimously agreed that when they refer a severe personality disordered individual to another practitioner for medication evaluation, it is significant to first investigate and clearly communicate the client's attitude about taking medication for their symptoms. The reason being, they have stated, is because many of these individuals are concerned about significantly altering their inherent 'self,' because they view their symptoms as a genuine manifestation of their self. This concern goes to the center of an individual's identity and therefore, may be of even greater concern for those individuals diagnosed with *Borderline Personality Disorder or Narcissistic Personality Disorder.* Therefore, when possible, this significant issue requires thoroughly being work or addressed in detail before referring them. *Histrionic* or dependent patients might in addition becomes resentful at a medication referral, because they widely dread giving up manifestation. Individuals diagnosed with BPD, may in addition view a referral for medications, as abandonment by a psychotherapist, whom has given up on them. Therefore, effective awareness is forewarned toward the initial stage now set for splitting between the therapist and the specialist.

By the same token, an individual suffering with severe symptoms, might soon come to realize that neither the counselor, who does not make a medication referral, is not obtaining, nor certainly proposing all the potential that is accessible.

Of course, the *paranoid* patient, nevertheless, may reject such for both reasons, *a) being referred for medications and (b) not being referred for medications.* Trust subsequently becomes the central issue and a 'strong dosage of frank, straightforward' discussion about the potential risks and the advantages for taking medications, should be a very beneficial approach.

Due to descriptive similarities found within the DSM IV plus *published by the* American Psychiatric Association, personality disorders were grouped into three clusters. *Cluster A,* which includes a Paranoid, Schizoid and Schizotypal Personality Disorders. According to the DSM IV, individuals with these disorders are described as odd, or eccentric. *Cluster B,* which includes the antisocial, the borderline, the histrionic, and the narcissistic personality disorders and these individuals were described, as dramatic, emotional, or erratic. *Cluster C,* which includes the avoidant, the dependent and the obsessive-compulsive personality disorders. Individuals with these disorders often appear anxious or fearful. Some mental health professionals, found that such clustering system could have significant limitations, particularly with those individuals with co-occurring personality disorders, who might tend to cross cluster. In addition researchers have found traces of scientific evidence, demonstrating that there may exist genetic possible relationship between paranoid personality disorder, schizophrenia and schizotypal personality disorder. And they have documented extensively about these individuals with paranoid personality disorder, whom often develop the Axis I disorders of substance abuse, obsessive-compulsive disorder and anxiety-based disorders, such as agoraphobia.

And have asserted that often they experience depression, because of their suspiciousness and distrust they are ego-syntonic, due to their worldview. That they are more likely to come to a clinic or office for treatment of associated anxiety mood or substance related disorders, trouble controlling their anger, or various personal, legal or situational problems attributable to poor interpersonal relationships and skills. Clinicians experienced with this type of client, have recommended that when discussing medication for treatment of related symptoms, it is better to be especially forthright and precise, so they do not feel that something is being withheld. Some evidence has proven that neuroleptics may be helpful if there is forthright and frank psychotic ideation. However, the more common presentation of non-psychotic suspiciousness does not appear to be responsive to medication; in fact, suggestions about medication use may cause the individual to feel that you are trying to suppress or control legitimate concerns. Clinicians have commented about their experiences when doing medication management with such patients and have realized that it could be an error to allow the individual to reveal too much during the initial interview. They have recommended we must instead allow several sessions in order to obtain enough information before determining whether or not the medication could be helpful. Other therapists have also confessed, they have found out the hard way that when rushing such process, the patient initially acts compliant within the interview, but tries to incorporate them into an aggressive worldview, or may tend to become suspicious about their real motivation for learning so much about them. Though it is not uncommon for a patient with paranoid personality disorder to fire his therapist before the end of the first session, or drop out of treatment shortly thereafter. Individuals with Schizoid Personality Disorder convey a sense of social detachment and restricted emotional expression.

This disorder does not tend to be genetically related to schizophrenia and may be better understood as a manifestation of extreme introversion, a temperament that is comprised with a genetic basis. However, because the main symptom is that of a very low apparent ability to experience positive affect, experts in the field of psychiatry and neuropharmacology have suggested that Schizoid Personality Disorder, represents the signs of sub-threshold negative symptoms of schizophrenia, and that schizotypal personality disorder represents a sub-threshold, positive symptoms of Schizophrenia. Therefore, schizoid personality disorder does not respond well even to the newer atypical neuroleptics, which are usually more effective than earlier medications, when targeting the negative symptoms of Schizophrenia. The major noted differences between Schizoid Personality Disorder and avoidant personality disorder appears, as an anxiety based symptom, such which appears in the form of absence in the desires for intimate social relationships in the person with schizoid personality disorder. These individuals can appear depressed at times, but most often this appearance really seems to reflect a detachment without depression.

Throughout my thirty plus years, experience of working with the mentally ill, while studying the mental health field, conducting research, questioning psychiatrist, psychologist, nurses, social workers, observing and employing previously earned law enforcement investigative skills to seriously investigate individuals with personality disorders. Noting that persons with Schizoid Personality Disorders, appear somewhat more responsive to staff and their peers, when they received antidepressant medications. When questioned 'why?' Psychiatrist, psychologist and nurses, have answered this question in conclusion, and usually in the same manner, "serotonin reuptake inhibitor!" although the exact mechanism of action of the SSRIS, is still unknown … curiously most have agreed, the patients themselves seldom reports feeling any better.

Noted often times during interviews, patient themselves appear not to have a clue of what we are talking about when we say to them "you have been looking much better these days." It is noted also that at such point, almost all of them would always want to discontinue their medications, but that they would still also want to remain in treatment. Recently, clients suffering with mental illness, have started seeking out natural approach to treatment, via neuropathy, homeopathic, remedies, etc. I have recently began to investigate and conduct research with a neuropathic treaters, whom deals in all natural, none chemical treatments and I do plan to continue my assessment following this publication. Many of the mental health professionals whom I have interviewed during this research, have also responded to this question in the same fashion. And have agreed that this phenomena is not being caused, due to the fact that these individuals do not desire intimate social relationships, but it is rather their difficulty conceptualizing, on how to go about having a relationship and what this might mean to their lives.

Schizotypal Personality Disorders.

Individuals diagnosed with schizotypal personality disorder actually, feel acute discomfort about close relationships. Researchers have found associated genetics between schizotypal personality disorder and schizophrenia. And have related their findings to be that of individuals diagnosed with either of these disorders, have a deficit in the cognitive process of attention and selection. This makes it very difficult for them to relate to their environment. Most naturally, they feel a great deal of discomfort in social isolations and therefore, they isolate themselves. Clinicians has also suggested that prior to diagnosing an individual with Schizotypal personality disorder, one must first make note of the differentiation between them and those suffering with frontal lobe epilepsy, nevertheless, it is not difficult, because the symptoms of epilepsy occur episodically. Schizotypal personality behavior could also be found in some patients whom have been diagnosed with borderline personality behavior. Although unlike those exclusively diagnosed with BPD, the individuals with schizotypal personality disorder, have enduring cognitive-perceptual aberrations that are not confined to periods of stress or intense anxiety. As noted in a series of studies, it has been found that schizotypal personality disorder can be thought of as a sub-syndromal manifestation of some of the positive symptoms of Schizophrenia and as such could respond to neuroleptic medication in low doses. Psychiatrists and other healthcare professionals has asserted this to be true, though in the lesser of the clinical symptoms such as social isolation, which is seen as anxiety based. They have recommended and cautioned about the risks of tardive dyskinesia and other side effects, therefore it being probably better to taper neuroleptics during times when the patient is less distressed. Several newer antipsychotic and antidepressant medications are currently also being studied for use in this condition.

Cluster B: Antisocial, Borderline, Histrionic, Narcissistic and Antisocial Personality Disorders

Individuals diagnosed with Antisocial Personality Disorders, are impulsive and display aggressive disregard for social norms. Impulsivity that leads to aggression is a dimension that is likely heritable. This is also seen in the Axis I disorders of DSM IV intermittent explosive disorder, as a bipolar affective disorder and as a conduct disorder. Evidence for a genetic factors associated with antisocial personality disorder appears stronger than most other psychiatric disorders, including bipolar disorder and schizophrenia. Literature shows these individuals to have a low baseline arousal level, especially when dealing with potential painful stimuli.

It has been postulated that they develop less fear and guilt surrounding the consequences of ignoring social norms. Two-thirds of persons with Antisocial Personality Disorders tend to have associated Substance Abuse Disorder and that this only helps to further decrease their impulse control. Therapist find individuals with antisocial personality disorder as being some of the most difficult personality disorders to treat, reason for which outpatient therapy is rarely successful. Most have agreed that therapy works best when it is backed up by the real consequences for their continued antisocial acts, especially for those individuals with psychopathic behaviors. Research have found that a practical approach which focuses on the value of a behavior patterns that conforms to social norm, are the best approach for most of these individuals, rather than using approaches that attempts to deal with fear, guilt or a building conscience technique. Because the individuals with antisocial personality disorder often do not readily accept responsibility for their behaviors and therefore rather place blame, or accept the idea that medications should control their symptoms.

Experts however, find this fact to have positive and negative conditions, such as depression and irritability, which could lead to aggression, anxiety, and substance abuse ... and that immediate medication intervention could indirectly reduce antisocial behavior and it's a propensity for violence. On the other hand, individual clinicians might argue that one should not have to excuse responsibility for behavior. Individuals with Antisocial Personality Disorders, who have been depressed, have responded well to antidepressant medication in terms of affect and their ability to control emotional outbursts and impulsivity. Recent findings, have suggested that antisocial personality disorder could be considered somewhat of a neurodevelopmental abnormality. Such which could also be associated with minor physical anomalies, hyperactivity and learning disabilities ... or more simply put, as being adults with a residual attention deficit disorder, with impulsivity, irritability, mood lability, difficulty focusing, and subtle learning disabilities, which are attributable to Attention Deficit Disorder.

Histrionic Personality Disorder

The individual with Histrionic Personality Disorder *HPD* display excessive emotional attention-seeking behavior. These persons have great difficulty delaying gratification. Histrionic personality disorder, may share a genetic disposition toward impulsivity or sensation seeking, which also characterizes persons with antisocial personality disorder. The Histrionic person's symptoms worsen, when they recognize a threat to physical attractiveness or bodily integrity, thus, medical illness and hospitalization can be especially difficult for these individuals. Mental health professionals, have also found this disorder difficult to treat with medication, moreover, they have agreed that some symptoms may respond to treatment with antidepressants, especially mood reactivity, hypersomnia and rejection sensitivity.

Narcissistic Personality Disorder

Narcissistic personality Disordered individuals, display a pervasive behavioral and thought configuration of grandiosity, a need for admiration and a lack of empathy with others. They idealize and then devalue others and are preoccupied with conflicts and insecurities toward their self-worth. They do seek treatment for substance abuse; intervention with medications may be helpful here, as they often present with depressive symptoms. Clinicians have also found antidepressant medications to be especially helpful for this group of patients. Although they must first consider whether to continue administering these medications when the depression is present and they has agreed to take them. They have also found that the depressed narcissistic individual is rather unpredictable and at times could represent a high risk.

Avoidant Personality Disorder

Persons with Avoidant Personality Disorder have an increased level of tonic sympathetic nervous system activity, higher levels of cortical arousal and slower habituation to new stimuli. Avoidant personality disorder and dependent personality disorders, may coexist with major depression and obsessive-compulsive disorder, symptoms of apparent avoidant personality disorder, may remit via treatment of associated axis disorders.

Dependent Personality Disorder

The individual with Dependent Personality Disorder experiences a need to be taken care of. This could later lead to submissive behavior and fear of separation. This disorder may be the result of an interaction between an anxious-inhibited temperament and an insecure attachment to a parental figure that can occur for a variety of reasons. *Dependent Personality Disorder is often seen in mentally retarded persons and also in others who have suffered since childhood from a serious general medical disorder.* Experts with this patient group have strongly suggested that taking a medical history is very important, when evaluating and treating these persons. Dependent personality Disorder is often associated with mood or anxiety disorders, treatment of these associated disorders may be helpful to the person, although there is no known pharmacological approach to treat the personality disorder itself. The relationship with the psychotherapist or pharmacotherapy, may become an end in itself for the patient. *This can be a problem if it results in the person becoming less than straightforward about symptom resolution or medication use. They have all agreed that it is important to set some limits on these patients at the outset, so that their expectations for contact does not exceed what members of the treatment team are able or willing to do for them over the long run.*

Studies has found these individuals to respond well to limit setting, once they've reassured themselves that they will not be abandoned. Clinicians, also has recommended that all treaters should explain up front that such continuance in their relationship be viewed as such and to not burn them up all at once. This should also be documented, viewed and discussed via the treatment plan among the treatment team.

Obsessive Compulsive Personality Disorder

Studies have shown us that obsessive-compulsive personality disorder differs from the Axis l, in that Obsessive-Compulsive Personality Disorder is not characterized by the presence of obsessions or compulsions. Thus rather it involves a more pervasive pattern of preoccupation with orderliness, perfectionism and control, which, begins in early adulthood. There may be genetically inherited traits of obsessionality, related to the development of this disorder. Obsessive-Compulsive Personality Disorder also involves rigid behavior patterns that are somewhat ego-syntonic to the individual. Patients with Obsessive-Compulsive Personality Disorder may be prone to anxiety, feelings of hostility and physical disorders related to a constant worrying. Depression may develop in middle age or if career problems do occur. These symptoms can be treated. Clinicians experienced with this group, highly recommend Pharmacological treatment, which should involve treatment of associated Axis I disorders involving anxiety or depression. Unlike the obsessions and compulsions of the Axis I disorder, which may respond to medication, the preoccupation with orderliness and perfectionism of the person with Obsessive Compulsive Personality Disorder does not respond to any known treatment with medication.

Borderline Personality Disorder

It should be noted that I have chosen to list this personality study for last and the reason for this, is simply because it has been one of the most challenging among all of the severe personality behaviors for mental health professionals and paraprofessionals to treat. Therapist usually cringe, when an individual diagnosed with BPD appears among their caseload. The reason being is because individuals diagnosed with Borderline Personality Disorder tend to display a pattern of impulsivity, mood instability, unstable and unsatisfying interpersonal relationships, and an unstable image. Researcher's belief toward such mood instabilities present in Borderline Personality Disorders is probably due to a genetic based trait.

Because these persons are impulsive, they have trouble controlling their quick intense anger and may do physically self-damaging acts. Their selective recall of emotion charged events may be related to their intense rage, which may distort their registration, thus clouding their memory of an event. Borderline Personality pathology plays a very significant role in the suicide of people in their 20's. The stressors surrounding these suicides are often fairly mild and it is postulated that this could reflect as lower threshold for suicide among borderline patients. Therefore, clinicians recommend that when treating depressive symptoms in these individuals, results are far better attained with serotonin reuptake inhibitors, than with antidepressants. There is some evidence that show injury behaviors to be reduced when treating borderline patients with serotonin reuptake inhibitors. Those patients experiencing decreased energy, hypersomnia and *hyperphagia,* sometimes respond best to the antidepressants known as monoamine oxidase inhibitors. They have found Benzodiazepines to not be a good choice because of the potential for behavioral *dyscontrol* and that Lithium reduces mood instability, which is associated with a decrease in aggressive acting out.

It is especially effective in those borderline individuals, who have a relative with Bipolar Affective Disorder. Anticonvulsants such as sodium valproate and carbamazepine are also helpful in stabilizing affective lability and increasing the capacity to delay impulsive action, and to some extent also improving brief psychotic episodes.

Patients with behavioral dyscontrol or physical and verbal aggression respond well to monoamine oxidase inhibitors and almost as well to a neuroleptic, or mood stabilizers, such as carbamazepine. Their symptoms worsen with benzodiazepines in terms of increased severity in episodes of behavioral dyscontrol. Some studies have revealed a substantial overlap between Borderline Personality Disorder and schizotypal personality disorder. Therefore, patients with both of these disorders, the atypical and typical, benefit greatly when given neuroleptics. This treatment appears equally effective for subtle psychotic symptoms such as suspiciousness and could also disperse its mood-stabilizing qualities in these individuals, reducing depression and interpersonal sensitivity. Throughout my years of observing and dealing with individuals who had been diagnosed with BPD, I noticed that clinicians throughout their practice, have found it useful to first determine, whether an individual with borderline personality disorder has predominantly affective or psychotic symptoms.

Once these are distinguished this emphasis, they then proceed to try to manage the most prominent symptoms. Many psychotherapists have chosen rather not to treat transient symptoms or those that can be ameliorated, or move on with supportive psychotherapy. Many psychotherapists, who have previously dealt with treatment resistance issues, including resistance to taking medications correctly, usually proceed toward teaching the patient coping skills management and reactions to life stressors.

Including teaching this group how to cope with feelings of identity diffusion, and improve interpersonal relationships. Henceforth, the birth of Dialectical behavioral therapy has been found to be especially helpful in persons with suicide-related behavior, as suicidal ideation, hopelessness and anger which is directed at self or others, dissociation, and risky behaviors. In a recent study done on the outcome of clients involved in DBT treatment, found that by the 4th month of treatment, only 25% of patients were still on medication, compared with 60% in the control group. Thus the use of the emergency room patient and psychiatric hospitalization both had also declined in great numbers.

Diagnosis Features for Borderline Personality Disorder

Individuals with Borderline Personality Disorder have a pattern of unstable and intense relationships

Criterion 2. Is clearly defined as the, *"you are the best thing that ever happened to me, or the best therapist I've ever met syndrome."* They may idealize potential caregivers or lovers at their first or second meeting, demand to spend a lot of time together and share the most intimate details early on in the relationship. However, they may switch quickly from idealizing other people to devaluing them, feeling that the other person does not care enough, does not give enough, is not 'there' enough, etc. These individuals can empathize with and nurture other people, but only with the expectation that the other person will be there in return to meet their own needs on demand. These individuals are prone to sudden and dramatic shifts in their view of others, who may alternately be seen as beneficent supports or as cruelly punitive. Such shifts often reflect disillusionment with a caregiver, whose nurturing qualities had been idealized, or whose rejection or abandonment is expected. There may be an identity disturbance characterized by markedly and persistently unstable self-image or sense of self.

Criterion 3: Shows us that there are sudden and dramatic shifts in self-image characterized by shifting goals, values and vocational aspirations. There may be sudden changes in options and plans about career, sexual identity, values and types of friends. These individuals may suddenly change from the role of a needy supplicant for help to a righteous avenger of past mistreatment. Although they usually have a self image that is based on being bad or evil. Individuals with this disorder may at times have feelings that they do not exist at all.

Such experiences usually occur in situations in which the individual feels a lack of a meaningful relationship, nurturing and support. These individuals may show worse performance in unstructured work or school situations. Individuals with this disorder display impulsivity in at least two areas that are potentially self-damaging

Criterion 4: indicates that these individuals may gamble, spend money irresponsibly, binge-eat, abuse substances, engage in unsafe sex, or drive recklessly. Individuals with Borderline Personality Disorder, often display recurrent suicidal behavior gestures, or threats of self-mutilating behavior

Criterion 5. Completed suicide occurs in 8 to 10% of such individuals and self-mutilative acts e.g., cutting or burning and suicide threats and attempts are very common. Recurrent suicidality is often the reason for which these individuals seek help. These self-destructive acts are usually precipitated by threats of separation or rejection or by expectations that they assume increased responsibility. Self-mutilation may occur during dissociative experiences and often brings relief by reaffirming the ability to feel or by expiating the individual's sense of being evil.

Individuals with Borderline Personality Disorder may display affective instability that is due to a marked reactivity of mood e.g., intense episodic dysphoria, irritability or anxiety, usually lasting a few hours and only rarely more than a few days.

Criterion 6: The basic dysphoric mood of those with Borderline Personality Disorder is often disrupted by periods of anger, panic or despair and is rarely relieved by periods of well-being, or satisfaction. These episodes may reflect the individual's extreme reactivity to interpersonal stresses. Individuals with Borderline Personality Disorder may be troubled by chronic feelings of emptiness

Criterion 7. its rather indicative to the persons with BPD that being easily bored, they may have them constantly seek something to do. Individuals with Borderline Personality Disorder frequently express inappropriate intense anger or have difficulty controlling their anger

Criterion 8. They may display extreme sarcasm, enduring bitterness or verbal outbursts. The anger is often elicited when a caregiver or lover is seen as neglectful, withholding, uncaring, or abandoning. Such expressions of anger are often followed by shame and guilt and contribute to the feeling they have of being evil. During periods of extreme stress, transient paranoid ideation or dissociative symptoms e.g., depersonalization may occur

Criterion 9, generally points to insufficient severity or duration to warrant an additional diagnosis. These episodes occur most frequently in response to a real or imagined abandonment. Their symptoms tend to be transient and lasting minutes or hours. The real or perceived return of the caregiver's nurturance may result in a remission of symptoms.

Diagnostic Criteria for Borderline Personality Disorder

Borderline patients usually display a pervasive pattern of instability toward their interpersonal relationships, self-image and affects, marked impulsivity. These, which appear at the beginning of early adulthood and remain present in a variety of contexts, as indicated by five or more of the following:

1. Frantic efforts to avoid real or imagined abandonment = this does not include suicidal or self-mutilating behavior, which is found in Criterion 5.

2. A pattern of unstable and intense interpersonal relationships, characterized by alternating between extremes of idealization and devaluation

3. Identity disturbance of markedly and persistently unstable self-image, or sense of self.

4. Impulsivity, in at least two areas that are potentially self-damaging e.g., erratic spending, sex, substance abuse, reckless driving, binge eating, etc. This also does not include suicidal or self-mutilating behavior covered in Criterion 5.

5. Recurrent suicidal behavior gestures, or threats, or self-mutilating behavior

6. Affective instability due to a marked reactivity of mood e.g., intense episodic dysphoria, irritability, or anxiety, usually lasting a few hours and only rarely more than a few days.

7. Chronic feelings of emptiness

8. Inappropriate intense anger or difficulty controlling anger e.g., frequent displays of temper, constant anger and recurrent physical fights.

9. Transient, stress-related paranoid ideation or severe dissociative symptoms.

CHAPTER V

A Long Awaited Birth … the Arrival of Dialectic Behavioral Therapy .

As if ancient wisdom is reintroduced into the modern world perspective

Historian Arnold Toynbee said it best, when he stated that: "the coming of Buddhism to the West may have been proven to be one of the most important events of the Twentieth Century." To the average individual this might have come across as *"whom, what, etc?" However realistically speaking, to the persons diagnosed with borderline personality disorders it has a whole new and different meaning.* Although Toynbee wasn't exactly talking about BPD, DBT Buddhism is actually credited with saving many lives. *While we might naively ask ourselves what do Albert Einstein, DBT, Buddhism and Marsha Leinahan has in common? Albert Einstein once wrote that, "The religion of the future will be a cosmic religion … that should transcend a personal God and avoid dogma and theology. Covering both the natural and the spiritual, it should be based on a religious sense, arising from the experiences of all things natural and spiritual, as a meaningful unity." Buddhism answers this description. Others have followed his statement, acknowledging that "If there is any religion best prepared to cope with our modern scientific needs, less blaming and finger pointing, it would be Buddhism." In reality what Albert Einstein, DBT, Buddhism and Dr. Leinahan have in common is that point in religion that is best known in the Buddhist tradition as the, (8 spoke wheel of interconnected links, which is directed at developing our wisdom, ethics and meditative awareness).* Buddhism has actually proven to the psychiatric community, major accomplishments in the treatment of borderline personality disorders through *Dialectic Behavioral*

Therapy. This was previously unattained with pharmacotherapy and all other therapeutic approaches no too long ago.

Dialectic Behavioral Therapy's interconnected links are directed at helping this group develop the essential values of life. It is also a direct link to the enhancement of self-worth, self-esteem and therefore provides a brighter understanding of our fellowman and ourselves. In turn, it is a direct link to all other religions, because it helps us to further understand and accept ourselves and others. It is my humble view and my hope that perhaps the reentry of Christianity and other religious and spiritual groups into the mental health arena through gospel and spiritual counseling could perhaps aid to reach even greater heights and find major break-troughs in treatment.

A Little History on the Successful DBT Research

Throughout the late 1980's, when most therapist scratched their heads, pulled out their hair in frustration and were about to throw in their towel and give up ... around this same time almost everyone thought that working with individuals diagnosed with borderline personality was hopeless and saw their attempts to treat to be no more than a long and exasperating losing battle. Dr. Marsha Linehan, was until then, an almost unknown university professor who would emerge with an innovative treatment to save the day.

She didn't merely just save the day, she would instead help breathe life back in to an entire generation and save countless lives. Armed with a grant from the National Institute of Health, Miss Linehan would open up shop and began testing clinical trials with her newly aggregative type of therapy, by first locating clients and assessing them for borderline personality traits and initiated therapy, while collecting data. However, it wouldn't be until the end of the decade, when her natural instinct, along with years of intellectual stimulating researcher's drive that of course, was awakened through God's power, wisdom and guidance. An awakened guidance that spiritually served her well grounded altruistic beliefs and inner instinct toward mindfulness. Although still and somewhat unsure about her findings, until the final data analysis, professor Linahan recalls often times sitting for countless hours at her desk at the University of Washington's computer center trying to conduct the research. Until that one time, she typed a few words, stroked several keys and minutes later, the words *Dialectical Behavioral Therapy* appeared on her screen. This new therapeutic approach would later come to outperform the run of the mill treatment by a hundred times over. She had been inspired by several dozen highly suicidal and self-destructive borderline individuals, whom she had been treating and encouraged not only by her faith in God and her new findings, but rather by the accomplish success she had seen in her clients, professor Linehan, would soon began introducing and presenting DBT workshops wherever she could.

Overwhelmed by the number of patients wasting away in locked inpatient hospital wards, where borderline clients were suspected of hostility for apparently ordinary actions, such as 'shrinking back self-confidence,' when faced with a room full clinicians, and other minor actions. She appeared and toured throughout hospitals across the country, her ultimate goal was simply to change the clinician's mindset toward borderline clients. To stop them from hating these individuals and to get them to start seeing them more as sick individuals, rather than as hateful people.

Miss Linehan gave one of her first memorable speeches, when she spoke in the fall of 1991, at a conference hosted by the North Carolina Psychological Association in Durham. After her presentation, many mental health professionals signed up to attend her first 10 day DBT intensive clinical training. The psychologists and other clinicians who attended this training then went on to teach it to others in the field, DBT then caught on and spread like wild fire shortly thereafter. One of the most recent completed studies on borderline personality disorders showed that by the 4th month of treatment, only 25% of patients were still on medication, compared with 60% in the control group, use of emergency room patient and psychiatric hospitalization also declined, and more importantly, the suicide rate had also dropped by an alarming percentage. Perhaps critics who are still bent on arguing the fact of whether or not God, faith, religion and spirituality does not belong in the field of mental health won't be so hard after comparing the remarkable improvement among this patient population. It is still not quite understood why God's name is not included within these treatments, when one could clearly see his actions throughout her teachings, "is it because of the separation of church and state perhaps?"

After spending years of working with this population and seeing the countless numbers of mutilations, self-destructive behaviors and so many successful suicides I don't really believe that these patient are much interested in political 'jargon' but rather in living successful lives. I believe that if we were to study the success of DBT a bit closer, private and state run psychiatric hospitals might reconsider opening their doors and letting God back in.

Prior to Dialectic Behavioral Therapy and throughout our many years of studying, researching and teaching coping skills and number of other approaches, we had seen little to no improvement in any of these individuals. Despite their five days per week psychodynamic talk, theralectroshock treatment, lithium, Librium, tricyclics, or any other anti-psychotics therapy. Many of these individuals had even given up trying to find ways to end their lives and some had even lost faith in their ability to kill themselves. "One of these individuals once told me that they had given up on pills because, they had been rescued so many times." A therapist turned DBT instructor, once told me that "studies still find guns to be rather foreign to many borderlines, although they remain in and out of hospitals. Hence more in than out, they cut and bang their heads, and become assaultive, or self-destructive, but in reality, they do not really wish to die."

The Origin of A Name for A Code Word That = 'Trouble.'

Long before the ambiguous term "*borderline*" was coined and placed upon women by mostly *heterosexual old man,* nearly a hundred years ago, individuals known to us today as 'borderlines' were considered public nightmares, *islands of intractable misery* and the annoyance of many a psychotherapist's lives. Centuries of shifting diagnostic labels and rising feminist sympathies, cannot paper over the entire mental health system, nor the treatment endured by these individuals. This is due in grand part to the ill-oriented therapy signaled by blind folded mental health professionals, whom have repeatedly failed them. Among individuals with borderline personality disorders, we find that nearly eighty percent of them are women and we have also found that about an equal percentage of all persons diagnosed as borderlines, tend to report the same repeated similarities. All share the same story and that is a history of childhood sexual abuse, over three times the rate of clients given other diagnosis.

Many repeatedly try to kill themselves and unfortunately over nine percent of them ultimately succeed. Among them, we find the volatile, traumatized and damaged individuals, which Freud then called *'hysterics'* and attempted to treat with very little success during the last century. Many others, got worse, deteriorated and went to the dogs during grand *classical psychoanalysis period*. Otto Stern later described this as being on the borderline between psychosis-neurosis. Individuals being treated by feminist therapists during the early part of the 1980's achieved equally, mixed result … although by now the derogatory 'borderline' label was being drop in favor of a less intimidating and more humane term, opted to instead call them *'trauma survivors.'*

The DSM-IV +, *today simply defines borderline Personality as an Axis I character disorder, marked by instability of interpersonal relationships, self-image, affects, of marked impulsivity. The enumerated symptoms of the disorder includes frantic efforts to avoid real or imagined abandonment, followed by episodes of depersonalization and dissociation, oscillation between idealizing and denigrating other suicidality, self-mutilation, loneliness, anger, inner emptiness and impulsivity in at least two areas that are potentially self-damaging e.g. bizarre spending, substance abuse, reckless driving, binge eating, etc.* Between therapists' frustration and secretive jargon, the term borderlines is also accompanied by much eye-rolling, which has long been the short-ended stick for those clients who never got beyond the crisis du jour-clients, alike the fragile alcoholic Blanche Dubois the character in the movie A Street Car Named Desire, who depended eternally on the kindness of strangers. Clients reminiscent of Marilyn Monroe, who was removed from the care of her psychotic mother and was repeatedly sexually abused during childhood, she remain ever wandering, in and out of exploitative relationships, thus unable to protect herself.

Actually the term 'borderline' was a 'code word' defined not for an individual, but rather for a relationship, *a therapeutic double drowning if we may*. It was meant to label practically any individual that terrified, enraged or repulsed their therapist, like Alex Forrest, the seemingly competent New York city's, career woman, life, whom is portrayed by Glen Close in the film *Fatal Attraction*. She flew into rages, slit her wrists and stalked her married lover, when he tried to leave her. Bob, the 'human crazy glue' played by Bill Murray in the film *What About Bob*. Who tracked his stuffy psychiatrist to his summer home and drove him crazy. The frustrated therapist later became set on trying to blow him up with dynamite. And of course, how can we forget Barbara Streisand's powerful character in the movie 'Nuts.'

Some of these real-life frustrated therapist interviewed went as far as considering and defining them as *'the therapeutic menace from hell.'* To many of the senior and veteran colleagues whom I have worked side by side in treating this population throughout my career, they were secretly known *as the seclusion room terrorists* back then. Several years ago, prior to the arrival of DBT, they could have easily been identified as the *Binladen's Taliban's* of the therapeutic world.

Although many of them were very likable, some therapist refused to work with them, claiming there was too much effort for such little result. I spoke with a clinician who clearly still remembers two clients who made her tear out her hair back in the early 1980's. One man frequently threatened suicide and called her office collect to say things like *"You descriptive+ explicit + descriptive … you don't give two descriptive about me. I'm just a paycheck to you … my illness means nothing more than a job to you."* Adding that that same client later threw hot coffee on her brand-new suit. Another client would simply put his fist through glass windows or tried punching through cinder blocks, *his right hand had more scar- tissue and sin fractures than a reptile has scales on its back.*

Throughout my many year- long career in the field of mental health, I have frequently witnessed and dealt with more borderlines diagnosed individuals than I could possibly remember, though out of all, one in particular comes to inevitably mind. One individual that will persistently top all of them. In these writings I will make reference to him as (Mr. B.G). Although this is not the men's real name due to accountability, confidentiality and the respect due to him as an individual person afflicted with a severe illness, whom have since passed on. Although his name had become synonymous throughout most state and private mental health facilities and hospitals throughout the Northeast.

Some of the mental health workers, who knew him, jokingly believe if officially approved, the DSM and Webster's Dictionary would have promptly placed a recognized copy of his photograph right next to the 'graphic borderline criteria.' After touring almost every psychiatric facility throughout the Northeast, he was sent back to the hospital where I worked at the time. Upon his second day of arrival, he plotted and unreservedly, encouraged another client, who'd also been diagnosed with BPD, to tie plastic bags around each other's feet and legs, strike a match, and together set themselves a blaze. A week later, he got out of control and punched a nurse, as she walked up to him with a glass of cold juice to soothe his thirst. He struck her so hard; she bounced back about three to four feet and banged her head up against the wall. To this day she remains paralyzed from her neck down, for this cruel act, he was later sent to a forensic institute for the criminal insane, (one of the strictest and most rigorous behavioral treatment centers in the region.) While there, he selfishly managed to accumulate the highest number of mechanical restraint hours recorded to this day, in the history of state psychiatric hospitals in the country. When totaled, these hours, would amount to over twelve hundred days in a little over four years. However, criminal charges had not been pressed nor filed against him for the assault on the nurse. Following years later, the (*PSRB*) Psychiatric Review Board was expertly developed, they subsequently pulled his file for a conduct review to realize that he could no longer be kept there if he wasn't actually convicted of committing a crime. Mr. B .G. was afterward, sent back to our facility; unfortunately, he landed on our ward. As luck would have it, I was selected and appointed as his primary care therapist. All staff members were concerned about his return again to the hospital, and they especially seemed to empathize with me about my faith in this patient, as if they could somehow measure the level of my internal anxiety, meter's gage. Throughout the weeks that followed and those long awaited days, all I thought about was exploring new avenues and try to successfully find practical ways in which to effectively work with this client. I sat and wondered that of all the available facilities throughout the state, why would it have to be our unit … our little quiet ward? I then realized that the fundamental rationale for his being sent to our ward was because we'd been chosen as the designated statewide pilot unit for the then newly released drug, Clozaril. Borderlines, as well as schizophrenics were also being tested back then on this new cure-all drug. At first I believed I was being set up to fail, but as I later reflected, spoke with my supervisor and was reassured that the reason I was designated for such, was due to my prior experience with borderline patients and my ability to be productive and keep them focus and constantly occupied. He would ultimately prove to be the most challenging individual I'd ever meet … so did the rest of the hospital. At times, we would be anticipating to having a good night, I'd make sure to dedicate him ten to fifteen minutes of individual attention each shift, work with him toward brief attainable goals, while proposing to him chores of his liking, etc. Made sure his immediate needs were met and openly interviewed him about targeted, particular specifics of his preference. Although the evening would've been moving right along quietly, with the remaining twenty three other patients either resting, in bed, socializing in the smoking room, or sitting in the lounge watching T.V., etc. Mr. B.G., would walk right up to the television set, yanked it from the wall and smashed it on to the floor, up against the wall or simply just pick up a chair and put it right through the screen. He just did not care, whether there were other clients sitting they're watching it or not. "To him it made no difference." On separate occasions he was confronted by other male patients, prepared to fight back and therefore, disrupt the entire ward. At times, he would jump, or punch staff and other clients without any provocation. One of the most bizarre of his memorable instances that come to inevitably mind is the one, which took place during a Christmas season, when the state legislators struggled over cutting the state's budget. In truth, the entire mental health system was being run far below budget, administration did not allot the required funds for the conventional special Christmas treats on these wards, nor did they purchase the items needed for the clients. The head nurse and remainder of unit staff together we dug into our pockets and funded a unit Christmas party. Staff baked Christmas cookies, purchased apple cider, candies and I brought in a karaoke machine … we played music, sang and together we celebrated Christmas. All the clients appeared to have enjoyed, even Mr. B.G. volunteered to help us clean up after the recreational activity. Once he'd finished, he decided to pick up a chair and smashed the nursing station's plexiglass window, after, he proceeded to take the chair and used it as a weapon, while threatening staff and patients. We then opted to put him in the seclusion room, which he then willingly walked in to, however, once in there, he immediately began banging his head on the concrete wall. My coworker, Joan and I went in to speak to him, while trying to discourage him from banging his head and further hurting himself … reluctantly he agreed to stop. Nonetheless, when we turned around to leave the room, he proceeded to jump her from behind.

Joan, who then had long hair, which sat midway down her back … she on a daily and regular basis received compliments on it and was very proud of her curly brunet hair, this patient was somehow able to wrap his entire hand around and in between each strand of it and absolutely wouldn't let go. We then called for a psych emergency and it eventually took about seven staff members to gradually peel each finger away, one at a time. Still he continued fighting and was later placed in to four-point restraint and I had to sit there and observed him, due to patients requiring to be monitored once placed into mechanical restraints. The man continued screaming, yelling pulling and cursing … "If I'd listen to, or heard the 'N word' remark once more that night;" I thought to myself. He had used it in excess of fifty times in less than an hour. In fact, he even began singing it out aloud. I just sat there quietly while I myself monitored him. Of course, he had in addition been medicated with intramuscular medicine shot. My supervisor later walked up to me and asked, "how can you tolerate this *explicit* and? Doesn't it bother you?" Before I could respond to his questions, he proceeded toward, Mr. B.G., who was strapped down in the bed, still swearing and screaming, he afterward stepped up to him and immediately started slapping him around, but this critical time instead of screaming, crying, or calling out for help, be spontaneously began laughing out hysterically, as if he was being tickled. In less than an hour, I had seen this man gone from singing karaoke and enjoying a Christmas party, to pleasantly assist with cleaning up the 'unit,' to being assaultive, to becoming psychotic and even driving a veteran psychiatric nurse over the edge. By the way that was Christmas eve-night 1993. Of course, the supervisor, regain control shortly thereafter, he was still in shock when he turned to me and asked that if I had seen anything. I myself was in surprise of such behavior stemming from the part of a professional and … I absolutely recommended that he wrote himself up that he completed an incident report and that he seek counseling and anger management groups, because he needed help in dealing with his out of control anger.

The Emergence of Light, Toward the Emotional Skin

Throughout the decades since most clinicians who had a choice to avoid, avoided borderline clients, while state and agency staff that could not, simply went through the motions with a sense of ineffective uselessness. Others chose to adopt a psychoanalytic view, blaming the disorder on the disturbances on mother-infant attachment or a constitutional excess of aggression. In simple terms, their therapy consisted solely of guarding against manipulation and hostility, versus the borderline's reactions to the therapist, who daily searched for clues to their fragmented inner world. It was hard on both clients-and therapists alike." We were accustomed to make too much of an assumption that if we directly understood the patients' conflicts and made correct interpretations, they would know how to say 'no,' or stand up to somebody or go through a job interview. At least that was the belief of many psychiatrists in those days that still followed the psychoanalyst, Otto Kernberg's theories. Who's views toward "Role-playing or teaching a behavioral skill, was considered a no-no, simply because he thought it would create a different type of transference, where the person would become dependent on their therapist and develop false hopes. Other clinicians adopted the 'feminist-trauma-focused' view, which concentrated more on client's histories of sexual, physical and psychological trauma.

Like Sigmund Freud and Burke, who had previously studied Anna O, nearly a hundred years earlier, clinicians would gradually began to come to their senses and realize that trauma, mounted with untreated trauma, the pain worsens, the rage gets worse and to those people whom they have not been thought adequate coping skills, the pain definitely worsen. Despite all, Dialectic Behavioral Therapy (DBT) treatment would not come to light until late 1991, after an article published this new study in the *Archives of General Psychiatry.*

Psychiatry's leading journals … the article did not give the treatment much creed in its initial report, perhaps in part because it wasn't authored by a white male psychiatrist, whom we still believed to hold the reigns as being the only leading authorities in the field. Perhaps, because it leaned more toward ones faith, which until then was still being heavily viewed as 'nontraditional.' Nevertheless, it did kindly pointed toward *a small National Institute of Mental Health indiscriminate fund for clinical trials that had showed dramatic improvement, amid two-dozen borderlines, suicidal and severely self-harming women.* To the amazement of many in the psychiatric and the psychology communities, who read the article, the lead author and researcher, was not even a psychiatrist, rather a behavior psychologist and Zen student at University of Washington; her name was Marsha Linehan. The treatment was being identified as Dialectical Behavior Therapy, or DBT. The article also indicated that of the women in Marsha's study, had tried to kill themselves at least twice, and many had practiced parasuicide. They addictively attacked their own bodies during flashes of emotional crisis. Slashing their forearms their tendons and wrists, they had burnt themselves with cigarettes and lighters and even strangled themselves severely enough to risk death, unconsciousness and hospitalizations.

The article also indicated that after only four months of treatment, fewer than half were still harming themselves, compared with roughly three quarters of control group of 22 equally self-punishing women given treatment as usual. *It was that the establishments began to pay closer attention.* The article concluded that during the course of one year, 'DBT women' steadily improved, spending significantly fewer days in mental hospitals and engaging in fewer suicide and parasuicide attempts. Although a small and limited stride, it was still a major improvement, compared to what had been previously available in the areas of treatment for individuals, diagnosed with borderline personality disorder. *The study had established DBT as the only treatment for borderline suicidality ever validated by a randomized clinical trial and published in such journal.*

Treatment is based on a set of behavioral techniques, which Doctor Linehan called 'a technology of change, balanced by a technology of acceptance.' It is a soft, gentle and semi-mystical, Asian emphasis on radical acceptance and exercises for calming the mind by following the breath. Clinicians teach these individuals how to tolerate difficult situations and their own intense emotions by using mindfulness-meditation practices and the cultivation of radical acceptance. Strangely enough, all of Marsha's clinical subjects consecutively had also had learned Western social skills, such as interpersonal effectiveness to meet their needs and behavioral chain analysis, which helped them to pinpoint exactly what triggered their desires of suicidality. However, DBT is no walk in the park. It requires a consistent treatment team approach; including weekly individual therapy, a yearlong skills training class, telephone coaching and supportive supervision. Nevertheless, the rewards are priceless for both the therapist and client alike … it offers both hope and peace of mind and a gentler way out of chaos. DBT is a systematic, clinical package that integrates the technical and analytical strengths of behaviorism subtleties of Zen training, the warmth and acceptance of relationship centered therapies and the often undervalued power of psycho-education. Although more importantly than all, DBT has help gave these individuals back their lives. Dr. Linehan's name will undisputedly be recorded in histories books as being not only the most articulate advocate for the borderline diagnosed individual to ever emerge in the mental health field, but rather undoubtedly the first to ever exist.

Her inimitable ability to explain the borderline's inner world in terms that professionals and laypersons could understand makes her far more valuable to the borderline individuals, their therapist and to our world. In her writings, she clearly display to us that these individuals previously had no emotional skin that they had been raised in families where their hypersensitivity had been routinely discounted. Therefore, this had bred self-distrust and created within them a tendency that leads toward extremes and pervasive 'emotional behavioral, interpersonal and cognitive deregulation.'

Throughout her writings she also noted how therapy recapitulates the invalidating family environment, when it offers insulting interpretations, ignored cries of distress and inadvertently rewards emotional explosions or suicidality with extra attention. An example of such is of those seen in patients who are constantly on 1:1 observation, or frequent hospitalization. And that at its worst, therapy instead becomes 'iatrogenic,' or medical. This treatment approach also helped us to reconfigure the borderline diagnosis in the behaviorists, by placing it in a more humane term, thus undressing and ridding it from direct verdict, indignity, and shame. Her approach virtually places the diagnosis under a softer and more feminine light than her male predecessors, who reign in the realm of psychodynamic theorists during the last century. Otto Kernberg, James Masterson and John Gunderson, are a few who come to mind. They engaged in shaping and pessimistically damning the field with their views. She reminded us that borderline individuals have huge deficits in life skills and rather not deficient personalities. In an area where male psychoanalysts, had previously seen 'a constitutional excess of aggression, primitive thinking and manipulation,' she saw terror, stress related difficulties in cognitive processing and despair. She prompted that it was far more feasible to rather teach BPD, diagnosed individuals, better ways to manage their moods to cope with the world and therefore, help remind them to reduce their self-destructive behavior. Writings found while researching her widely popular, 1993, *Skills Training Manual* for Treating Borderline Personality Disorder. She also suggests and provided us with ways in how such new approaches could be accomplished. In these she handed us a wide blend of guidance toward assertiveness and mindfulness. Throughout her books we find deep, inspiring and spiritually uplifting, quotations written and made popular by the Vietnamese Buddhist monk, Thich Nhat Hanh and several other spiritual teachers.

Her straight forward approach type of language, so clearly written, the texts drew immediate attention and praises from conventional psychiatrists and psychologists schools alike. Therefore, gradually managing to convert those who otherwise would have dismissed any type of cognitive behavioral approach and remain ignorant to prayer, or meditation in any form. Although traditional clinicians throughout the years had been engaged in the application of the same old borderline diagnosis used for years, which had already proven to be rather blameful, nevertheless, Dr. Linehan came out of nowhere to rescue it from the blame-tradition and began describing it as an understandable response to the way in which these individuals grew up. Her standards gave patients great coping skills, meanwhile clinicians also benefited from it as well as her training organization of the Behavioral Technology Transfer Group. Since her 1991 article appeared in the psychiatric journal, her books published by the Guilford Press, have gone on to become professional bestsellers. An estimate of over 70,000 therapists throughout the world has purchased and used her books, which has since been translated into French, German, Italian, Dutch, Swedish, Spanish and soon to be translated into several other languages. At this point I do not yet have a clear estimate of numbers, but it is well in the tens of thousands of clinicians whom have attended introductory DBT trainings and more than 500 government and nonprofit agencies has since, provided intensive DBT training for their staffs. To feed our intellectual voracious curiosity, the name for this Dialectical Behavior Therapy treatment, is a reference to the philosophical proposition popularized by Immanuel Kant, Friedrich Hegel and Karl Marx. In essence, dialectics presumes that there are two sides to every coin. *Every extreme in thought and in the world calls forth its opposite and points the way to a synthesis or reconciliation. Though wide enough to cope with the paradox, dialectics sometimes simply holds contradictions in balance rather than integrating them ...* "You have to change, yet you are as perfect as you are." That is the essential dialectic of the treatment. DBT therapists, she says, should continually question themselves about "what they are leaving out as an important part of the treatment?" Under the DBT's broad umbrella stands a cluster of therapeutic tactics that require a head-spinning degree of gut honesty, self-assurance and flexibility from the therapists.

Dr. Marsha Linehan still teaches at the University of Washington. She studied Zen Buddhism with the German Benedictine monk, Willigis Jager. Her life's work with DBT consisted of confronting numerous challenges. Instead of confronting DBT, she broke down the borderline dilemma into bite-size pieces and resolved them one by one until her therapy included everything, including the bathroom cabinet and the kitchen. In order to stop current emergencies from overwhelming the attempts at the behavioral changes, the skills training class was later created, therefore hypothesizing the self-injury halted neurobiological cascades of unbearable feelings. The research also pointed toward delayed gratification and questioned of friends on how they have gotten through difficult times. The result lead to a handout on distress tolerance and simple tips for self-soothing and self-distraction, such as taking a bath, thinking of someone more miserable than ourselves, or lighting a candle and watching the flame.

Clients throughout the research also discovered that holding ice and letting it melt often quelled their urge to cut themselves and this too was incorporated and it all became part of skills training tips. Throughout her research, Dr. Linehan found that even those among her most competent looking clients, often did not know the basics of negotiating with others, or acting independent of current mood. Her syllabus later grew to include sections on interpersonal effectiveness and emotion regulation, observing current emotions, as well as acting despite of them. The therapeutic package became tightly organized, but nothing resolved the central paradox that had tripped her up in the early 1970s: the difficulty of maintaining a good therapy relationship and getting behavioral change at the same time. Then in 1986, when she was 42 and suffering from a dryness in her own spiritual life, Linehan impulsively took a year's leave of absence to train in Zen monasteries in California and Germany and then committed herself to following instructions, rather than given them and it was there in the monasteries, where Linehan meditated in solitude and found the spiritual grounds for the foundation of DBT.

Frequently Asked Questions, About DBT = DBT-S

A) DBT stands for Dialectical Behavior Therapy.

B) DBT was developed as an outpatient therapy for patients with Borderline Personality Disorder

C) DBT has now been adapted for use in inpatient residential and day treatment settings. What are the therapeutic modes of DBT?

D) Individual therapy that is focused on a list of treatment targets.

E) Skills training focused on helping patients learn new skills and replace the old, maladaptive skills.

F) In Real-time coaching to help patients use skills in particular situations.

G) Contingency management to use the power of reinforcement and punishment to help shape and maintain behavior.

What are the targets for treatment with DBT?

H) Developing and maintaining a commitment to treatment … decreasing parasuicidal and life threatening behaviors.

I) Decrease assaultive or destructive behavior.

J) Decreasing therapy interfering behavior.

K) Decreasing behavior that interferes with high quality of life.

L) Increasing adaptive, skillful behavior. What new skills do patients learn from DBT?

M) Core mindfulness skills which focuses primarily on taking hold of ones mind.

N) Interpersonal effectiveness skills, which focuses on dealing with other people.

O) Emotion regulation skills, which focuses on identifying modulating and dealing with the emotions.

P) Distress tolerance skills that focus on how to get through a crisis.

How is DBT adapted for an inpatient environment?

Q) Treatment targets may be modified to focus on behavior that causes or prolongs hospitalization.

R) The inpatient environment provides many opportunities for coaching patients on the use of skills, cheerleading when they do use their skills and consulting with the patient on how to handle issues that come up with other patients and staff.

S) Patients join the Skills Training groups at any place in the cycle of modules being taught.

T) There is increased emphasis on orientation and commitment strategies, since many patients are being introduced to DBT for the first time.

U) DBT-S is a treatment program that extends standard DBT to treat patients with BPD and substance abuse. ***How Does DBT-S Differ From The Standard DBT?***

V) Substance abuse behaviors are targeted earlier in the treatment. DBT-S includes new strategies for enhancing the patient's motivation to stay in treatment.

W) Specific skills on coping with urges and tendencies to abuse substances are taught in Skills

Training Groups Designed for DBT.

X) A new "case management" mode is added to the standard DBT modes of therapy.

Z1) A specific pharmacotherapy mode is added to the standard DBT modes of therapy.

Journey Spiritual Counseling. Theologians Suggested Guidelines To Counseling The Emotionally Ill From The Pulpit

Although throughout the years working with the mentally ill was seen as a responsibility only for psychiatry and the psychological communities ... In recent years, theologians, Christians and faith counselors, have since emerge and have shown through research that counseling the emotionally and mentally ill spiritually, also have great benefits. Although, mental health remains primarily of special psychological and psychiatric concern, they've suggested that a combined approach between the highly skilled psychiatric, psychological and theological fields, could perhaps bring out even better results. Studies have shown that it is a team effort, in which all concerned individuals play a vital role.

Christian, Jews, Muslims and all other spiritual counselors can also offer untold help. They have in fact demonstrated in many cases shared responsibility and successful result, which has stemmed from a privilege and duty in their lives as faith healers, while visiting and helping the individual who suffers with mental distress.

Faith Healers Suggested 9 talents to helping.

All spiritual counselors should first pause and recognize their limitations. When a case is beyond their training and their ability, they should refer their counselee to another specialist such as a medical doctor, clinician, therapist, psychologist or a psychiatrist. "For no one counselor is competent enough to handle all cases placed before them." It is a sign of maturity when a counselor knows they are not capable of making all of the necessary diagnosis and is therefore willing to refer a client to one who maybe better suited to meet that individual's particular needs. And step aside!

1) To accept the individual's illness as their natural condition:

Whenever talking with an individual whom is suffering emotionally or is mentally ill, one must first realize that their behavior is caused by their illness. What they do and how they think, is primarily a natural outgrowth of what is going on in their lives. If a counselor could obtain an accurate mental picture of the individual's inner self and grasp all of their experiences entering their lives through such illness, they would then realize that the individual's behavior, fits their life pattern. If you could know their true physical condition, you would readily understand why they think, talk, react and why their thought process, functioning is as such. Although as a counselor you may immediately not have all of the information, and perhaps neither would their physician have all of the facts, however, it is recommended that you conduct yourself on the basis that there are real causes for their illness and therefore their behaviors. A positive attitude, and being well informed, could avoid and therefore prevent us from being overly perplexed and confused, about the experiences through which they now deal. In return, we will be far more at ease and relaxed if the client could also sense your understanding and therefore produce a more positive result.

2) To refrain from arguing with a person whom is seriously disturbed:

An argument form a counselor, is a rather emphatic way of telling the client that we cannot accept their behavior and that we aren't quite ready to accept them as they are. The client's already senses their differences from the norm, hence when confronting or disagreeing with them, arguably it only serves their rapid withdrawal. It therefore, destroys any trust we might have gained, rapidly pushing them into further isolation. Though as rational, or scene individuals, it is rather natural to argue, when we talk with someone whom does not understand our point. In fact, it may often be the only way to make them clearly see the light. However, in the case of the mentally ill individuals, argumentation will not change their attitudes. Discounting their feelings offers no solution and disagreements, breaks bonds of confidence and friendship. In many cases, it does little good to argue, with a person who is well and therefore much less with one whom is suffering from mental illness. They already senses that they might be seriously troubled, they expect you to help them out. Furthermore that you, their counselor, someone whom they've since considered to be a so-called friend also does not understands them, is might be a lot more than they could bear.

3) To encourage the clients to express themselves:

We must first keep in mind that the first step toward their recovery, starts with their voicing how they feel. We could perhaps remind them that talking things out, is just another way of thinking things over. Hence, therefore, think as we talk. In talking, we clarify our feelings, as we seek new directions throughout life. One of the best recommendations the experts have indicated, is to encourage the client to talk, to reflect on what they just told you, and to ask them to further elaborate. An example of these could be used, when the client tells you "I feel terrible. Sometimes I feel like I would like to die." Your professional reflection, could then be the following. "Do you feel sometimes that life is not worth living?" One of my favorite, was to promptly ask a client. "Which part of you really wants to die?" Though it is a bit outdated, but it usually engaged them into conversation and often times, brought them back to a present state of mind. This last one, however, is built on trust. You must have first developed some sort of therapeutic ease, prior to attempting such intervention. Client must also be in a kind of relaxed state of mind.

These responses, naturally leaves an open door for them to make a broader statement. They may in fact even say something like, "well sometimes I don't feel so badly, but sometimes I just feel terrible!" You might even encourage them to continue talking by simply saying, "at this time you're feeling better, but sometimes you don't." they might be likely to volunteer further information by using an effective technique. Again, all of these approaches, are primarily built on trust. The clients, would then also feel that they are free to talk about the things that are bothering their minds and might soon discover other hidden feelings, currently affecting their lives. Discourage them from talking about other people and any gossip, pauses are also very important. It is not necessary to keep the conventional ball rolling all the time. A person dealing with mental illness, often need some silent moments to think about things. They might take long pauses to breath and then they would reinitiate their conversation. Patience, then becomes an extremely important gift for counselor.

4) To not always expect that persons dealing with mentally illness, will respond to us in a "normal fashion." If police departments throughout the America were to understand this concept, implement it in their training, and follow such protocol, life would be much easier for individuals in our communities with mental illness, for taxpayers and for the police officers themselves.

As counselors, we must keep in mind that the strange responses of individuals suffering from mental illness, is rather a clear indication that they are not doing well. So, if their answers and ideas seem to be unusual accept them as they are. If they pay little attention to you, you must then realize that this is normal for a person in this condition. After they begin to get well, they will react more enthusiastically to your visits. Often times, we've seen the unexperienced clergy, or clueless lay persons visiting patients in hospitals, whom are not doing well, hence they do not receive a cordial or normal reception, and they do not return. Unfortunately, this indicates that such people do not understand the nature of mental illness. When counselors visit someone that is ill in a psychiatric setting, they cannot expect the same normal reactions, as if when visiting a person whom is mentally well or dealing with mere physical complaints. Ministers, clergy, church members, parishioners, via church committee, perhaps need to designate a family member, or church person knowledgeable in pastoral care, or someone whom has the best approach with the individual and perhaps become acquainted with hospital policies, regarding visits, a) call the psychiatric unit and ask for the clients primary care persons, stability, ability to entertain visits, etc. .

5) Implement the reassurance approach by reassuring the patient that they will get welt.

Some patients whom are mentally ill and suffering another relapse, may tend to believe their recovery is impossible. Therefore, the simple act of expressing confidence and reassurance toward their getting well, counselor helps becomes rather immeasurably, this could often mean the difference between hope and despair. One of the best fortifiers of health is encouragement. It is like a balm to our soul. Encouragement also serves as healing remedy, when a client realizes that others have suffered from the same sort of difficulty and that they have recovered completely. Pastoral Counselors need to reassure the mentally ill persons that undoubtedly they will, in time, feel much better. A well versed counselor should be able to share his encouragement with confidence, since countless research resources has shown that most mentally ill people do recover with proper treatment.

6) To show genuine concern and interest in the person.

Sometimes we make the mistake of not telling people how much we really do care about them, and how much God cares about us. As theological counselors, it is rather important that we do this, when first arriving and right before leaving. This is especially needed when dealing with those whom are suffering with mentally illness. We should also do this, when visiting friends suffering with mental illness of this type, we should let him know we are interested in them, in their health and that we do care. In fact, this might help to counteract the unbearable isolation, which they may currently be experiencing. We should also use gentle remarks as, "we've certainly been missing you, Dorothy. All of your friends at church are praying for you, and we are all anxious to see you well again," bring much encouragement. Make certain to call them by their first name. It is also important that you reminded them about their coworkers and colleagues, whom might have perhaps asked about them. Important that you may talk to them about your friendships, about your friends, your job, and about your family, when you visiting them. This offers them an important bond that they will cherish from one visit to another.

7) To try encouraging them to follow their treatment as indicated.

People receiving impatient psychiatric care, sometimes grow to dislike their doctors. They may become discouraged, feel-that the doctors and nurses are not doing all they should be doing for them. They may even transfer their hostilities from family members or from others to their physicians. It is your responsibility as a Christian counselor, as a theological visitor as clergy, to help the patient gain more confidence in those who are clinically treating them. Try encouraging them to express themselves, while at the same time reassuring them that their doctors, are doing the best they can and that they do have an interest in their wellbeing. Sometimes patients tend to blame their doctors for their being hospitalized. These resentments can be very deep. Therefore, your encouragement as a counselor, fellow church member and a friend to follow their doctor's orders, will help that ill person to place more confidence in those whom are treating them. Try being sensitive to their needs and to the demands you might want to place on someone who is mentally ill.

Often times, some Christian and spiritual counselors do not feel content unless they leave a sick person's room, having assigned considerable amounts of reading materials. As an effective counselor, you must refrain from doing such. We must first keep in mind that an ill person may not be up to this. They may just want rest ... they're unable to tax themselves to the extent of picking up books and reading. During each visit we might instead want to read to them from the Bible or from a chosen book. Although we might instead just want to stick to current events that are pleasing, not political, not frustrating, neither stressful. You might ask things like, "I'd like to share a wonderful portion of God's Word with you and I thought you might like to hear it." Your reading will help to bring comfort. The Scriptures could mean much to them and help with a much quicker recovery. It is also recommended that as counselors, we must be discreet in the use of scriptures. God's true Words are very important to those whom are mentally ill, but remember that they may not be able to absorb too much at one time. So when you are visiting one who is mentally ill, use only a few verses at a time. Continue to repeat them as the months go bye. A man who had been in a mental institution, once ask his pastor, visiting him at the time, "if he had ever had the experience of being mentally ill?" The pastor replied, "no." The man then said. "Let me just give you a word of advice. When counseling the mentally ill, don't throw the whole Bible at them just give, them only a verse or two at a time, then keep using the same scripture week after week." As he continued, "while I was hospitalized, there were groups that came to visit our unit and they used too much scripture. They got us all confused." He was right! We've seen so many ministers and theological counselors, visiting the mentally ill and deciding to set up church on a psychiatric ward. While most patients, aren't really ready for long sermons. The patients I have talk to about this, in fact do prefer only a few verses of scripture, rather than large portions. This simple plan of repetition, is not overwhelming and it leaves a single spiritual impact. Besides, too much could also be disruptive to other patients on these unit, whom do not understand, do not want to be bothered, currently in distress and would rather it be quiet.

8) To use devotional materials wisely, when counseling

If a mentally ill person feels well enough to read, there are Jewish, Islamic, Buddhist and Christ-centered devotional materials, which could help them. The *Moody Colportage* series and spiritual journals, there are also a number of excellent books. Try focusing primarily on devotional materials that are short and easy to read. Try using materials that are from the heart and those that brings new hope and victory to those whom are disturbed. All who counsel with the emotionally and mentally ill should also visit Christian and spiritual bookstores pertinent to their beliefs and carefully select materials that are especially suited. In addition to reading materials, splendid devotions are available on recordings. These combine music Scripture speaking, poems and prayers in combination are ideal for those who are not well. Try to emphasize God's love and comfort. The greatest comfort is God's comfort. *God is the author of all love and mercy. As much as people may care for one another, in a Christian faith, human love never equal God's love.* When people are mentally ill, they sometimes feel that God has forgotten them. So when you visit them, tell them about God's love. Give them Scripture verses as, *"Casting all your care upon them, through a creator whom careth for us."* Let them know that God is truly interested in them.

9) To try not to cut your visits too short.

People who are ill do not like to be rushed. So give them enough time. This tells them that you are genuinely interested and that they are worthy of your love and respect. It also allows sufficient time to talk things out. This added time will help them share their true feelings. Patience on your part, will help you gain a better standing of them, thus contribute to a faster recovery. Mental illness can strike anyone, anywhere and at any time. It is not only the Christian counselor's duty but his privilege to visit and counsel the mentally ill. Recall once overhearing a former patient wisely advising his friends, "Your visits and true understanding may very well mean the difference between my recovery and the further prolonged of my illness."

CHAPTER VI

Defining Anxiety Disorders (Such spectrum could be easily defined as follows)
Listed Associated Disorders To MDD (Major Depressing Disorders)
Defense Mechanisms
The Stages
The Oedipal Crisis
Freud's Therapy
Dialogue
What Are The Positive Aspects of Freud's Theory

Defining Anxiety Disorders

The spectrum of anxiety disorders could be easily defined as follows …

Anxiety = Symptom +Definition = Fear.

History of anxiety disorders, atypical depression, hyperventilation DaCosta's syndrome, hypochondriacal, neurosis, hysterical neurosis, etc.

Autonomic Nervous System: Sympathetic = *Flight \ Fight*

Parasympathetic = *Feed \ Breed*

The psychological symptoms of anxiety could easily be found within the following categories: *anxiousness, impatience, tense, edgy, fear, alarm, panic, mental disintegration, etc.*

The cognitive symptoms of anxiety are as follows:

Impaired attention, frightening visual images, poor concentration, forgetfulness, blocking of thoughts, injury, decreased perceptual field, ruminations, and hyper-vigilance.

Stages of Anxiety: *mild anxiety, moderate anxiety and severe anxiety, panic.*

Types of Anxiety: *Acute stress disorder, generalized anxiety, panic disorder, anxiety disorder due to a medical condition, substance induced anxiety disorder, panic disorder, panic with or without agoraphobia, agoraphobia without history of panic.*

Avoidant Anxieties: *Specific phobia, social phobia, obsessive-compulsive disorder, posttraumatic stress disorder.*

Listed Associated Disorders to MDD

Major Depressing Disorders

Panic disorder without agoraphobia, panic disorder with agoraphobia, agoraphobia without history of panic disorder, specific phobia, social phobia, obsessive-compulsive disorder, posttraumatic stress disorder, acute stress disorder, generalized anxiety disorder, anxiety disorder due to a general medical condition, substance-induced anxiety disorder and anxiety disorder not otherwise specified. Because panic attacks and agoraphobia occur in the context of several of these disorders, criteria sets for a panic attack and agoraphobia were listed separately at the beginning of this section.

A panic attack is a discrete period in which there is the sudden onset of intense apprehension, fearfulness, or terror often associated with feelings of impending doom. During these attacks, symptoms such as shortness of breath, palpitations, chest pain or discomfort, choking or smothering sensations and fear of "going crazy" or losing control are always present. *Agoraphobia* is in reality an anxiety about, or avoidance of places or situations from which escape might be difficult or even embarrassing, or perhaps of being in a place, in which help may not be available in the event of having a panic attack or panic-like symptoms.

Panic Disorder without Agoraphobia is characterized by recurrent unexpected panic attacks about which there is persistent concern.

Panic Disorder with Agoraphobia is characterized by both recurrent unexpected panic attacks and agoraphobia.

Agoraphobia without the history of panic disorder is characterized by the presence of agoraphobia and panic-like symptoms, without a history of unexpected panic attacks.

A specific phobia: is characterized by clinically significant anxiety provoked by exposure to a specific feared object or situation, often leading to avoidance behavior.

A Social Phobia: is characterized by clinically significant anxiety provoked by exposure to certain types of social or performance situations, often leading to avoidance behavior.

Obsessive-compulsive disorder: is characterized by obsessions, which cause marked anxiety or distress and/or by compulsions (which serve to neutralize anxiety).

Posttraumatic Stress Disorder: is characterized by the re-experiencing of an extremely traumatic event accompanied by symptoms of increased arousal and by avoidance of stimuli associated with the trauma.

Acute Stress Disorder: is characterized by symptoms similar to those of posttraumatic stress disorder that occur immediately in the aftermath of an extremely traumatic event.

Generalized Anxiety Disorder is: characterized by at least 6 months of persistent and excessive anxiety and worry.

Anxiety Disorder Due to a General Medical Condition: is characterized by prominent symptoms of anxiety that are judged to be a direct physiological consequence of a general medical condition.

Substance Induced Anxiety Disorder: is characterized by prominent symptoms of anxiety that are judged to be a direct physiological consequence of a drug or abuse of a medication, or toxin exposure.

Anxiety Disorder Otherwise Not Specified: is included for coding disorders with prominent anxiety or phobic avoidance that do not meet criteria for any of the specific anxiety disorders defined in this section or anxiety symptoms about which there is inadequate or contradictory information. Because *Separation Anxiety Disorder,* which is characterized by anxiety related to separation from parental figures usually developed during childhood. It is included in the "disorders usually first diagnosed in infancy, childhood or adolescence." Phobic avoidance that is limited to genital sexual contact with a sexual partner, is classified as *sexual aversion disorder* and is included in the *"sexual and gender identity disorders." Anxiety* "life is not easy!" The ego the 'I' sits at the center of some pretty powerful forces: *in reality, society is represented by the superego and biology is represented by the id.* When these make conflicting demands upon the poor ego, it is understandable that you will feel threatened, fell overwhelmed and that you will feel as if you are about to collapse under the weight of it all. This feeling is called anxiety and it serves as a signal to the alert and also to protect the ego. It is its survival and the survival of the whole organism when it's in jeopardy.

Throughout his writings, Freud mentions three different kinds of anxieties: The first being realistic anxiety, the kind you and I calls fear. Actually Freud did too, although he did it in German, but his translators thought the word fear was too mundane. However, if you were pushed into an alligator's pond, I believe you might definitely experience a great deal of realistic anxiety, don't you think?

The second is moral anxiety. This is what we feel when the threat comes not from the outer physical world, but from the internalized social world of the superego. It is in fact just another word for feelings like shame and guilt, and the fear of punishment.

The third is neurotic anxiety. This is the fear of being overwhelmed by impulses from the id. If you have ever felt like you were about to lose control of your temper, your rationality, or even your mind, you have felt neurotic anxiety. The word *neurotic* actually means in Latin *nervous,* so this is nervous anxiety. It is this kind of anxiety that intrigued Freud the most, though we usually just call it anxiety, plain and simple.

Defense Mechanisms

The ego deals with the demands of reality, when placed on the id and the superego as best as it can. But when the anxiety becomes overwhelming, the ego must defend itself. It does so by unconsciously blocking the impulses, or distorting them into a more acceptable and less threatening form … 'these techniques are called ego defense mechanisms.'

Denial involves blocking external events from awareness.

Listed are some real life descriptions of how they actually work:

If a situation is just too much to handle, the persons automatically refuses to experience it. As one might imagine, this is a primitive and dangerous defense, no one disregards reality and gets away with it for long. This mechanism can operate by itself or more commonly in combination with other more subtle mechanisms that supports it.

Several years ago, while working as a case manager in a state run community base program one of our clients committed suicide. Throughout the last seven years prior to his unfortunate untimely death, I had work closely with him and came to know him rather well. From the day of his first admission to the state hospital in Middletown, Connecticut, I was assigned to his case as a translator and had aided him in a number of legal, financial and therapeutic services, between him, his psychiatrist and different other advocate outlets in a span of about seven years. Throughout most of this critical time, I was one of the only bilingual mental health workers employed at the hospital and had become pretty much his legal, and therapeutic lifeline. In the last weeks prior to his committing suicide, his treatment had become critical, as he grew clinically depressed, had been refusing medications and essential treatment. On this particular evening after returning from a recreational activity, basketball in hand, he passed by me as he walked into the office, I greeted him, and he did not respond. I thought nothing about it. "Some patients tend to shut the world off when they are depressed." He had been angry with his therapist and of course with me because I was transferring him over to his new therapist and was perhaps, viewed as an extension to his problems. He came in and returned the basketball and walked right back out the office without saying anything to me, or to anyone else. About ten minutes later, we heard a hurried knock by someone at the office door. When I opened it, there was a woman standing her voice shaking, trembling telling us that "one of your clients just jumped off the roof." This young man had just left the office, headed right up to the roof and plunged himself four floors head-first on to the asphalt and on to his death. I immediately ran down and my first instinct was an attempt to initiate cardio pulmonary resuscitation (CPR), though as I got closer to him, I realized it was impossible.

His scull had been completely crushed due to the impact on the pavement he also had several fractured bones shooting out his skin from all four limbs. Vas number sharp points off of the broken bones, were visibly protruding through torn skin, all throughout his body. The paramedics had already been called and they arrived shortly after. I provided them with all the needed data and assisted with hooking up the resuscitation devices. While my colleague, though terribly affected attempted to follow emergency procedure by collecting charts, head count and initiating to proceed with debriefing and counseling the other fifteen clients. As program protocol, dictated, I later went around the building with a Mobil Crisis psychologist, debriefing and talking with several other tenants who'd appeared emotionally affected. My struck colleague and I worked throughout that evening, completing our shift, almost as if it was business as usual. Nevertheless, the following morning, it was a whole different experience. I felt dispirited, angry, guilty, insignificant, stupid, drained, etc. It appeared as if all of my emotions had suddenly come down on me like a Mack truck loaded with tons of bricks.

I then shed a few tears and refused to eat, my sleep was also interrupted. I then realized that I had to eventually pull myself together, if I were to be of any good to the rest of the clients, whom depended on us, and on our program to keep them safe. I took two additional days off from work and spent the time taking my home-recording studio asunder, cleaned each piece of equipment, while I blasted and sang to the beat of my favorite reggae tunes. Realizing perhaps that I had done all that was humanly possible. That was my defense mechanism at its best.

By the following Monday, I was able to reluctantly tolerate and deal with it somewhat better, and move-on … Only then I was able to understand his death by taking a professional standpoint, rather than making it personal. I have since noted and observed little children sort of glancing over, when confronted by circumstances they rather not be confronted with. I have also since researched and studied case studies about people fainting at the site of autopsies being performed. People have been known to deny the reality of the death of a loved one, we also hear about students who have been known to fail to pick up their test results for fear; this is denial 101.

Repression, also called '*motivated forgetting,* 'is just that. Not being able to recall a grim situation, person, or event, is also dangerous and it plays a great part in most of our other defenses. As a pet lover and myself owner of three cats, I have heard of and seen people with a rather strong fear of cats, especially long-haired cats, like my Persian and my Himalayan. A friend whom I wasn't aware she suffered from such fears came to visit me one evening and of course my very friendly cat ran down the stairs to greet her. He was innocently running up to her and she took off running; she tripped, skinned her arms and her knees, and almost broke her legs. She was crying in hysterics and it wasn't from the fall, but rather from the fear ... though I had already put my cats in a room and closed the door behind them. Several months later she told me about a dream she'd been having and that she was seeking professional counseling for. She told me they were helping her to get over her fears with a technique called *systematic desensitization,* though she still had no idea where this fear had come from. Several years later, I saw her again

and again she brought up this dream thing. This time I paid close attention and listened. She explained how this particular dream, clearly involved her getting locked up in her grandmother's basement by some older cousins when she was very young. The basement was small, dark and had unfinished dirt floors covered with fresh cut sheep wool and they would throw their neighbors four long-haired cats in there with her and lock the door. According to the Freudian analogy and understanding of this phobia is that: She had repressed a traumatic event the cats and sheep wool incident, but seeing long hair cats aroused the anxiety of the event without arousing the memory. Other common examples of these phobias are: "A young girl guilty about her rather strong sexual desires tend to forget her boy-friend's name, even when trying to introduce him to her relatives and friends." Or "an alcoholic is unable to remember his suicide attempt and claims to have blacked out." Or perhaps someone almost drowns as a child, but is unable to remember the event even when people try reminding them of it, but they do have a fear of open water. Note: *to be a true example of a defense, it should function unconsciously.*

My son had a fear of dogs, when he was a little boy, but there is no defense involved. He was bitten by one as a child and wants very badly not to relive the experience. Usually, it is the irrational fears we call phobias that derive from repression of traumas.

Asceticism, or the renunciation of needs is one, which most people haven't heard of, but it has become relevant with the emergence of the disorder called anorexia. Pre-adolescents when they feel threatened by their emerging sexual desires may unconsciously try to protect themselves by denying not only their sexual desires, but also all desires. They get involved in some kind of *ascetic monk-like lifestyle* wherein they renounce their interest in what other people enjoy. In boys nowadays, there is a great deal of interest in the self-discipline of the martial arts. Fortunately martial arts don't hurt you as much, in fact, they may actually help you.

Unfortunately, girls in our society often develop a great deal of interest in attaining excessively and artificially thin standard of beauty. In Freudian theory, their denial of their need for food is actually a cover for their denial of their sexual development. Our society conspires with them. After all, what most societies considered a normal figure for a mature woman is considered in ours a 20 - 30 pound overweight.

Isolation, which is also known as intellectualization, involves stripping the emotion from a difficult memory or threatening impulse. A person may in a very cavalier manner acknowledge that they had been abused as a child, or my show a purely intellectual curiosity in their newly discovered sexual orientation. Something what should be a big deal is treated as if it were not. In emergency situations, many people find themselves, completely calm and collected until the emergency is over, at which point they fall to pieces. Something tells you that during the emergency, you can't afford to fall apart. It is common to find someone totally immersed in the social obligations surrounding the death of a loved one. Doctors and nurses must learn to separate their natural reactions to blood, wounds, needles and scalpels, and treat the patient, temporarily, as something less than a warm, wonderful human being with friends and family. Adolescents often go through a stage where they are obsessed with horror movies, perhaps to come to grips with their own fears. Nothing demonstrates isolation more clearly than a theater full of people laughing hysterically, while someone is shown being dismembered.

Displacement is the redirection of an impulse onto a substitute target. If the impulse, or desire is okay with you, but the person you direct that desire towards is too threatening, you can displace it to someone or something that can serve as a symbolic substitute. Someone who hates his or her mother, may repress that hatred, but direct it instead towards women in general. Someone who has not had the chance to love someone may substitute cats or dogs for human beings. Someone who feels uncomfortable with their sexual desire for a real person may substitute such with a fetish. Someone who is frustrated by his or her superiors may go home and kick the dog, or beat up a family member, or engage in cross-burnings and racial slurs. Turning against the self is a very special form of displacement, where the person becomes his or her own substitute target. It is normally used in reference to hatred, anger, and aggression, rather than more positive impulses and it is the Freudian explanation for many of our feelings of inferiority, guilt, and depression. The idea that depression is often the result of the anger we refuse to acknowledge, is indeed accepted by many people, Freudians and non-Freudians alike.

Projection, which Anna Freud also called displacement outward, is almost the complete opposite of turning against oneself. It involves the tendency to see your own unacceptable desires in other people. In other words, the desires are still there, but they're not your desires anymore. We should be aware that whenever we hear someone going on and on about how aggressive everybody is, or how perverted they all are one ought to wonder if this person doesn't have an aggressive or sexual streak within themselves that they'd rather not acknowledge. Here are a couple of live examples: A husband, a good and faithful one, finds himself terribly attracted to the charming and flirtatious lady next door. But rather than acknowledge his own, hardly abnormal, lusts, he becomes increasingly jealous of his wife, constantly worried about her faithfulness, and so on. Or a woman finds herself having vaguely sexual feelings about her girlfriends. Instead of acknowledging those feelings as quite normal, she becomes increasingly concerned with the presence of lesbians in her community.

Altruism surrender is a form of projection that at first glance looks like its opposite: Here, the person attempts to fulfill his or her own needs vicariously, through other people. A common example of this is the friend, of one who while not seeking any relationship themselves, is constantly pushing other people into them and is particularly curious as to the 'what happened between you and your date last night' and 'concerned about how are things going between you and?' The extreme example of *altruistic surrender,* is the person who lives their entire life for and/or through another. Like some parents who've place their entire savings toward their child's college, wedding, purchases them their first home and then expects to live the young couple's lives.

Reaction formation, also known as *believing the opposite,* is changing an unacceptable impulse, into its opposite. So, a child angry with his or her mother may become overly concerned with her and rather dramatically shower her with affection. An abused child may run to the abusing parent. Or someone who can't accept a homosexual impulse may claim to despise homosexuals. Perhaps the most common and clearest example of reaction formation is found in children between seven and eleven or so: Most boys will tell you in no uncertain terms how disgusting girls are and girls will tell you with equal vigor how gross boys are. Adults watching their interactions, however, can tell quite easily what their true feelings really are.

Undoing, involves *magical* gestures or rituals that are meant to cancel out unpleasant thoughts or feelings after they have already occurred. Anna Freud mentions for example, a boy who would recite the alphabet backwards whenever he had a sexual thought, or turn around and spit whenever meeting another boy who shared his passion for masturbation. In 'normal' people, the undoing is, of course, more conscious and we might engage in an act of atonement for some behavior, or formally ask for forgiveness. But in some people, the act of atonement isn't conscious at all. Consider the alcoholic father who after a year of verbal and perhaps physical abuse, puts on the best and biggest Christmas party ever for his kids. When the season is over, and the kids haven't quite been fooled by his magical gesture, he returns to his bartender with complaints about how ungrateful his family is and how they drove him to drink. One of the classic examples of undoing concerns personal hygiene following sex: It is perfectly reasonable to wash up after sex. After all it can get messy! But if you feel the need to take three or four complete showers using gritty soap, perhaps sex just doesn't quite agree with you.

Introjections sometimes called *identification,* involves taking on the personality and characteristics of someone else, because by doing so, might aid in solving some emotional difficulty. For example, a child who is left alone frequently may in some way try to become "mom" in order to lessen his or her fears. You can sometimes catch them telling their dolls or animals not to be afraid. And we find the older child or teenager imitating his or her favorite star, musician, or sports hero in an effort to establish an identity. A more unusual example is that of a women whom husband, dies and she begins to wear his clothes, albeit neatly tailored to her figure. She then began to take up some of his habits, such as smoking a pipe. Although the neighbors might find it strange and even referred to her as *the man-woman,* she might not be suffering from any confusion about her sexual identity. In fact, she might even remarry and still retain to the end her men's suits and pipe routine. Identification was very important to Freudian theory as the mechanism geared in the developing of superegos. Identification with the aggressor is a version of introjections that focuses on the adoption, not of general or positive traits, but of negative or feared traits. If you are afraid of someone, you can partially conquer that fear by becoming more like them. This could be seen in the classic gangster movies and in the patterns of young gang members who fear their leaders, only to later engage in wiping them out to take control. A more dramatic example is the one called the Stockholm syndrome. After a hostage crisis in Stockholm, psychologists were surprised to find that the hostages were not only not terribly angry with their captors, but also often downright sympathetic. A more recent case-study is that of Patty Hearst, of the wealthy and influential Hearst's family. She was captured by a very small group of self-proclaimed revolutionaries called the Symbionese Liberation Army. She was kept in closets, raped and otherwise mistreated. Yet she apparently decided to join them, making little propaganda videos for them and even waving a machine gun around during a bank robbery. When she was later tried, psychologists strongly suggested that she was a victim, not a criminal.

Nevertheless, she was convicted of bank robbery and sentenced to 7 years in prison. President Carter, however, then commuted her sentence, after 2 years. Introjections might have been perhaps the same rationalization attorneys for the defense of John Walker Lynd, the 'so called' *American Taliban* consider using when explaining his taking up arms against the United States.

Regression is a movement back in psychological time when one is faced with stress. When we are troubled or frightened, our behaviors often become more childish or primitive. A child may begin to suck their thumb again or wet their bed when they need to spend some time in the hospital. Teenagers may giggle uncontrollably when introduced into a social situation involving the opposite sex. A freshman college student may need to bring an old toy from home, or sleep with their favorite stuffed animal. A gathering of civilized people may become a violent mob when they are led to believe their livelihoods are at stake. Or an older man, after spending twenty years at a company and now finding himself laid off, may retire to his recliner and become childishly dependent on his wife. Many of us could still remember widely televised news pictures of the Reverend James Baker crouched into a fetal position. Although some might argue about it being his trump card in a sympathy search game. Where do we retreat when faced with stress? To the last time in life when we felt safe and secure, according to Freudian theory.

Rationalization is the cognitive distortion of "the facts" to make an event or an impulse less threatening. We do it often enough on a fairly conscious level when we provide ourselves with excuses. But for many people with sensitive egos making excuses comes so easy that they never are truly aware of it. In other words, many of us are quite prepared to believe our lies. Even though, sometimes they may come across as delusions of grandeur. A useful way of understanding the defenses is to see them as a combination of denial or repression, with various kinds of rationalizations. All defenses are of course "lies," even if we are not conscious of making them. But that doesn't make them less dangerous, in fact it makes them more so.

As your grandma may have told you, "Oh what a tangled web we weave …" Lies breed lies and tend to take us further and further away from the truth and from reality. After a while the ego can no longer take care of the id's demands, or pay attention to the superegos. The anxieties come rushing back and then you break down and might even lash out in their defenses. And yet Freud saw defenses as necessary. You can hardly expect a person … especially a child to take the pain and sorrow of life full on. While some of his followers suggested that all of the defenses could be used positively, Freud himself suggested that there was one positive defense, which he called sublimation.

Sublimation is the transforming of an unacceptable impulse, whether it is sex, anger, fear, or whatever, into a socially acceptable or even productive form. So someone with a great deal of hostility may become a hunter, a butcher, a football player, or a mercenary. A good example of this could be taken back to the days of the Romans and the triumph of the victory of slaves turn Gladiators in the arenas. Someone suffering from a great deal of anxiety in a confusing world may become an organizer, a businessperson, or a scientist. Someone with powerful sexual desires may become an artist, a photographer, or a novelist, and so on. For Freud, in fact, all positive, creative activities were sublimations, and predominantly of the sex drive.

The Stages

As we have seen early on while studying Freud, we realized that for Freud, the sex drive is the most important motivating force. In fact, Freud felt it was the primary motivating force not only for adults but also for children and even infants. When he introduced his ideas about infantile sexuality to the Viennese public of his day, they were hardly prepared to talk about sexuality in adults, much less in infants. It is true that the capacity for orgasm is there neurologically from birth, but Freud was not just talking about orgasm.

To Freud, sexuality meant not only sexual intercourse, rather all pleasurable sensation our skin experiences such as touch, caresses, kisses, and so on. Freud noted that at different times in our lives, different parts of our skin give us greatest pleasures. In later years, theorists would call these areas erogenous zones. It appeared to Freud that the infant found its greatest pleasure in sucking, especially at the breast. In fact, babies have a penchant for bringing nearly everything in their environment into contact with their mouths. A bit later in life, the child focuses on the anal pleasures of holding it in and letting go. By three or four, the child may have discovered the pleasure of touching or rubbing against his or her genitalia. Only later in our sexual maturity do we find our greatest pleasure in sexual intercourse. In these observations, Freud had the makings of a psychosexual stage theory. The oral stage lasts from birth to about 18 months. The focus of pleasure is of course the mouth. Sucking and biting are our favorite activities. The anal stage lasts from about 18 months to three or four years old. The focus of pleasure is the anus. Holding it in and letting it go, are greatly enjoyed.

The phallic stage usually lasts from three or four to five, six, or even seven years old. The focus of pleasure is the genitalia. Masturbation is common. The latent stage lasts from five, six, or seven to puberty that is somewhere around 12 years old. During this stage, Freud believed that the sexual impulse was suppressed in the service of learning. I must note that while most children seem to be fairly calm, sexually, during their grammar school years, perhaps up to a quarter of them are quite busy masturbating and playing 'doctor, nurses, etc.' In Freud's repressive era, these children were at least quieter than their modern counterparts.

The genital stage begins at puberty and represents the resurgence of the sex drive in adolescence although focusing more specifically of pleasures received in sexual intercourse. Freud felt that masturbation, oral sex, homosexuality and many other things we find acceptable in adulthood today, were immature. This is a true stage theory, meaning that Freudians believe that we all go through these stages in this order, or that we're pretty close to these ages.

The Oedipal Crisis

According to Freud, each stage has certain difficult tasks associated with it, where problems are more likely to arise. For the oral stage, this is weaning. For the anal stage, it is potty training. For the phallic stage, it is the oedipal crisis, named after the ancient Greek story of king Oedipus, who inadvertently killed his father and married his mother. Here is how the oedipal crisis works, according to Freud's theory: The first love-object for all of us is our mother. We want her attention, we want her affection, we want her caresses, and we want her in a broadly sexual way. The young boy, however, has a rival for his mother's charm, 'his father' His father is bigger, stronger, smarter, and also he gets to sleep with mother, while junior pines away in his lonely little bed. Dad is the enemy. About the time the little boy recognizes this archetypal situation, he has become aware of some of the more subtle differences between boys and girls, the ones other than hair length and clothing styles. From his naive perspective, the difference is that he has a penis and girls do not. At this point in life it seems to the child that having something is infinitely better than not having something and so he is pleased with this state of affairs.

But the question arises, *where is the girl's penis?* Perhaps she has lost it somehow; perhaps it was cut off. Perhaps this could happen to him. According to Freud's theory, this is the beginning of castration anxiety, a slight misnomer for the fear of losing one's penis. To return to the story, the boy, recognizing his father's superiority and fearing for his penis, engages some of his ego defenses: He displaces his sexual impulses from his mother to girls and later to women, and he identifies with the aggressor, 'his dad' then attempts to become more and more like him that is to say, a man. After a few years of latency, he enters adolescence and the world of mature heterosexuality. The girl also begins her life in love with her mother, so we have the problem of getting her to switch her affections to her father before the Oedipal process can take place. Freud accomplishes this with the idea of penis envy. The young girl too has noticed the difference between boys and girls and feels that she somehow doesn't measure up. She would like to have one too and all the power associated with it. At the very least, she would like a penis substitute, such as a baby. As every child knows, you need a father as well as a mother to have a baby, so the young girl sets her sights on dad, but dad, of course, is already taken. The young girl displaces from him to boys and men, and identifies with mom, the woman, who got the man she really wanted. Note that one thing is missing here. The girl does not suffer from the powerful motivation of castration anxiety, since she cannot lose what she doesn't have. Freud felt that the lack of this great fear accounts for fact (as he saw it) that women were both less firmly heterosexual than men and even somewhat less morally inclined.

Do not rush to conclusions just yet and before you get too upset by this less-than-flattering account of women's sexuality, rest assured that many people have responded to it. I recommend you ask questions and do your research, sit with a group of women and ask about all the specifics. *Freud felt that traumatic experiences had an especially strong effect. Of course, each specific trauma would have its own unique impact on a person, which can only be explored and understood on an individual basis. But traumas associated with stage development, since we all have to go through them, should have more consistency. If you have difficulties in any of the tasks associated with the stages, weaning, potty training, or finding your sexual identity, you will tend to retain certain infantile or childish habits. This is called fixation. Fixation gives each problem at each stage a long-term effect in terms of our personality or character.*

If the first eight months of a baby's life, is often filled with frustration in their need to suckle, perhaps because mother is uncomfortable or even rough with them, or tries to wean them too early, then they might develop an oral-passive character. An oral-passive personality tends to be rather dependent on others. They often retain an interest in *oral gratifications* such as eating, drinking and smoking. It is as if they were seeking the pleasures they missed during infancy. When we are between five and eight months old, we begin teething. One satisfying thing to do when while are teething is to bite on something like mommy's nipples. If this causes a great deal of upset and precipitates to an early weaning, then these babies could develop an *oral-aggressive personality.* These people retain a life-long desire to bite on things, such as pencils, gum, and other people. They have a tendency to be verbally aggressive, argumentative sarcastic and so on, etc. In the anal stage, we are fascinated with our 'bodily functions.' At first, we can go whenever and wherever we like. Then, out of the blue and for no reason we cannot yet understand, understand the powers that be 'our parent' want us to do it only at certain times and in certain places; our parents seem to actually value the end product of all this effort. Some parents put themselves at the child's mercy in the process of toilet training.

They beg, they cajole they show great joy when they have done it right and they act as though their hearts were broken when it isn't done right. The child is the king of the house and he knows it. This child will grow up to be an anal expulsive (a.k.a. *anal aggressive*) personality. These people tend to be sloppy, disorganized and generous to a fault. They may be cruel, destructive and given to vandalism and graffiti. The Oscar Madison character in *The Odd Couple* is a nice example. Other parents are strict, they may be competing with their neighbors and relatives as to who can potty train their child first, *(early potty training being associated in many people's minds with great intelligence)*. They may use punishment or humiliation. This child will likely become constipated, as they try desperately to hold it in at all times and will grow up to be an anal retentive personality. They will tend to be especially clean, a perfectionist, dictatorial, very stubborn and stingy. In other words, the anal retentive is tight in all areas. *The Felix Unger* character in The Odd Couple is a perfect example. There are also two phallic personalities, although no one has given them names. If the boy is harshly rejected by his mother and rather threatened by his very masculine father, he is likely to have a poor sense of self-worth when it comes to his sexuality. He may deal with this by either withdrawing from heterosexual interaction, perhaps becoming a bookworm, or by putting on a rather macho act and playing the ladies' man. A girl rejected by her father and threatened by her very feminine mother is also likely to feel poorly about herself and may become a wallflower or a hyper-feminine "belle." Meanwhile if a boy is not rejected by his mother and is rather favored over his weak, Milquetoast father, he may develop quite an opinion of himself (which may suffer greatly when he gets into the real world, where nobody loves him like his mother did), and may appear rather effeminate. After all, he has no cause to identify with his father. Likewise, if a girl is daddy's little princess and best buddy and mommy has been relegated to a sort of servant role, then she may become quite vain and self-centered, or possibly rather masculine. These various phallic characters demonstrate an important point in Freudian characterology: Extremes lead to extremes.

If you are frustrated in some ways or overindulged in others, you might have problems … and although each problem tends to lead to certain characteristics, these characteristics can also easily be reversed. So, according to Freud an anal retentive person may suddenly become exceedingly generous, or may have some part of their life where they are terribly messy. This is frustrating to scientists, but it may reflect the reality of personality.

Dr. Freud's Therapy

Throughout the years Freud's therapy remains one of the most influential among any other within the Western mental health field … though some might disagree, but not until we opened the doors and our minds to other alternative ways, his theory will remain the most influential among the scientific therapeutic communities.

Relaxed atmosphere: Means the client must feel free to express anything. The therapy situation is in fact a unique social situation, one where you do not have to be afraid of social judgment or ostracism. In fact, in Freudian therapy, the therapist practically disappears. Added to that, is the physically relaxing couch, the dimmed lights, soundproof walls and hello; the stage is set.

Free association: Means the client may talk about anything at all. The theory is that with relaxation, the unconscious conflicts will inevitably drift to the fore. It isn't far off to see the similarities between Freudian therapy and dreaming. However, in therapy there is the therapist, who is trained to recognize certain clues to problems and their solutions that the client could easily overlook.

Resistance: Means when a client tries to change the topic, draws a complete blank, falls asleep, comes in late, or skips an appointment altogether, the therapist then says "aha!" These resistances suggest that the client is nearing something within his free associations that they may unconsciously find threatening, of course.

Dream analysis: According to Freud, when asleep we are somewhat less resistant to our unconscious and we will allow a few things *in symbolic forms,* in order to come to the point of awareness, of course. These wishes from the id provide the therapist and client with more clues. Many forms of therapy make use of the client's dreams, but Freudian interpretation is distinct in the tendency to find sexual meanings.

Parapraxes: Means the 'Parapraxes' is a slip of the tongue, often called a Freudian slip. Freud felt that they were also clues to unconscious conflicts. Freud was also interested in the jokes his clients told. In fact, Freud felt that almost everything meant something almost all the time, dialing a wrong number, making a wrong turn and even misspelling a word, were serious objects of study for Freud. However, Freud himself noted in response to a student who asked what his cigar might be a symbol for? "Oh, that" Freud replied. "Sometimes a cigar is just a cigar. " Or is it? Other Freudians became interested in projected tests, such as the famous Rorschach or inkblot tests. The theory behind these tests is that when the stimulus is vague, the client fills it with his or her own unconscious themes. Again, these could also provide the therapist with clues.

Catharsis: *Is the sudden and dramatic outpouring of emotions that occurs when the trauma is resurrected. The box of tissues on the end table is not there for decoration. Insight is being aware of the source of the emotion, of the original traumatic event. The major portion of the therapy is completed when catharsis and insight are experienced.* What should have happened many years ago, because you were too little to deal with it, or under too many conflicting pressures, has now happened. *Freud said that the goal of therapy is* simply to make the unconscious conscious.

Dialogue

A more general criticism of Freud's theory is its emphasis on sexuality. Everything, both good and bad, seems to stem from the expression or repression of the sex drive. Many people question that and wonder if there are any other forces at work. Freud himself later added the death instinct, but that proved to be another one of his less popular ideas.

We must first remember to observe that, in fact a great deal of our activities, are motivated in some fashion by sex. If we were to take a good look at our modern society, we will find that most advertising use sexual images and our perception perhaps is that movies and television programs often won't sell well if they do not include some flirting, sexual gestures or explicit languages.

But this is meanly our perception and we have not matched it with nothing else. Recently several of the highest rated TV series involved more Christian philosophy and Christian teachings and did rather well. Another common practice seen in the fashion industry is primarily based on a continual game of sexual hide-and-seek, this, which suggest that we all spend a considerable portion of our everyday playing the mating game. Yet we all still do not feel that life all about being only sexual.

Although Freud's emphasis on sexuality was not based on the great amount of obvious sexuality in his society; but rather based on the intense avoidance of sexuality, especially among the middle and upper classes and most especially among women. What we appear to have easily forget is that the world has changed rather dramatically over the last one hundred years. Although we forget that back then doctors and ministers recommended strong punishment for masturbation, 'leg' was consider to be a dirty word and that any woman whom felt sexual desires, was automatically considered a potential prostitute, and that a bride was taken completely by surprise on her wedding night, and could well faint at the thought. "Although we still might disagree with Freud, but it is to Freud's credit that he managed to rise above his culture's sexual attitudes." We might have to go back and reexamine Ana O, to realize that even his mentors Burke and the brilliant Charcot, could not fully acknowledge the sexual nature of their clients' problems. Freud's mistake was more a matter of generalizing too far and not taking cultural changes into account. Although it is ironic that much of the cultural changes in sexual attitudes were in fact due to Freud's work. His unconscious accounts for some of our behavior, but rather how much and what is the exact nature of the beast. Behaviorists, humanists and existentialist all believe that *(a)* the motivations and problems that can be attributed to the unconscious are much fewer than Freud thought, and *(b)* the unconscious is not the great churning cauldron of activity he made it out to be. Most psychologists today see the unconscious *as whatever we do not need or do not want to see.* Some theorists do not use this concept at all. One theorist that comes to mind is Carl Jung, who proposed an unconscious that makes Freud's look puny.

What Are the Positive Aspects of Freud's Theory?

People have the unfortunate tendency to *throw the baby out with the bath water.* If they don't agree with ideas *a, b, and c,* they figure *x, y, and z* must be wrong as well. But Freud had quite a few good ideas, so good that they have been incorporated into many other theories, to the point where we forget to give him credit. First, Freud made us aware of two powerful forces and their demands they place on us. Back when everyone believed people were basically rational, he showed how much of our behavior was based on biology. When everyone conceived of people as being individually responsible for their actions, he directed us toward the impact of society. Back when everyone thought that the male and female roles were determined solely by nature, he also showed how much they also depended on our family dynamics. And that the id and the superego which serves our psychic manifestations to biology in our society will always be with us in one form or another. Second is the basic theory, going back to Burke's study on certain neurotic symptoms, being caused by psychological traumas; although most theorists no longer believe that all neurosis can be so explained, or that it is necessary to relive the trauma to get better, it has become a common understanding that a childhood full of neglect, abuse and tragedy tends to lead to an unhappy adult life.

Third is the idea of ego defenses. Even if you are uncomfortable with Freud's idea of the unconscious it is clear that we engage in little manipulations of reality and our memories of that reality to suit our own needs, especially when those needs are strong. "My recommendation to you is that you learn to recognize these defenses." And you would find that by having names for them would help you to notice them in yourself and others. Finally, we come to realize that Freud has, largely set the basic form of therapy. Except for some behaviorist therapies, most therapy is still *the talking cure,* and still involves the use of a physically and socially relaxed atmosphere. And even if other theorists do not care for the idea of transference, the highly personal nature of the therapeutic relationship is generally accepted as important to success.

Some of Freud's ideas are clearly tied to his culture and era. Other ideas are not easily testable. Some may even be a matter of Freud's own personality and experiences. But Freud was an excellent observer of the human condition and enough of what he said has relevance today that he will be a part of personality textbooks for years to come. Even when theorists come up with dramatically different ideas about how we function and how we work, they still compare their ideas with Freud's.

CHAPTER VII

Problem Solving the Study on Illicit Drug ... Educational Research

Stems from a typical advertisement for Coca Cola in 1890, Coca Cola was one of the dozens of colas and tonics sold in the United States containing cocaine at the turn of the century. This was the intrinsic part of the first Cocaine Explosion. Syrup and extract for soda water and other carbonate beverages.

History and Glamour

The coca plant and the ancient practice of chewing the coca leaf have been around for a long time. It could be traced as far back as the ninth century, since ceramic remains from that era; thus specifying that the Mohican people used coca at least throughout the eighteenth century. In Europe and in many other parts of the world, coca leafs were in addition being chewed as stimulant and pleasant derives. Around 1860, the scientist Albert Niemann, isolated the chief alkaloid of coca and named it cocaine and in 1884, Sigmund Freud, used while conducting experiments and immediately started writing extensively about it. Around that same time Park Davis and Company began a mass cocaine production and cocaine became a popular American drug. Several years later, Chemist Pemberton introduced Coca-Cola, as a new soft drink syrup containing cocaine. And the soda fountain became an intrinsic part of the American scene *the new wave*. People at all levels of society started using cocaine, as it was for sale in pure form. It was besides being used as a major ingredient in an endless list of medical tonics and elixirs. Not long after, the newspapers began to report the inevitable addiction and credibly linked horror stories and the government finally stepped in to put an end to the spreading epidemic. After 1906, the marketing of cocaine-boosted tonics was no longer allowed in America and the *Drug Act* was passed, directing all drug manufacturing companies to list their ingredients on the product labels. In 1914, the *Harrison Act* was passed, identifying cocaine, as a narcotic and basically requiring that all transactions involving the use of cocaine be reported. By the 1930's, cocaine had gone underground and its popularity was mainly among small selected group of musicians, pimps, entertainers and a limited number of writers. It wasn't until about 1970 that cocaine regained its popularity, shortly after by 1971, the Drug Enforcement Agency, was seizing more cocaine than heroine. Once again America had begun experiencing the second great cocaine explosion. With five to six million individuals regularly, using cocaine, 'perhaps history was repeating itself.' Consensus among authorities throughout the 1980's was that about forty-five, to fifty million people had tried cocaine and speculated that six to seven million were using it regularly. Estimates previously noted and also showed us that everyday five to six thousand individuals were trying it for the very first time.

Approach to Alcoholism and Narcotic Addiction

As in other fields of medicine and behavioral science, an interactional approach to the etiology, epidemiology, psychopathology and treatment of narcotic addiction, implies the operation of multiple causality within the person and their cultural environment. In such interactions, we must first consider two significant factors.

1), the long term predisposing factor, 2) the more immediate precipitating factor. The most immediate precipitating factor in narcotic addiction, is the degree of easy access to illicit drugs. This first factor, demonstrates in part that narcotic addiction rates are higher in the urban slums, housing projects and sleazy zones, etc., than in the middle class suburbs. Although with the advent of modern high speed technology, online social media, easy access from the countryside, to the suburbs, to the inner cities, much have changed in recent years. This factor gives us an example of why during WWII, reportable incidents of narcotic addictions approached zero levels. "When normal commercial channels within the illegal drug trades are disrupted, the demand will decrease," regardless how great the cultural, attitudinal tolerance for addictive practices, or how strong an individual's personality predisposition to illicit drugs might be ... "no one can become addicted to drugs, without having access to them!" Hence the logic of law the enforcement component prevention.

The second most important predisposing factor in the etiology of narcotic addiction, is the prevailing degree of attitudinal tolerance toward the standard practice in the individual's culture, subculture ethnic, racial and social milieu. This factor explains differences in incident rates between lower class and middle class groups; between Europeans, Americans and Asians, and between members of the medical and allied health professions and other occupational groups. Contributory factors in the developmental of this syndrome are probably genic, polygenic in the origins and are undoubtedly fostered by social class membership. This has been observed particularly in families that have been on welfare for one or more generations. Most of whom, (later youths certainly are not motivationally inadequate), tend to be occasional narcotic users, who do not become either psychologically, or physiologically dependent upon the drug in question. Epidemiological studies conducted by the New York University Research Center for Human Relations in 1975 developed various behavioral, familial and socioeconomic criteria between these groups. Discovering that euphoric properties found in illicit narcotic drugs obviously triggers certain effect in the depression of the self-critical faculty and the positive pleasure. Other continuous scientific investigations also shown that addicts received an immediate unearned form of gratification of ego enhancement. These same euphoric properties are also obviously adjustive for persons with history of recent reactive depression.

Advanced studies conducted throughout the 1980's and early 90's on endogenously produced opiates and endorphins found that in some instances, mental deficiencies in the production of the substances that contribute to our normal optimism in the face of life vicissitudes, consequently have evolutionary survival value for the natural species. Unfortunately this also contributes toward the incidence of narcotic addiction. Other studies done on psychologically disabled addicts, discovered that lower working class addicts, tend almost exclusively to develop critical anxiety state and reactive depression, when under emotional or environmental stressors. There findings, thus indicating where addicts from urban slums and welfare backgrounds, developed almost invariably schizophrenic symptoms under comparable circumstances.

This obvious difference in clinical outcome probably reflects some insidious internalization of mature motivational traits by lower middle class addicts and the working class ones, despite the overt domination of inadequate personality. The cognitive style of a person, whom uses and abuses drugs, is viewed as a pivotal factor in the individual's moving from drug experimentation, to drug abuse. There is a current trend in behavior therapy, emphasizing cognitive approaches and the major tenets of cognitive of cognitive behavior. Human behavior is mediated by unobservable that intervene between a stimulus and the response to that stimulus. Belief's sets of competitive strategies and expectations are the examples of the types of mediating, currently considered crucial to the thorough understanding of emotions and behavior's. The way the individual label, or evaluate a situation, determines his, or her emotional and behavioral response to it. Another basic assumption is that thoughts feelings and behaviors are casually interactive, to tie the cognitive to drug abusers. This theory posits the abuse process, with the conflict, as a predisposing factor of individuals having difficulty in meeting demands, or expectations placed upon them by work, society, friends and themselves. The direct result of stress is anxiety.

Anxiety is a universal feeling. It is something that we experience to some degree each day.

Nevertheless, it is not the extensive experience of anxiety in question rather the way each individual interprets the state of anxiety that makes the situation so crucial to the overall theory. Underlying the anxiety of drug abusers is the simple belief that they cannot significantly alter, or control the situation that they are powerless to their environment and cannot eliminate, or decrease the source of stress. The beliefs that they are powerless to cope with stresses, is the major cognitive disposition of the drug abusers. A consequence for such behavior, is the intense feeling of low self-esteem, which is a well-known clinical entity among drug abusers. A feeling of self-deprecation, which forms the beliefs that he is powerless, is the experience of anxiety. This is of course, uncomfortable and creates a means for a necessary anxiety reduction. The primary pharmacologic effect of heroine, is anxiety reduction, because not only does the drug provide a relief of anxiety, but the individual also obtains a temporary ecstatic feeling. Under the influence of the drug high, the individuals temporarily experience an increased sense of power, self-worth and control and a sense of wellbeing. The sense of powerlessness, immediately replaced by an exaggerated sense of being all-powerful, no task is too great and no feat is impossible, while he/she is high. Thus drug can do for the abusers what they cannot do for themselves. Unfortunately for the drug abuser, the effects are short lived and any temporary gains, turned into long term losses. Inevitably, after the high wears off, some internal or external source of stress will rekindle the conflict and anxiety. Thus, not only does the feeling of lack of control returns, but they are also likely to be stronger than before. And realizing, however that anxieties do not have to be tolerated, because there are drugs right around the corner. Knowing that such drugs have been successful in the past by removing tension and producing good feelings, the process of use, almost immediately graduates to abuse! It is therefore expected for the use of drugs to increase in frequency and by the number of different situations, in which it's employed e. g. Argument with parents, loss of jobs', conflicts with spouse, maybe just a few primary sources of conflict and anxiety for the young, currently experimenting with illegal substance for the very first time. *Each time drug users relies on an illicit drug to relieve tensions, gain unearned euphoria and feel good about themselves, they become less capable of coping on their own. By using drugs to cope, the individual biologically cut's himself off from using his natural adaptive mechanisms to cope with the situation and becomes less tolerant of pain and anxiety. This is a proven fact, regardless of the individual user and the type of drugs or alcohol. Biblically or naturally speaking, we interfere with God's creation for our bodies have already been designed to cope with life stressors. Of course, the need for a physician is imperative when we are ill, but this involves in-depth understanding of the person's metabolism, physical and cognitive functions. A caption from a 1970's cartoon indicates where a man is sitting at a bar requesting another drink, the bartender then looks at him and asked. "Thought you said you only drink to drown your sorrows?" The man then turns to him, slurred speech, then replies, "yes but my sorrows have developed into excellent swimmers since last spoken."*

Cocaine

Ear, Nose and Throat: Cocaine is readily absorbed through the nasal mucosa, after intra-nasal administration of 1.5mg of cocaine to thirteen surgical patients, cocaine was detected in the plasma within three minutes; and peak plasma concentrations were reached in 15 to 60 minutes. In addition, cocaine was still detectable on the nasal mucosa up to three hours after its application. The peak plasma levels attained are dose dependent with higher intra-nasal doses of cocaine. Because of its pronounced vasoconstriction properties, cocaine can cause acute and chronic rhinitis and chronic sinusitis, and ulceration and perforation of the nasal septum. Reports have also been found on cases of cerebral spinal fluid leakage from the nose and concomitant inability to smell, after sniffing cocaine. This is presumably due to changes in the bony portion of the skull (in this area) and the nerve responsible for the sense of smell. Cocaine sniffing may also produce a profound, rebound redness and congestion of the nasal mucosa. Chronic cocaine snifters, are also prone to develop upper respiratory infections and tend to use a variety of nasal sprays i.e., Salt, or tap water, glycerin and vitamin E oils to prevent and soothe the irritation of the nasal mucosa. In retrospect, the adulterant and dilutions used to cut cocaine may also play a role in damaging the nasal mucosa, (Siegel 1980). Throughout his studies on chronic free-base smokers, Siegel also reported chronic dry lips and sore throats. He also found that cocaine drops repeatedly instilled in the eye might cause clouding of the cornea. Which is the primary reason

Cocaine, is no longer used in eye surgery. Affirming that acute glaucoma may occur after topical application of cocaine to the eye and that nausea, vomiting and vertigo have been caused by application of cocaine to the middle ear. Klough, 1982, has commented on potential danger of aspiration, when cocaine is applied to the nose and runs to anesthetize the pharynx and larynx.

Respiratory: Smoking cocaine, as (pasta), or paste cocaine, or as free-base, is an extremely efficient way to quickly achieve substantial blood levels. However, there have been extensive reports on the phenomenon of coca paste. In Peru, the cocoa paste is a crude form of cocaine, containing several other substances, such as kerosene, methanol, sulfuric acid, etc. The paste contains 40 to 85% of cocaine sulfate and is usually mixed with tobacco, or marijuana in a cigarette.

The smoking binges may last for several days and the smokers may consume as many as 50 cigarettes in one night. As a result of this prolonged use and high dose administration of cocaine, the users experience euphoria, followed by dysphoria, hallucinations and cocaine psychosis. Studies conducted on the central nervous system of addicts, has shown us that effects of plasma cocaine levels as high as 975mg. can be achieved within five minutes of smoking 0.5grams of high grade cocaine. Experiments conducted throughout 1982 on cocaine paste mixed with tobacco, concluded that plasma cocaine concentrations as high as 462ng\ml., were obtained only three minutes after subjects smoked similar combinations of high-grade cocaine paste and tobacco. These levels were still obtained, although only an average of 6.1% of cocaine free-base was recovered from the mainstream smoke of burning cigarettes. The average relative bioavailability of cocaine is only 70% of that obtained by the nasal route. The main half-life of cocaine by this route was 38 minutes, which is slightly shorter than has been reported for other routes of administration. The above levels and time frames are roughly equivalent to those obtained by the intravenous route.

Cocaine free-base smoking, has been practiced in the United States since early 1970's, this method of administration is probably due to the decrease in efficiency. By which it allows significantly greater quantities of cocaine to be consumed than possibly through either the nasal or intravenous route. Seigel has reported that individuals may consume up to 30g, per twenty-four hours, or up to 150, in seventy-two, hours. In addition users may smoke without interruption for extended periods of times 'a run.' The longest reported run was, fourteen days, but cocaine free-base smokers, always experience a progression from paranoia and psychosis. Users reported a number of concurrent physical problems, including dry, chapped lips, sore throats, wispy voices, chest and back pains; and occasionally black and bloody sputum. It would be reasonably to assume that users also have increased incidence of bronchitis, due to the number of pulmonary complications reported by cocaine free-basers e.g., pneumomendiastinum of pmneumothorax. However, similar complications have also been reported after the use of marijuana. The possibility that frequent and prolonged valsalva maneuvers, and attempted forced expiration with the glottis closed, is significant in the reduction of the users, pulmonary carbon monoxide, thus diffusing its capacity. However, it is hypothesized that the damage may be caused by direct vasoconstricting effect on the pulmonary vasculature. Nevertheless, it hasn't been proven whether this effect was acute, or did it in fact persist to a highly unusual complication. Cocaine sniffing was reported, when cellulose granulomas were found in the lungs of a fatal case of pulmonary edema, on a twenty-six year old man who injected cocaine free-base.

Cardiovascular: Small doses of cocaine may slow the heart rate, as a result of central vagal stimulation, but large dose increases both, heart rate and blood pressure. According to proven studies done by the American Heart Association, the effects appear to be dose related, e.g. 8mg. of cocaine, administered intravenously to normal, healthy volunteers, increased their heart rate to 21%; and 16 - 32mg, increased their heart rate to 30 and 37.5%. Respectively, increases in blood pressure were less striking with an 8mg. dosage. A 16 - 32mg. injection of cocaine showed a peak increase of approximately 15%. Such increases were the direct result shown on the central, sympathetic stimulation and from peripherally mediated sympathetic vasoconstricting. Conversely, a large intravenous dosage of cocaine may cause immediate death from cardiac failure, due to a direct toxic action on the heart muscles. Clinically speaking, in addition to hypertension and tachycardia, cocaine has been reported to cause accelerated ventricular rhythm, ventricular heart ectopic beats, angina, subsequent subendocardial, myocardial infractions, ventricular fibrillation and death. Though there is no consistent or definite dosage at which any of the above toxic effects may occur, researchers have shown that volunteers took up to 244mg. of cocaine intravenously with no evidence of cardiac arrhythmia, nor any other signs of cardiovascular toxicity. However, cases have been reported fatal reactions with as little as 22mg injected submucously. *After many years of failed and repeated clinical trials and a wide variety of therapeutic interactions and scientific drawbacks, Script Research in the 1990's discovered a vaccine designed to deposit a four-month cocaine barrier into the brain. The vaccine is yet to be approved by the Food and Drug Administration, but it's function is designed to prevent addicts from relapsing, and could also be given to the would be user to keep them from ever becoming addicted. But we're not quite yet in the clear.*

Approach To Neurobiology ... (Neuroscience Teaching Models for Young People)

The Neurobiology of Drug Addiction: Our attempt here is to bring available valuable information that enables us to better discuss the effects of drug abuse on the brain so that it is easily understood. It is important to convey how the neurobiology of drug addiction plays a crucial role in mental health and psychiatric deficiencies.

This series is designed to teach patients, students, parents, family members and the average individual interested in learning about how the various street drugs impact the brain and body. As caregivers, counselors and educators, it is also rather crucial for us to share this valuable information as to why these drugs are harmful to human beings and the impact they place upon the individual user and society as a whole. Included here are brief studies on marijuana, nicotine, opiates, inhalants, hallucinogens, anabolic steroids, stimulants, and methamphetamine. *Our main goal within this series in addition to helping students understand the impact of drug use on the brain and body is to generate their interest and curiosity in neuroscience.* Since these models are tools that could also be used to provide teachers with present information on various aspects of drug abuse and addiction to middle, high school and college students understand the biology of addiction as well as specific abused drugs … *this information can also be very useful in the classroom or other teaching settings.*

The following include a list of drugs the brain and the actions of cocaine, opiates, and marijuana; the neurobiology of drug addiction; understanding drug abuse and addiction and neurobiology of ecstasy.

Marijuana … Common Street Names for Marijuana

Marijuana, although you may have heard it called pot, weed, grass, ganja or skunk, nevertheless, don't kid yourself regardless of the funky name it may be given, and its recent fruition toward legalization, marijuana is still a drug and it does affect the brain. Albeit, perhaps not long term, but just like all other street drugs, its effects varies from person to person's predisposition regarding addictions, etiology, etc. Marijuana is a mixture of the dried and shredded leaves, stems, seeds, and flowers from the hemp plant … hemp's scientific name is Cannabis sativa and it's colors can be a mixture of green, brown, or gray. Although a bunch of leaves may appear harmless to us, we must keep in mind that marijuana contains a chemical called tetrahydrocannabinol, better known as THC. Although THC is the main active ingredient, research has found many other chemicals are also found in marijuana, actually about 500 of them and many of these, are known to cause lung cancer. Though the research is currently in its infancy regarding the positive outcomes toward our medicinal usage. It might be rather wise for someone dealing with a substance abuse issues or any kind of mental deficiencies to stay clear of marijuana until these, just like its name has been settled and all cleared up. There are more than 200 street names or slang terms to describe marijuana, which vary from city to city and neighborhood to neighborhood. Some of the most common names are: *pot, grass, herb, weed, Mary Jane, reefer, skunk, boom, gangster, kif, chronic, and ganja.* Marijuana is used in many ways. Some users brew it as tea or mix it with food. Others smoke blunts-cigars hollowed out and filled with the drug. And sometimes marijuana is smoked through a water pipe called a bong. The most common method for smoking loose marijuana, is rolled into a cigarette called a joint or nail. It might be rather prudent for anyone suffering with mental illness or drug addiction to stay away from marijuana, unless under the care of a board licensed and highly qualified physician a psychiatrist and a psychologist.

About How Many Teens you've been lead to believe use Marijuana Today?

Bet you've often heard the lame line excuse "well everybody's doing it?" Well, now you could tell those individual to please check the facts. A recent researchers study funded by National Institute on Drug Abuse (NIDA's), on teen drug use results, indicated that when researchers in the field actually asked teens if they had used marijuana or *hashish* in the past month, *hashish* is another form of marijuana? The research found that only 8.4% of all the 8th graders surveyed said yes, only 17.9% of 10th graders had used or tried the drug for the first time in the past month and just 21.6% of 12th graders had ever used it. ***What do you think are the most common effects of marijuana to our bodies as a recreational drug?***

Imagine yourself as a soccer player and you're the center forward. A striker who receives the ball and sends you a pass right inside the penalty box, while the keeper is on the ground, but when the easy ball reaches your feet you're too psyched and forgets what to do with the ball? So instead of kicking it into the net, you deliver it to the keeper in a slow motion, thus completely blowing off your dreams of glory.

This loss of coordination, is caused by smoking marijuana, under the influence of marijuana, you could forget your own phone number, your best friend's street's name, what test where supposedly studying for, as you sit in a classroom and watch your grade point average drop like a hot potato into rain water, or perhaps worst. Lose concentration while driving and get into a car accident ... and these are just a few of the many negative side effects caused by daily and frequently use of marijuana in a developing brain. Even worse, since smoking marijuana in high doses have been found to also cause paranoia, anxiety, panic attacks and extreme withdrawals especially in young people.

Okay, okay, lets just back up a bit before we look at all the damages caused marijuana, let us just pause for a second and discuss a tricky truth. Because you will also hear some people tell you that smoking marijuana makes them feel very good. Now let me tell you why that happens and what happens to the brain in order to achieve such high. Within minutes of inhaling marijuana, users starts to feel *high*, or a pleasant sensations and this is because *THC* the chemical found in marijuana triggers brain cells to release the chemical dopamine. Dopamine is responsible for creating short time good feelings ... reasons as to the cause of addiction. Now here is the real fact ... keep in mind that once the dopamine starts flowing, users feel the urge to continue smoking marijuana again, and again, and again. The continuous and repeated use could lead to addiction, and addiction is a brain disease. Due to strict, federal law enforcement crackdowns on marihuana dealers, this often lead recreational weekend marijuana users in desperate search for stronger and quicker drugs, in order to achieve their level of starting point high.

Though in recent years several states have since enacted laws, thus legalizing it, lowering these restrictions and creating guidelines, regarding quality and minimizing the need of "THC spike," creating several other measures by which it could be administered with far lesser negative side effects. Marijuana has since also been implemented in therapies and natural medicinal usage, while it wages on in battle throughout a court system, which varies from state to state. However according to the federal government, marijuana remains illegal, though changes appear to be on the horizon.

Opiates

What are they, what's their purpose and how do they work on our organism.

When you think of opiates, think of the drugs called heroin, morphine or codeine. These are examples of opiates. Anyone whom use opiates regularly, their brain will very likely become dependent to them … hence the addiction to opiates.

Opiates are powerful drugs which derive from the poppy plant. Throughout history they have been used to relieve pain. Included within the opiate families are, opium, heroin, morphine, and codeine. Despite all of the technological advances in the medical field and although its been centuries since the discovery of opiates effective role in pain management, opiates remains the most available and most prescribed pain relievers by physicians, when treating pain today. Most of the opiates families are used in medical procedures, e.g. morphine and codeine are used in the treatment of pain related illnesses such as cancer, dental, postsurgical and other medical and procedures. When used appropriately or as prescribed by physicians, opiates are safe and generally do not produce addiction. However, opiates possess strong reinforcing properties related to pleasures this can quickly trigger addiction if used improperly. Heroin is the only one of the opiate families that has no medicinal use.

Opiates … their mechanism of action and how they work

Opiates bring forth to elicit their powerful effects by activating the opiate receptors widely distributed throughout the human body; once an opiate reaches the brain, it quickly activates the opiate receptors, distributed within brain regions. It then produces an effect that correlates with the area where the brain is involved. The two most important effects produced by opiates, are *morphine,* which involves *pleasure or reward* and *pain relief.* However, our brain also produce a substance known as *endorphins,* these endorphins also serve to activate the opiate receptors. Meaning that we could normally regulate and modulate our pain, when at normal levels … although research also indicates that endorphins are involved in many other functions in our body, including respiration, nausea, vomiting, pain modulation, and hormonal regulation.

Opiates are prescribed by physicians for the treatment of pain and is taken by following the prescribed dosage are safe. In recent years researchers actually though, challenged and debated this fact in open court, "there is very little chance of anyone becoming addicted if they follow the doctor's indications." This however is clearly no longer the case. Due to the high demand, and increased illicit and prescription drug value, greedy and unscrupulous physicians being manipulated by pharmaceutical industry, whom in tern respond directly to their greedy investment firms, demanding a higher profit for their investors and stock holders, have created a run-amok, perfect storm that has resulted in recent increased, American addictions, drug overdose and deaths.

However, if opiates are abused and if taken in excessive doses other than prescribed, addiction is definite to occur. Recent research findings in the study of animal control groups has also indicated that opiates can also activate their brain reward system, just like cocaine and other abused drugs. NIDA's research findings have also indicated that when an individual injects, sniffs, or orally ingests heroin or morphine, the drug travels quickly to the brain through the bloodstream. Once in the brain, heroin then is swiftly converted to morphine, which in turn activates opiate receptors located throughout the brain, including within the reward system.

How Addictions Are Triggered, it's Quick and Rather Simple

Cyclic Amp or CAMP, is a protein messenger present in many different types of cells, which activates CAM P dependent protein, kinases, causing them to transfer phosphate groups from molecules of adenosine triphosphate ATP. In biochemistry, ATP, is a molecular currency of intracellular energy transfer used in the transfer of various proteins in to cells. The increased *CAMP* produced in post-synaptic cell in a closer view, shows how this affects the function of the post-synaptic cell. Since there is more dopamine released; there is increased activation of dopamine receptors. This is very similar to the effect of cocaine, which causes increased production inside the post-synaptic cell. This alters the normal activity of the neuron and shows that there are increased impulses leaving the nucleus accumbens to activate the reward system point to the frontal cortex. As with any kind of drug over use, or abuse … continued use of opiates, cocaine, etc. makes the body rely on the presence of the drug to maintain rewarding feelings and other normal behaviors. The person is then no longer able to feel the benefits of natural rewards, such as food, water, sex, etc. This then means that they can't function normally without the drug being present in their system.

Researches within the clinical trials shows that the reward system and morphine activates the opiate receptors in the ventral tegmental area (VTA), nucleus accumbens and cerebral cortex. Major nucleus accumbens, include the prefrontal cortex, amygdala, hippocampus, and dopamine neurons located in the vta, via the mesolimbic pathway, suggesting then that stimulation of opiate receptors by morphine results in feelings of reward, which intern activate the pleasure circuit by causing greater amounts of dopamine to be released within the nucleus accumbens. This causes an intense euphoria, or rush, that lasts only briefly and is followed by a few hours of a relaxed, contented state. The excessive release of dopamine and brief stimulation of the reward system is an indicative clear pathway that leads to addiction. The hippocampus, is thought responsible for our emotional, learning, memory, and our automatic nervous system.

It should be noted that due to its chemical structure, heroin penetrates the brain faster than any other opiates this could be an indicator as to why many addicts drug of choice is heroin. The prolonged continued stimuli to this most important part of our brain, might be compared to the continuous pounding with a sledge hammer on your fingers, this might lead to a clear explanation of an addict rapid catastrophe.

Individuals should take note that opiates also affects directly the respiratory center within the brainstem, where they engage in activity slowdown … of course this then triggers a decrease in our breathing rate. Continuous use of excessive amounts of opiates especially heroin, causes the respiratory centers to shut down breathing altogether. Therefore, when an individual overdoses on heroin, it is the direct action of heroin in the brainstem respiratory centers that causes them to stop breathing and die.

We must keep in mind that the brain itself produces endorphins that often play an important role in the relief or modulation of pain. Therefore it is not an oldwife's tale when people talk about the body actually healing itself. Ever noticed the pain one feels when returning to the gym, running or playing a sport after being inactive for a long period of time? The only cure for such types of pain is hit to the gym again the following morning, or to remain active until relieve. "Granted you didn't overdue it that first day back and caused physical injury to the muscle tissue." However, when there is injury, surgeries, trauma and the pain too severe, the brain cannot produce enough endorphins to provide relief for this level of pain. It is then and only then that we would need a prescription, fortunately enough we'll be able to have insurance and could visit a physician that could prescribed one, since humans cannot produce strong, opiates, morphine or codeine, powerful enough to provide relief to severe pain. One should remember that when these used properly and under the care of a physician, opiates can effectively relieve severe pain without causing any type of addiction.

How Does Opiates Work On Our System?

Discomforts and feelings of pain are produced when a special set of nerves are activated by trauma to some part of the body, either through injury or illness. These specialized nerves are designed to carry pain messages to the spinal cord, for such ease in transportation they are located throughout our bodies. Once the pain message reaches our spinal cord, the message is then relayed to other neurons, whose exclusive job for these particular neurons is to carry and deliver pain messages to the brain. Opiates help to relieve our pain because it acts in both the spinal cord and brain. Opiates first role is at the level of the spinal cord, where it interferes with the transmission of pain messages between neurons, therefore preventing them from reaching the brain. Such interference or messenger pain blockage, serves to protect us from experiencing too much pain, or in certain cases, completely numbing the pain … this is known as *analgesic*.

Opiates also plays another important role by acting within the brain to help relieve pain, however, such is accomplished in a different way than it does when operating within the spinal cord. There are several areas in the brain involved in interpreting pain messages and subjective responses to pain. These brain regions are responsible for notifying us and allowing us to know, when we are experiencing pain and its unpleasant feelings. Opiates acts in these brain regions, nevertheless, they don't block the pain messages themselves. Instead they rather serve to change the subjective experiences received in the brain thus indicating the pain. Reason as for the meaning when a hospice's nurse talks about keeping the patients comfortable … *If we ask an individual receiving morphine therapy if they still feel pain, they'd say that they still feel the pain but that it no longer bothers them.*

Humans and animals naturally produced endorphins may not be adequate to relieve severe pain, but they are very important and they also play a vital role within the realm of our survival. When an individual or even an animal is severely injured and swiftly needs to escape from a harmful situation, it would be rather difficult to do so if we're experiencing severe pain. The amount of endorphins that are immediately released following an injury are often enough to provide the needed relief to allow us to escape a harmful situation. At a later point when we feel safe, our endorphin levels are again decreased, then intense pain is perhaps felt. If the endorphins continued to reduce our pain, it then becomes rather easy to ignore an injury and not even seek medical care.

Our brain contains several types of opiate receptors, the delta, the mu, and the kappa. These receptors maintain specific individual brain functions, each with a different control factor. E.g. opiates and endorphins block pain signals by attaching and binding on to the mu receptor site. Within recent years, scientists have been able to copy the genes that make each of these receptors. The advent in modern technology has allowed cloning in turn researchers are now conducting laboratory studies to better understand the opiates functions in our brain. Furthermore, research scientists are now able to study and focus on how opiates interact with each opiate receptor to produce such effect. *The purpose for collecting this valuable information may eventually lead us to find better treatments for individuals suffering with chronic pain and far more effective ways to combat opiate addictions.*

On a personal note, I could attest that the battle of physical pain is real, since I have personally undergone three separate back surgeries in the last twenty eight years, dating back to 1989, yet I remained drug free and have never developed a narcotic addiction. I underwent a discectomy of the lower back in 1989, recovered and then reinjured in back at work on an acute psychiatric unit back in 2003, had another surgery in 2008. This time a spinal cord stimulator was implanted, with two (RL) leads weaving through my vertebrates, travelling from my lower back, up to the up upper mid back. A generator, transmitter, controller, was also implanted in my upper right buttocks. This device, was designed to block the pain signals traveling through my nervous system via the spinal cord, by sending pulsating like vibrations that interrupted the pain circuit breakers throughout my body. It was battery operated, and the batteries were charged via a wireless wand that I had to tape to my outer skin over the generator, then plug it in to a 110 wat electrical outlet ... remain steady for about an hour, until it was fully charged.

It kind of help when the pain was really intense, sometimes it did not. Nevertheless, the wires came asunder and seven years later, the wires disconnected and implanted pulse generator (IPG) broke while inside of my back. Dr.'s suggestion, was to go in and repaired it, remove the broken parts and reconnected it. I opted to have it removed and deal with the challenges day by day. Twenty nine staples on my outer skin and an untold number of inner stitches, I decided it was time to get off all narcotics and deal with my pain a la natural. My doctor his assistant and PA, could not believe it when I gathered all of the prescribed of the tablets of oxycontin, percocet and other narcotics, returned them to their office, signed them off and requested a receipt. Doctor perhaps thought and questioned, whether the stressors from the ongoing pain had began to affect me psychologically? He opted to give me a standby prescription slip in case I needed it later. That was nearly three years ago. I have since relay on daily dosage of smoothies, teas, natural remedies, eating a healthy diet and the gym. Of course I do have flare ups from time to time that may require my need for a spinal cord injection, although even that has reduced from four, three times a year, to two and counting. My wife Damaris put it best when she looked at me and said. "You have really taken your recovery into your own hands!" I have known addicts whom still blame their doctors, thus holds them accountable for their addictions!

Inhalants. What Are They? How Do They Affect Us, and Why?

Inhalants are hair spray, gasoline, spray paint, finger nail polish remover, turpentine, glue and even magic markers ... they are all inhalants, and so is a long list of other everyday household goods found at the corner store and regular supermarkets, among these, we'd also found poppers, which became famous during the 70's and early 80's during the Studio 54, Saturday Night Fever disco era. Poppers, I believe is made of eyeglass cleaning liquid solution, concentrate and compressed into a styrofoam package that was usually popped and immediately inhaled, hence the name, 'poppers.'

Based on early childhood observation, global travels, this and several other research's, we realized that many individuals throughout the world like to inhale the vapors on purpose ... here I'll try to explain why. Although most inhalants are common household products that, when inhaled, cause a psychoactive mind-altering effect. There are literally hundreds of inhalants, including everyday products such as nail polish remover, glue, gasoline, household cleaners, and nitrous oxide *laughing gas*, which can be found in whipped cream dispensers and is often inhaled via a balloon. Inhalants also include fluorinated hydrocarbons found in aerosols such as hairspray and spray paint. There is also a wide range of chemicals found in different products that can all have different effects, however, inhalants generally fall into three categories, which are solvents, gases, and nitrites. Among the solvents we include certain industrial or household products, such as *paint thinner, nail polish remover, degreaser, dry-cleaning fluid, gasoline, glue,* and a few art or office supplies, such as *correction fluid, felt-tip marker fluid, and electronic contact cleaner.* Among the Gases we equally include household and commercial products, such as *butane lighters, propane tanks, whipped cream dispensers, refrigerant gases, etc.* There are also certain household aerosol propellants, such as those found in spray paint, hair spray, deodorant spray, and fabric protector spray. Among the Nitrites we find them primarily geared to the medical field, included are the anesthetic gases, such as *ether, chloroform, halothane, and nitrous oxide,* a*myl nitrite* etc. Except cyclohexyl nitrite, which is a substance used in hotel room deodorizers and butyl nitrite, previously used in perfumes and antifreeze, which is now banned and labeled as illegal substance. Although not an inhalant and not harmful, via acquired knowledge of science and medicine, nurses, doctors, mental health workers and other hospital workers have long put in practice the imbedding or inhalant of oxygen into their lungs to sober up, after a night of partying and their starting up their morning shift. Years earlier, during each change of shift during census on the units, lead mental health workers and nurses often had to check the gauges on our oxygen tanks, prior to accepting an official shift change, thus assuring complete hospital and patient safety in case of a lifesaving emergency. "Therefore, during the 1980's, 90's, throughout my tenure, it wasn't uncommon to run down the halls of a psychiatric ward during and emergency to collect a 'crash-cart,' emergency kit, only to realize the oxygen tank was empty or rather almost empty."

How Many Teens Do We Estimate Frequently Use Inhalants?

A recent NIDA survey on drug abuse, reported that more than 23.5 million Americans had abused inhalants at least twice in their lives, this number doubles, however, when we think in broader terms. Inhalants abuse often starts at very early age, according to NIDA's latest report conducted between 2004 and 2005, which showed that some young people used inhalants, due to its easy access in homes and stores, thus in many cases, its being used as a substitute for alcohol, obviously the precursor to other illicit drugs. Other surveys during recent years, also found that 3.5 percent of 4th-graders had used inhalants at least once in a year. Of course these numbers vastly increase if we were to conduct a research on the street children in Latin America, who sniffed glue and gasoline in the open on the streets of Tegucigalpa, San Pedro Sula and other major Latin American cities, on a regular basis. According to other NIDA-funded survey on drug use among 8th, 9th, 10th, 11th and 12th graders, the students in the 8th grade regularly reported the highest rate of inhalant abuse, when compared to their senior counterparts. This is perhaps an example to access versus availabilities. A noted, but gradual and persistent use of inhalants among teens was on the rise throughout the United

States from 1975 to 1996. After the mid 1990's it began to show a steady decline, the ten '10' year drop lasted until recently. The research and survey conducted by NIDA in 2004 - 2005, reported another increase in the use and abuse of inhalants among 8th and 9th graders; a steady increased not previously experienced in America by such young population . The two year report also showed that an 18.2 % of 8th graders, 13.1 % of 10th graders, and 12.5 % of 12th graders had now tried inhalants at least once in their lives and just as the Latin American street children, many American kids where now using it regularly. The study also found that between 2002 and 2005, over 250 deaths among teenagers throughout the United States were associated with inhalant abuse.

Hallucinogens

Hallucinogens, we always hear about them, but what do we know about hallucinogens? In reality, they cause people to experience hallucinations, or imagined experiences that seem real, when they're unreal.

Hallucinogens are a type of drugs that produces altered state of perception and feeling that can produce flashbacks long after the effects of the drugs has wear off. Among them we find natural substances, such as mescaline and psilocybin, which is naturally produced by the *cactus and mushroom* plants. We also find the chemically manufactured type of hallucinogens, such as LSD and MDMA *ecstasy*. Lysergic acid is used to manufacture LSD this acid is found in ergot, a fungus, which grows on rye and other grains. MDMA is a synthetic mind-altering drug that contains both stimulant and hallucinogenic properties. PCP, although not recognized as an hallucinogen in the pharmacological sense, PCP causes many of these same effects as hallucinogens, reasons why it is so often mistaken and included with this group of drugs. Hallucinogens powerful mind-altering effects, can change how our brain perceives time, our everyday reality, and our environmental surroundings. Hallucinogens also affect regions and structures in the brain that are responsible for coordination, our thought processes, our hearing, and our sight. People who use hallucinogens can start hearing voices, see images, and feel sensations that do not exist. According to researchers, scientists are still not certain if our brain chemistry could permanently change by using hallucinogen. Other research have since shown that some people who've used certain types of hallucinogens regularly, do develop chronic mental disorders. PCP and MDMA are usually very addictive, whereas LSD, psilocybin, and mescaline are not. Research has clued us in, as to how hallucinogens functions on our brain to cause such powerful effects, nevertheless, due to there being three different types of hallucinogens acting differently, all with their specific diverse effects, there is still much yet unknown about them.

Anabolic Steroids

What are anabolic steroids? Anabolic Steroids are actually the artificial version of *testosterone*, a human growth hormone that is naturally produced by each and every one of us. Some people take anabolic steroid pills or injections to try to build muscle faster.

In reality, anabolic steroids are synthetic substances related to the male sex hormones, called androgens, which have a number of physiological effects on the individual. The most notably, anabolic effect promotes the growth of skeletal muscle and androgenic effects that foster the development of male sexual characteristics. Although the proper term for these compounds are anabolic-androgenic steroids, they commonly are called anabolic steroids. Anabolic steroids, are legally available only by prescription in the United States. Doctors use these drugs to treat delayed puberty, impotence, and body wasting in patients with AIDS and other physical illness. Illicit abuse of steroids, are most often obtained from clandestine laboratories, smuggled, or illegally diverted. Traditionally the abuse of steroid has been higher among males than females, however there is a noted rapid increase among young women, now using steroids. According to previous NIDA funded survey on drug abuse among adolescents, researchers found an estimated 3.2 % of 8th graders, 4.5 % of 10th graders and 5.5 % of 12th graders had taken anabolic steroids at least once in their lives. These figures represented large increases since their 1990's to early 2000's surveys. That indicated approximately 80 % among 8th graders and over 75 % among 10th graders and 12th graders.

The abuse of anabolic steroids is propelled in most cases by fashion, followed by the need and desire to build muscle, reduce body fat and look good among their peers. These are all of course are perhaps followed by the need to improve sports performance, while applying for spots on the teams that'll place them in the position as competitive student athletes to earn college scholarships, or as college students, hoping to get noticed by NBA, NFL, NHL, baseball and other professional competitive sports leagues.

Abuse is estimated to show increase among competitive bodybuilders and is now widespread among many other lazy athletes who refused to put in the hard work, time, yet still want to look 'buff!' Some men who abuse steroids, perceive their own bodies to be small and weak, even if they are large and muscular. Some women who abuse these drugs, think they look obese or flabby, even though they are actually lean and muscular. Anabolic steroids are usually taken orally as tablets or capsules, by injection into muscles, or as gels or creams that are then rubbed into the skin. Studies have indicated that dosages taken by this type of abuse can be up to 150 times higher than any recommended therapeutic treatment in medical a condition. Steroid abusers, often take anabolic steroids in combination with oral and intravenous steroids in a practice called *stacking*, by which the abuser mixes both types of anabolic steroids. Abusers of the drugs often also stack *pyramid* compounds in cycles of 6, 8 to 12 weeks. Individuals gradually increase dosages, then slowly decreases them back to zero levels. Their belief is that such practice produces bigger muscles, while allowing the body to adjust and recuperate from high doses of steroids. Although in reality such theory has not been scientifically substantiated. Except, but to prove their negative side effect.

What Is Nicotine?

Nicotine is the drug found in tobacco leaves … whether you smoke it, chewed it, or sniff tobacco, you are actually delivering nicotine to your brain. When tobacco is smoked, nicotine is absorbed by the lungs and quickly moved into the bloodstream, one of the most rapid process by which nicotine is circulated throughout the brain.

Each cigarette contains about 10 milligrams of nicotine. Nicotine is the property that keeps people smoking despite the harmful effects imposed upon the human body. Although a smoker inhales only some of the smoke from a cigarette and not all of each individual puff is absorbed in the lungs, a smoker gets about 1 to 2 milligrams of the drug from each cigarette. Nicotine is lethal and very poisonous in its pure form ... a single drop of pure nicotine could easily kill a person if swallowed. As a matter of fact nicotine is powerful enough that it could easily be used as a pesticide on agricultural crops with a vast significant results to farmers.

The most popular ways of administering tobacco, although harmful, is usually by smoking it via cigarettes, cigars, or pipes. Tobacco can also be chewed or sniffed in a powdered form. Another alternative to cigarettes is *bidis*, bidis are originally hand rolled and packaged in India. Bidis are currently popular in America among teens, due in part to their colorful packages and flavored choices. Often times, smokers believe bidis to be less harmful than regular cigarettes, but in reality, bidis actually have more nicotine than cigarettes, which tends to make them smoke more, therefore they are more harmful to the lungs than cigarettes.

Cigarettes are very addictive and their addiction grapples rather fast ... According to recent research findings, more than 4 million teens between the ages of 12 and 17 have used tobacco at least once ... these same studies also later showed that about 16% of teens that same age who first tried it continued using it. A more recent study conducted on over 1500 six-graders showed that 30% of kids who smoke, become addicted within one month of taking that first puff. Dreadfully so, 10% of them get hook after only two days of smoking. The research also discovered that smoking just a few cigarettes during an entire month can lead to nicotine withdrawal, making it that much harder to kick the addiction. *At the time of these writings, over 67.5 million Americans or about 30% of the population, used tobacco daily.*

Methamphetamines.

Methamphetamine comes in a variety of forms accompanied by many different ways for administering or abusing it. Whether it is snorted, swallowed, injected, or smoked, methamphetamines could cause lots of harm to our organisms, including an inability to sleep, paranoia, hallucinations and aggressive behavior.

So what is methamphetamine you might ask? Methamphetamine, is a drug ... it is a very addictive stimulant that activates certain systems in the brain, its chemical components are related to amphetamine, though at comparable dosages, the effects of methamphetamine are far more potent, additionally more harmful and its harmful effects far longer lasting to our *CNS* or central nervous system.

Within the scientific research, medical or therapeutic communities, methamphetamine is viewed as a *schedule II stimulant*, meaning that it is of high potentiality for abuse, it is therefore available only through a physician's prescription. Although most of the illicit substance found on the streets, is surely being produced in small, illegal laboratories. Such productions endangers not only the individuals working in these laboratories as well as, neighboring businesses residential neighborhoods and the environment, but the users as well. This powerful stimulant shares a variety of ways for abuse. And there are also many names for it on the streets. Among the street known names by which methamphetamine is referred to we include; speed, meth, and chalk. Methamphetamine hydrochloride, which is a clear chunky crystals resembling ice, and can be inhaled by smoking, is called ice, crystal, glass, tina, etc.

The most popular ways of taken methamphetamine is orally, intranasal or *snorting* the powder form, intravenous or needle injection and by smoking it. Abusers tend to quickly become addicted, therefore, requiring higher dosages and more often intervals to curve such craves. Currently the most effective treatments for methamphetamine addictions are behavioral therapies, such as cognitive behavioral and contingency management interventions.

The health hazards found within such drug abuse are the following ...

Methamphetamine normally increases the release of the neurotransmitter dopamine, at very high levels this neurotransmitter is in charge with stimulating our brain cells, thus enhancing mood and body movement. Continuous research studies conducted on animals dating back to over 35 years has repeatedly shown us that chronic methamphetamine abuse, significantly changes how the brain functions. Furthermore, these studies have also shown that high doses of methamphetamine use does damaged neuron cell endings; although dopamine and serotonin containing neurons does not die after prolong use of methamphetamine, their nerve endings or *terminals* are cut back, thus preventing and limiting their re-growth. Noninvasive human brain imaging studies have shown alterations in the activity of the dopamine system. These alterations are associated with reduced motor speed and impaired verbal learning. Recent studies in chronic methamphetamine abusers have also revealed severe structural and functional changes in areas of the brain associated with emotion and memory, which may account for many of the emotional and cognitive problems observed when treating chronic methamphetamine abusers.

A small dosage of methamphetamine can result in increased insomnia, increased physical activity, decreased appetite, increased respiration, rapid heart rate, irregular heartbeat, increased blood pressure, and hyperthermia. Other known effects reported by the methamphetamine abusers, were irritability, anxiety, insomnia, confusion, tremors, convulsions, cardiovascular collapse and death.

The noted long-term effects conducted on chronic methamphetamine abusers were clinical paranoia, aggressiveness, extreme anorexia, severe memory loss, visual and auditory hallucinations, delusions, and severe dental problems.

Within this population we also found a high level of transmission of *HIV*, hepatitis B and C as a possible direct consequence of methamphetamine abuse. Our studies also showed a number of documented cases among abusers who inject the drug, though infected with HIV and other infectious diseases they still shared contaminated syringes, *needles* and other injecting equipment with more than one person. Due to the intoxicating effects caused by methamphetamine, whether injected, orally or via the nasal passages, it does alter our judgment and lower our inhibitions, which may lead the individual to engage in unsafe behaviors. Methamphetamine abusers contaminated with HIV, may actually worsen the progression of the virus and its consequences on their organisms. Recent studies conducted on methamphetamine abusers with HIV, have indicate that the HIV causes greater neuronal injury and cognitive impairment, when compared with HIV positive tested individuals who do not abuse such drug.

This data collected from the National Institute on Drug Abuse NIDA and National Institutes of

Health, DHHS, funded research study, showed that there were no statistically significant increases in methamphetamine abuse among 8th, 10th, and 12th graders in the year 2005. Methamphetamine abuse among 8th graders remained stable and was lower than for 10th and 12th graders ... furthermore, 10th and 12th graders reported significant decreases in lifetime methamphetamine abuse and 12th graders reported significant drop in annual and 90 day abuse.

Stimulants

What are they? Stimulants are a type of drugs. Cocaine, *crack*, amphetamines, and caffeine are substances that help to speed up activity within our brain and spinal cord. These often influence the individual to become more talkative, anxious and to experience feelings of excitement. Stimulants are a class of drugs known as mood elevators, or increase feelings of well-being, and increase energy, alertness, vigilance, etc. They often produce feelings of unearned euphoria among users. Among the listed stimulants we include cocaine, crack cocaine, amphetamines, methamphetamine, methylphenidate or *Ritalin*, nicotine, and methylenedioxy *MDMA*, better known as Ecstasy.

Cocaine is a hydrochloride salt, made from the leaf of the coca plant, and comes in the form of a white powder. Crack is a smoked form of cocaine, which is processed with ammonia, baking soda, water, and heated to remove the hydrochloride. Amphetamines are sometimes prescribed by doctors for physical problems, nevertheless, these pills are often abused for their effects on the brain. Methamphetamine is a powerful form of amphetamines that comes in clear crystals or powder and easily dissolves in water or alcohol. It is often made in illegal laboratories with inexpensive and readily available ingredients *such as drain cleaner, battery acid, and antifreeze.* Methylphenidate *Ritalin* is a medication prescribed for individuals *usually young children* with attention deficit hyperactivity disorder *ADHD.* Numerous studies have shown its effectiveness, when used as prescribed, in the treatment of ADHD. When it is abused or not used as prescribed, however, methylphenidate can lead to many of the same problems experienced with other stimulants. Nicotine and ecstasy *MDMA* is also considered as a stimulant and are covered extensively in separate topics throughout this study.

The Common Known Names for Street Drugs Are the Following ...

Cocaine is generally sold on the streets as a fine, white, crystalline powder. Out on the streets, it is known as *coke, C, snow, flake, blow, bump, candy, Charlie, rock, toot, etc.*

Crack, appears in a rock form, called 'piedra' in Spanish. It's a street name for the smoked form of cocaine, the name crack is due to the crackling sound made when it is being melted down. A speedball is cocaine or crack combined with heroin or crack and heroin smoked together.

Some of the known street names for amphetamines include: *speed, bennies, black beauties, crosses, hearts, LA turnaround, truck drivers, and uppers.*

The street name for methamphetamine is commonly known as speed, meth, chalk, and tina. When being sold or purchased in a smoked form, it is then often called ice, crystal, crank, glass, fire, and go fast. The street names for methylphenidate are rits, vitamin R, and west coast.

These stimulants can be taken in a variety of ways ... they can be swallowed in pill form snorted in powder form, through the nostrils, where the drug is quickly absorbed into the bloodstream through the nasal tissues. They can also be injected, using a needle and syringe, to release the drug directly into a vein, heated in crystal form and smoked or inhaled into the lungs. Stimulants that are swallowed or snorted, when compared to those that are injected or smoked are at a faster rate absorbed into the bloodstream, therefore intensifying the effects of the drug. It is also important to note that sometimes these drugs are diluted with other toxic substances. Cocaine is often snorted or injected via a process called *mainlining*, or it is also rubbed onto mucous tissues, such as the gums. It is also known that street dealers generally dilute cocaine with other substances such as cornstarch, talcum powder, or sugar; and other active drugs such as *procaine*, which is a chemical that produces local anesthesia; or with other stimulants such as *amphetamines*. Crack cocaine is smoked in a glass pipe. Among the stimulants, we defined cocaine as one of the most powerfully addictive drugs. The powdered, hydrochloride salt form of cocaine can be snorted or dissolved in water and injected. Crack is cocaine that has not been neutralized by an acid to make the hydrochloride salt. This form of cocaine comes in a rock crystal that can be heated and its vapors smoked *One must keep in mind that regardless of how cocaine is used or how frequently, a user can experience acute cardiovascular or cerebral-vascular emergencies, such as a heart attack or stroke, which could result in sudden death. Cocaine-related deaths are often a result of cardiac arrest or seizure followed by respiratory arrest ... the human body can never be trained toward cocaine use, or abuse. Amphetamines are usually swallowed in pill form. Methamphetamine is swallowed, snorted, injected, or smoked. Ice, the smoked form of Methamphetamine, is a large, usually clear crystal of high purity that is also smoked like crack, in a glass pipe.*

How many teens do we believe use this type of drugs today?

According to the 2004 - 2005 NIDA-funded study among the following percentages of 8th, 10th, and 12th: 3.4 % of 8th graders, 5.4 % of 10th graders, and 8.1 % of 12th graders had tried cocaine at least once. Meanwhile 2.4 % of 8th graders, 2.6 % of 10th graders, and 3.9 % of 12th graders had tried crack at least once. Among the amphetamines users, the research showed that 7.5 % of 8th graders, 11.9 % of 10th graders, and 15.0 % of 12th graders had tried the drugs at least once. Although the numbers showed tremendous drop among methamphetamines use, where only 2.5 % of 8th graders, 5.2 % of 10th graders, and 6.2 % of 12th graders had tried these drugs at least once. Throughout the research, twelfth-graders regularly reported the highest rate of use for all three drugs. Conversely, eighth-graders reported a drop in use for all three drugs, with a significant drop in Methamphetamine use, from 3.9 percent in 2003 to 2.5 percent in 2004.

Cocaine's Health Hazards To Our Bodies.

Cocaine is a strong stimulant. The use of cocaine interferes with the re-absorption process of dopamine on our central nervous system. Dopamine is a chemical messenger that is associated with pleasure and movement. The buildup of dopamine causes continuous stimulation of receiving neurons this is associated with the euphoria commonly reported by cocaine abusers.

Physical effects of cocaine use include constricted blood vessels, dilated pupils, and increased temperature, heart rate, and blood pressure. The duration of cocaine's immediate euphoric effects, which include hyper-stimulation, reduced fatigue, and mental alertness, depends on the route of administration. The faster the absorption, the more intense is the high. On the other hand, the faster the absorption, the shorter the duration of action. The high via snorting cocaine, might last 15 to 30 minutes, while a high via smoking might last 5 to 10 minutes. The increased use of cocaine also reduces the period of time a user feels high, therefore increasing the risk for addiction. Research conducted on cocaine users, have reported feelings of restlessness, irritability, and anxiety. Many have also reported that when tolerance to the *high* develops, they seek, but fail to achieve as much pleasure as they did from their first exposure to the drug, thus demanding addict's desire try to increase their doses in an attempt to intensify and prolong the euphoric effects. Although tolerance to the *high* can occur, users can also become more sensitive to cocaine's anesthetic and convulsing effects without increasing the dosage taken. This increased sensitivity may explain some deaths occurring after administering very low dosages of cocaine.

During a weekend cocaine binge, where the drug is taken repeatedly and each dosages are regularly increased, such behavior could lead to a state of increased irritability, restlessness, and increased paranoia. This behavior could easily result in a period of full-blown paranoid psychosis, at clinical levels to which, the user loses touch with reality and experiences visual and auditory hallucinations. There are many other complications associated with cocaine use; such may include disturbances in the heart rhythm and heart attacks, chest pain and respiratory failure, strokes, seizures, headaches, and gastrointestinal complications such as abdominal pain and nausea. Chronic users can easily become malnourished, due in part to cocaine's tendency to decrease a want for food or appetite. *The many different ways of administering cocaine can also produce different adverse effects. E.g. habitual cocaine snorting can lead to the loss of one sense of smell, regular nosebleeds, problem with swallowing, hoarseness, and chronically runny nose. Ingesting cocaine can cause severe bowel gangrene due to reduced blood flow. Addicts who inject cocaine usually experience severe allergic reactions and are at increased risk for contracting HIV and other blood-borne diseases. This however is the risk for all injecting or intravenous drug users.*

Other Added Dangers Found Within the Use and Abuse of Cocaine "Cocaethylene."

Most recent NIDA-funded researchers have found that when people mix cocaine and alcohol consumption, they are compounding the danger each drug poses, therefore unknowingly forming a complex chemical experiment within their own bodies. This happens when the human liver combine's cocaine and alcohol it manufactures a third substance, known as *cocaethylene*, this mixture tends to swiftly intensifies cocaine's euphoric effects, thus potentially increasing the risk of sudden death.

Future Treatments ... The widespread abuse of cocaine throughout the years has stimulated extensive efforts to develop treatment programs for this type of drug abuse ...

One of NIDA's research priorities is geared to find a medication that blocks and could significantly reduce the effects of cocaine ... such will be used in the upcoming years, as part of a comprehensive treatment program. Meanwhile other researchers are also looking at medications that will help alleviate the severe cravings individuals involved in cocaine addiction treatment, often experience.

There are several medications that are currently being investigated for their safety and efficacy in treating cocaine addiction. In addition to treatment medications, behavioral interventions, they have also found that cognitive behavioral therapy, could particularly and effectively be used in decreasing the drug use by patients involved in the treatment for cocaine abuse. Providing an optimal combination for such treatment and services of each individual is critical to future successful outcomes. Throughout this latest research, the study noted that the annual, and 30 day cocaine use remained stable among all three grades during the middle to later 2010 and 2015, thus perceived harmfulness of occasional use also remained stable.

The study measured at 65.3 % among 8th graders, 72.4 % among 10th graders, and 60.8 % among 12th graders. This data was collected from the 2015 monitoring. The future studies funded by the National Institute on Drug Abuse, National Institutes of Health, DHHS, study tracked teenagers' illicit drug abuse and related attitudes among, 8, 10 and 12th graders.

The Illicit Drugs and Your Mental Health. *How A Young Pothead Contracted AIDS.*

Yes, of course smoking pot could be a gateway that could also lead to other drugs and therefore addictions and other destructive behavior to some. Specially, if you already have mental health issues. As we carefully investigate and study these factual cases we could easily reflect upon present day behavior and produce a file, enumerating the number of individuals whom have ignored the warnings, believing they could regularly smoke marijuana each and every day, without facing any consequences. Just as in everything in life, there are also those very lucky individuals, who's brain and other circumstances, are perhaps strong enough, fortunate enough, or perhaps wired well enough to weather the storms!

It is believed and often discussed that young people whom end up with similar fates as many of these cases we have just read about. Many of them being diagnosed with personality disorders, drug induced schizophrenia, AIDS dementia, etc. realized

Today after nearly thirty years ago, I could still reflect upon and vivid recall the real life story of one of our young clients at a state hospital. It is perhaps one of the saddest, if not the saddest cases I've personally encountered in the field of mental health, throughout my career. This story is about a very young person's short, tragic encounter, as recreational weekend pot smoker. Scary thing is that it could've been any of us growing up during the 70's and coming into adulthood during the 80's … his typical story was that of me, my shipmates, classmates and friends. I had only been employed in state services for a couple of years, when a young man in his early twenties of Puerto Rican descent, was admitted to the state psychiatric hospital, where I worked at the time. He was very angry, combative at every turn, shared violent hostility toward his peers, by taunting and getting into physical fights. He was constantly threatening, challenging and verbal abusive to the staff.

He allowed no one to get close to him and quite frankly no one actually appeared to want to. He had been recently diagnosed with AIDS, contracted via the use and sharing of dirty needles. Of course this was during the earlier part of the mid 1980's. People did not necessarily understand much about AIDS and they actually feared everything about it. Of course EZT and no other medications was yet available. Individuals diagnosed with the contagious decease, in psychiatric facilities, were dying fast, often simply being seen as 'the living dead,' we had no way to treat them. Specially, once they'd decompensated and had to be quarantine from the population. This was a sad and grim reality, but we were actually on the frontlines in this battle, with little to no knowledge and no weapons to actually fight back, not even in our defense. "We were all very scared."

This gentleman however, continued getting into trouble and was repeatedly put into mechanical restraints at least twice per week. Although he wasn't on my unit, I was often floated onto his unit to cover. I then understood sufficiently about his psychiatric and medical history and on several separate occasions tried to connect with him when he was calm, but he'd ignored me, and simply told me to get out of his face that I didn't care. Basically that I didn't know him and that it wasn't any of my business nor my concern. He was always furious at the world and permitted no one to enter into his space.

One day though I wasn't as scheduled to work on his unit, I offered to volunteer to take the turn floating up there, specially knowing that they had 2 1:1 sitting and could use the help. As I entered the door I witnessed him and he was in the process of escalating, by actually picking a fight with another patient on his unit. He was then ordered into timeout by of his unit staff, whom advised and later threatened he'd be placed in lock seclusion if he'd keep it up, undoubtedly, this is precisely what he wanted to hear to rave up his level. As I began doing my scheduled rounds indicated on the assignment sheet, I immediately checked out the time out room, to no surprise to realize he was in there psyching himself up, shadow boxing head banging against the window, in preparation for a fight with staff. He then started punching the walls, swearing and gradually beginning to escalate. Ignoring the staff warnings and his rather awful, threatening and nasty demeaning attitude, I calmly approached him at the door, as I opened it to observe him closer, as hospital close observation, time out, following the every 15 minutes, constant observations protocol indicated. At first I greeted him by his name, he did not answer. I then asked if he was alright. His answer, rather unexpected, far from displaying the usual combative brash, bravado defensive attitude, he'd always put up front, this time he was a bit argumentative, and ready negotiate a response. Taking advantage of this once in a lifetime therapeutic opportunity, I suggested to the head nurse on the unit that perhaps she might want to call and request a constant observation order via the on-call psychiatrist on duty? That allowed me to sit and engaged him in positive conversation that might help to create a therapeutic break through toward his behavior. As I returned, I approached the door to the time out room with my chair, Roberto was still rather chatty, and surprisingly, much calmer and very pleasant. "I've always been happy throughout life, look at what they've done to me? They turned me into an angry person?" What do you believe they did to you that turned you into such? Whom turned you into an angry person? "They did, the doctors and nursing supervisors in this place did this to me." The doctors did what to you? Do you believe these doctors travelled all the way to New Haven, Connecticut, picked you up off the streets and brought you here to this hospital and placed you into this time out room, Roberto? (Roberto took a very long pause as if searching for an answers. Perhaps finally realizing that his health was rather serious.) I took the opportunity to remind him that I was there to help him in any way I could, as I proceeded to point out some of his strength to him. Primarily that we were similar in age, since we were both, in our mid-twenties, both of Latin American background, while asking him if perhaps he'd like to share a little of his upbringing and time spent growing up in Puerto Rico?." Strangely, he immediately began crying uncontrollably, "You don't understand, I was told today that I am here to die! I contracted something that I wasn't quite ready for its brutally killing him. I do not care about anyone else, someone got me infected and am going to seek my revenge!" I was astounded when I asked. "What's really happening with you, what is going on?" this was perhaps his first time admitting to himself or anyone that he'd been tested positive for HIV AIDS and it was rather difficult. So I gradually insisted he talked more about it. "What are you talking about, Roberto what did you contracted and how did you contracted this that you're telling me about?" Expecting that engaged in a deeper extended conversation that might provide not merely answers, but rather help him regain control, while shedding his machismo and stepping into a covered layer of his humanity.

He instead began uncontrollably sobbing like a little boy, as tears rolled down his eyes. As he gradually began narrating his story, "right after completing high school in New York, I went to visit my grandparents in Puerto Rico, when I returned to NYC, I relocated to CT, where I was attending the University of New Haven. I was a good student, although I worked part-time, I was obtaining good grades. I believe I was a typical college student, but I must admit, I was an occasional pot smoker." Stumbling when I asked him "I'm not accusing you, but how much did you smoke, how often you smoked, marijuana?" "Oh, not much. Not too often … just weekends mostly. I didn't even smoke while in high school!" He appeared sincere, as he continued. "Although, it was on this particular night about two years ago, I was out with my friends and I wanted to smoke some pot. No, I dint just want to, it was a craving … a very strong desire. I really, really." I swiftly intervene, "and then, what happened?" "I went to look for weed and couldn't find any. Apparently the cops had been making major sweeps throughout the city, all pot dealers had been arrested and no one had any around." "So what did you do?" "I ended up going to visit a friend, who'd taken me over to his friends' house later that evening, whom, we knew would always had weed, but he was also out of the stuff. The guy had a bunch of other people over, and they were all doing intravenous shit, I was invited to try it. At first refused, but the urge of definitely wanting and wishing to get high, though reluctantly, I agreed, and that that one time I injected anything into my body, it was via a dirty needle." After offering him a sip of water, I proceeded. "is that how you believe to have contracted the virus?" almost leaping out of his skin, he abruptly responded. "Yes and it was that one time that I contracted HIV that has since turned to AIDS and now look at me? I now have a terminally illness, not only that I'm dying." In that moment of clarity, he assured me, "just look at me now, I have been reduced to acting far worse than humans. Don't you think I realized that I'm more like an animal? My life is now locked away in a mental hospital, just warehoused here to die." I had continuously been struggling hard to contain my tears. As I fought to remain professional, and relay back to prayers, as in "there by the grace of God goes I." it shook me to the core. It was perhaps that very insightful lesson, learned that evening from this individual that would become the most significant one in my career, that'll really shocked and scared me straight! I since visited him frequently, couple of times a week, with a piece of fruit, fruit juices, Spanish foods and some comic books. He'd gradually began to trust me, I used this approach as a therapeutic tool and behavior modification. Meaning that if he threatened staff or fight with his peers, I just wouldn't reward his behavior with a visit, and it worked. Upon my visits to his unit, I would sit and listened to him talk, based on his improved behavior, I was able to approach his treatment team to obtain him a closed in courtyard pass for fresh air to get him off the unit with staff. These visits later also helped to obtain him grounds pass. Unfortunately, his dementia rapidly deteriorated his cognitive process, he also physically decompensated rapidly getting sicker and were we would become unable to provide any more care. He was soon discharged and sent home to die.

Ever since that day, I feel the need to speak up and realize that I must share Roberto's lesson, which I'd learned from his tragic story, with as many young persons, whom remains oblivious about the powerful connections to marijuana and any other types of drugs, with the society and our community at large … this is of course, if they'd sit and listened to it … particularly, mostly with all whom are still in the dark, blinded by the misconception and believing still that marijuana is totally safe and causes no harm.

How I Loss My Merchant Marine Buddy To Alcoholism

To this day I still recall the lesson learned early on in life on aboard the merchant ships, when I was about sixteen years old. At the time I worked as a quartermaster on board the S/S Rubbens.

The Rubbens was registered in Panama and flew a Panamanian flag sailing throughout Central America, the Caribbean, Mobile Alabama, Tampa, Pensacola; Florida. I had signed on a 10 month contract aboard the ship, about three months prior to Francisco's joining the ship, as an apprentice deckhand, a seaman's position seen back then, as an assistant (A\B) or able body seaman. Though he was much older, having sailed two previous ships, obtained quarter master, currently attending deck officers training, besides two and a half years on the high seas experience under my belt, I qualified, as his captain designated mentor, his immediate boss on wheelhouse and we would soon become close friends. Throughout the months, my ship buddies and I would invited him when going ashore, while in Trinidad and Tobago, Barbados, Martinique, Saint Martin and all of those other exotic Caribbean ports, but he'd always declined, and refused without a valid excuse, at least one strong enough to convince this seventeen years young, hardworking, energetic, responsible, party boy mariner. I'd also wondered why he never drank any type of alcohol, even while ashore in Mobile, Miami, Tampa, Canada or even New York, but paid little attention and didn't bother asking any questions. I guess I wasn't particularly curious about other people's lives, was rather too busy just trying to work and support my four younger siblings, a couple on nieces and nephews, and my mother back home in Honduras. This was as fretting enough while trying to help get them through school. Considering my daily anxieties of being still a teenager and my own personal worries as a young man, whom was being hunted down for recruitment by the military, each time my ship dropped anchor or docked alongside a Honduran seaport. After our government privatized its public high school and tripled its tuition, id then realized that the opportunity for my dreams of studying and perhaps obtaining an education had literarily and figuratively leaped out of my hands and was far out of reach. Worried of how each day our country, was being flushed down into a deeper economic hole from which it might not recover during my lifetime. My option was to study hard at sea, and accomplish as much as I possibly could, as I taught the new sailors in preparation to carving out my future far away from the country of my birth..

Several months after teaching Francisco to stare the ship, deck and ship's maneuvering safety, flags, the basic and fundamental principles of navigations, etc. Francisco then confided in me on the navigation bridge one evening that he had a drinking problem and those were the reasons why I never saw him drinking and hanging out with the guys. Although I had very little understanding, if any at all about what he was talking about, he requested I swore him the secrecy to anonymity, since it was highly requested by AA during those days, though I had not a clue. Francisco would later tell me the story behind the founding of Alcoholic Anonymous and the importance of their need to remain anonymous. More importantly, he'd slowly shared his story, which he'd laid upon me like a burdened guilt of confession, as I'll turned out to realize later, it was.

As shared deeper his most intimate fears, I then understood and agreed to end up offering to accompany him to AA groups in any English speaking seaports and countries, since he spoke only Spanish, which was still very limited throughout America, Europe and most Caribbean countries back then. This turned out to be one of the most eye opening decision of my young life and our friendship would soon blossom into a brotherhood at sea.

The year was early 1977, and back then Alcoholic Anonymous wasn't just a catch-phrase word used on a daily basis, without any significance as it is today; it was a significant step and those involved adopted every possible measure to consciously maintain themselves and their sought recovery activities anonymous for fear of sabotage and emotional taunting and constraints from those still actively drinking. Francisco told me he'd been a former lieutenant in the Honduran secret police that his entire adult life revolved around drinking and that he had once hit rock bottom. That he had again recovered and again been fired due to his uncontrollable drinking. Dropping his head and avoiding eye contact, as he carefully and slowly explained in detail that if he were to ever pick up another drink, he might as well go ahead and bought himself a coffin. This time around I really listened to what he was saying, it same significant at the time, but far from what I could have ever imagined. I agreed to accompany him to AA groups and scheduled meetings throughout some Caribbean islands and assisted him to get to some meetings in Mobile Alabama and other American seaports. Didn't attended too many with him in the states, but at those that I attended I heard some of the most dreadful and frightful, horror stories, unable to even imagined at the time.

The one that still remains most vivid in my mind is, perhaps the one I heard at an AA group in Trinidad and Tobago by a man in his early forties, whom attended the recovery group that evening. He told us he had been on a run with alcohol for about three straight weeks that he had been out there whoring and drinking, barely making it home to get a clean suit of clothes and head back out. He told us he had eventually tried to stop and returned home two days earlier and that on the third day he was trying to go through detoxification in his home, but was awaken one night believing that he was in bed with a prostitute, but instead, it was his teenage daughter who's bed he had mistakenly climbed in to. That it had been two years since he had not had a drink, but still felt shame and couldn't bear to look at his daughter straight in the face. His wife had since divorced him and neither of his other children trusted him any longer. One of the lessons I learned that night, was that alcohol, was a lot stronger than our own will power, in a person with strong addictions.

The news surrounding Francisco's death was tragic, dreadful and to this day, still unbelievable. We never wrote to each other and I'd not seen nor heard from him in a few years. It had been several years since I had switched from working the cargo ships and had moved on to working on board the cruise ships, and Francisco had gone on to work the tanker ships out in the Persian Gulf. He sailed through the Middle-east and I continued sailing throughout the Caribbean. My mother had told me in her letters that Francisco, was back home that he had saved up all of his money and bought a successful restaurant downtown, right across from 'el parquet central,' in Puerto Cortes. .

When I took my vacation off the cruise ships and decided to spent some time on dry land back home that year, my first evening home I invited mother and my younger brothers and sisters to dine at his restaurant. "What a beautiful place?" I thought out aloud, as he showed me around. It was enormous, a great menu, and well decorated, virtually bordering on extravagant. Lots of youthful looking beautiful waitresses all around, I mean it was something to see! I was very proud of my friend and though not jealous, but felt somehow that perhaps I'd had something to do with his success; although not really, since he was my brother, and I instead felt proud, thankful and blessed. However, it was the overall fearful feeling, I walked away with, as we shook hands and give each other a pleasant hug that night haunted me still to this day. I visited his place a few more times before returning to sea and still felt bothered and concerned, but couldn't really remember nor specify the basic reasons why. A few months later it hit me and I remembered what he had told me years ago on that bridge, about his involvement with alcohol. I remember that his restaurant primarily served top-shelf alcohol, I later wrote to mom back home concerned, asking about him. Mother then told me he had since broken up with his longtime girlfriend whom was a bit older than he, and he'd recently begun dating one of his young waitresses that she'd visited his restaurant, he appeared happy and he was doing fine. I tried calling him several times, afterward wrote to him, but got no reply. Several months later I received a letter from mother where she expressed he'd since he started drinking that his restaurant wasn't doing well and she thought he might be facing financial difficulties. In another letter about a month later, I received from mother shortly after, she told me he had lost his business and had been seeing frequently sleeping in park benches and eating out of the garbage. I believe Francisco must have died perhaps, as mother's letter was on its way, because when I called her from Miami, she told me they'd had found him dead on the streets that same week. I sat and I cried for hours, he wasn't just a close friend, but rather a combination of father figure, brother and a very good friend.

Years later, as I initially began to work with drug and alcohol, studied and gained maturity and more knowledge about the chronic disease that is associated with drinking, I credit him each day, as I say a solemn prayer, because only God, could have created such a miracle.

I still believe to this day that perhaps God had delivered my brother Francisco through divine powers to teach me about the dangers of alcohol. You see I was a young boy at the time, earning lots of money and spending it wildly and living dangerously. Closing down bars and buying booze for everyone inside, was a sort of a sports for many of us sailors while in port. During these times we cared very little about the money and even less about ourselves. We were young, full of youth, negative options and indestructible attitudes. I genuinely believed that by agreeing to accompany him to those meetings, was a maximum test of faith, where I since learned to share what I have took away from those meetings so long ago with my clients, my children and my friends, and perhaps help to save some of their lives in the process. God had manifested himself through Francisco and I since grew to have great respect for alcoholic drinks and the life it could lead if not careful.

Modern-day Approach to Co-occurring Substance Abuse Disorders

Some of the most recent changes in treatment conducted by SAMHSA throughout the new millennium and posted toward the end of the year 2007, shows the availability of funding for screening, brief intervention, referrals and enhanced treatment programs to combat substance abuse. The Substance Abuse and Mental Health Services Administration (SAMHSA), began accepting grant applications for Cooperative Agreements for Screening, Brief Intervention, Referral and Treatment (SBIRT) programs at the state and tribal level. SBIRT programs are proactive approaches that provide early identification and early intervention for persons at risk for, or diagnosed with, a substance use disorder. This is one of the key program elements of the National Drug Control Strategy, and promise to expand and enhance the effectiveness of state and tribal substance abuse service systems by:

Expanding their continuum of care to include screening, brief intervention, referral and treatment in general medical and other community settings, such as community health centers, nursing homes, schools, occupational health clinics, and hospitals; Supporting clinically appropriate services for persons at risk for, or diagnosed with, a substance use disorder (i.e., substance abuse or dependence); and Identifying systems and policy changes to increase access to treatment in generalist and specialist settings.

It is expected that approximately $10 million will be available to fund up to 4 grants. The average annual award amount is expected to be about $2.5 million per year for up to five years. The actual award amount may vary, depending on the availability of funds. The grants will be awarded by SAMHSA's Center for Substance Abuse Treatment.

Eligibility to apply is limited to the immediate office of the Chief Executive (for example, Governor) in the states, territories, and the District of Columbia, or the highest ranking official for federally recognized American Indian/Alaska Native tribe or tribal organizations. For applications for No. TI-08-001 are available by calling SAMHSA's Health Information Network at 1-877-SAMHSA7 [TDD: 1 800-487-4889] or by downloading at http://www.samhsa.gov . Applicants are encouraged to apply online using www.grants.gov.

Additionally, ten states and Puerto Rico has recently received SAMHSA funding for pilot programs to enhance transformation of mental health systems. This program supports an array of infrastructure and service delivery improvement activities to further the vision of Transforming Mental Health Systems for the 21st Century.

The states selected were Alabama, Florida, Iowa, Illinois, Kentucky, Minnesota, North Carolina, North Dakota, Pennsylvania and Tennessee. Each of these states and Puerto Rico will receive an award for up to $105,000 for one year.

The Transformation Transfer Initiative will support new and expanded efforts to improve the capacity and effectiveness of mental health systems that fosters recovery and meet the multiple needs of consumers.

The pilot programs will also explore new ways of getting mental health care services to everyone in need – a critical public health challenge. For example, according to the latest National Survey on Drug Use and Health, among the 24.9 million adults aged 18 or older with serious psychological distress, only 10.9 million (44 percent) received treatment for a mental health problem in the past year. The Transformation Transfer Initiative's pilot programs will implement a number of innovative approaches to meeting these mental health challenges, including:

Developing new, comprehensive peer support services for adults with serious mental illness and for youth with serious emotional disturbances. It will also enhance juvenile forensic mental health services by providing courts with alternative ways of conducting mental health evaluations. Instead of requiring all juveniles involved in the criminal justice system to undergo involuntary examinations performed at traditional inpatient settings, such as hospital psychiatric wards, new systems would be established to offer the courts the discretion to have juveniles undergo mental health screening and pretrial evaluations in outpatient settings, such as community mental health centers. The goal here, is to develop strategic plans to better address the continuing needs of individuals with mental illnesses and co-occurring substance abuse disorders.

It is believed that "The Transformation Transfer Initiative will build a wealth of experience in the steps it takes to improve mental health services for consumers and their families," said SAMHSA

Administrator, Terry Cline, PhD. "The knowledge gained through these individual awards will be shared with other states and territories working to provide more coordinated and effective care."

The State-of-the Art Approach to Treatment for People with Co-Occurring Disorders

The Substance Abuse and Mental Health Services Administration (SAMHSA) recently provided an overview of three new papers, containing information about how epidemiology, services integration and systems integration research and practices can be best utilized in helping people with co-occurring substance use and mental disorders.

These overview reports were the final in a series developed by SAMHSA's Co-Occurring Center for Excellence (COCE), a leading national public health resource in the field of understanding and disseminating crucial information about addressing this problem. The series is based on the best available science, research and practices and is primarily geared for a wide array of mental health and substance abuse treatment service professionals, although they provide useful information to the general public as well.

The newly overview papers are now available, included are the following: *Services Integration: Overview Paper 6* defines and explains how services integration practices can help merge previously separate substance abuse treatment and mental health clinical services provided at the individual level to people with co-occurring disorders. Combining and coordinating these treatments at the level of direct contact with individual clients can better ensure that their full range of treatment needs are addressed. This approach emphasizes that successful treatment of co-occurring disorders is very often based on providing all the client's treatment needs as concurrently as possible. *Systems Integration: Overview Paper 7* outlines the benefits of developing public health infrastructures that systematically integrate mental health and substance abuse treatment programs to better meet the full needs of people with these disorders. The paper encourages integrated system planning, continuous quality improvement analysis activities and other practices that lead to more effective, comprehensive public health services for meeting the health needs of this client community. *The Epidemiology of Co-Occurring Substance Use and Mental Disorders: Overview Paper 8* is presented in two parts. Part 1 provides the general public with a basic understanding of the field of epidemiology and how it has been used to shed light on the problem of co-occurring disorders. In particular, it focuses on three major studies that are regularly referenced as prime sources of information on the nature and scope of this problem. Part 2 is geared more to the scientific community and provides more detailed technical information on these three studies.

SAMHSA is creating these training materials as part of the plan outlined in its *November 2002 Report to Congress on the Prevention and Treatment of Co-Occurring Substance Abuse Disorders and Mental Disorders*. Previously published short papers address a wide range of other issues and practices related to the needs of people with co-occurring disorders. More information about the Co-Occurring Center for Excellence and the short papers can be found at www.coce.samhsa.gov .

Global Suicide Prevention Protocol

In the short time that it takes the average person to watch a television program, go for a jog, and do a load of laundry, vacuum or wash their cars, about 100 Americans would have tried to end their lives. According to researchers estimate, about a million suicide attempts take place each year in the United States ... unfortunately approximately 30,000 of them are successful.

Rolando was an eight-year old bright talented kid growing up in Honduras, Central America, back in 1968. His family consisted of his mother, himself and seven brothers and sisters. Hard work, eight children, mental and physical abusive relationships had taken an emotional profound toll on his mother. She had apparently gotten sick and tired of everyone using her, as means to an end when needed, then repeatedly disregarding, ignoring and kicking her to the side, once they'd gotten through with her. She came home one night from an extraneous day of work, as a domestic employee, one of the few jobs available to women in their early forties, in Honduras back. Upon her arrival, she suddenly discovered that her 15 year old daughter, one of the eldest, had taken off, neighbors told her that she'd run away, with her boyfriend from earlier during the day. After sobbing and pacing back and forth in desperation, she paused for a short while, turned to Rolando and asked him to go to the store and buy her a can of lye, then swiftly going back to the course of grieving. The consistently obedient, Rolando took his little sister by the hand and headed out to the neighborhood stores, and promptly began looking for the stuff without even questioning his reasons for buying it. After failed attempts at the first two corner stores, he opted to make one last attempt at the third and if he didn't find it, he would go back home and try again the following day. Of course, being only eight years old and, naive, not knowing what he was purchasing, or even the reasons for its intended use, its particular purpose, nor its high powered and fatal capabilities, certainly made him even more vulnerable.

Nevertheless, on his third attempt he succeeded, and after going back home and handing over the package to his mother, he went inside the house to finish up his homework. A couple of minutes later, he stepped back outside to the backyard, where he'd last left his mother. As he approached her, he could overhear Don Martin, the store owner at the first corner store, pleading with her. Don Martin being a neighbor and the first shopkeeper who had rejected to sell him the can of lye, perhaps his instinct kicked in based on the fact that he knew their home, actually had an outhouse and not sewerage, thus requiring no need for unclogging a toilet. Additionally, perhaps he'd realized his mother had been under stress and as an excellent shopkeeper and good neighbor, he kept a close eye on everyone.

By the time Rolando reached her, his mother had already poured the lethal content into an aluminum drinking-glass, mixed it with water and was about to put this bubbling and steaming concoction to her mouth to drink it, as Don Martin, rapidly intervened, gently placing one of his hands on her shoulder and with the other he gradually approached the poisonous glass. Meanwhile he continued pleading to her in a lower softer voice going almost into a quiet mourn. With tears rolling downs his face, Rolando confided to me in my office that years later those same words still resonated in his mind as he often remembered, "I still clearly remember him pleading with her and begging her not to drink the stuff, to slow down to sit back, to pause and give consideration to all her other young children that she'd be leaving behind and how much they were going to suffer without her being around to protect them and help them grow up." (He strongly believes that God had sent Don

Martin, there that night, as her guardian angel to virtually preserve and spare his mother's life …
and that he was certain that only God could have been looking over their shoulders in such a way).

His affectionately attentive mother, was a very strong and proud woman and perhaps she had
essentially recognized that she was heading for a nervous breakdown and had preferred to take her
life, rather than endure the inhumane and cruel punishment, she would have received in a Honduran
government operated psychiatric hospital. Thirty-five years later, while interviewing him, Rolando
cried when he told me, "to this day, I still implore to the Almighty in prayers each day, while I
strongly proffer God thanks for placing that wonderful man in our path. That man, Don Martin
religiously saved my mother's life!" His memory to such darkened times during his young life had
persistently remained suppressed for many years, but somehow had reawakened, resurfacing about
twenty years later, when he thought about the disagreeable, feelings of guilt he would have carried
around throughout life. He often imagined having himself to blame for being the cause of his mother's
death. Due to his being raised to be morally upright and to stand up, and speak up for his beliefs, to
be trustworthy and honest and to always, always do the right thing, nonetheless years later, he asked
his mother for an apology. At first she refused and tried to brush it aside, but he instead demanded
it and it was granted.

In closing, he expresses to me, "I still count my blessings each day, for we were very fortunate and
moreover, very blessed, because whatever Don Martin told my mother that night actually worked …
never again did she made another suicidal attempt." "Though she is no longer with us, she lived a
lengthy and wholesome, productive life." She was able to finish raising all of her children and even
lived long enough to witness and sees some of her children and grandchildren become doctors,
lawyers, professional athletes and hardworking valuable citizens in their communities, and throughout
the world, as they aptly accomplished amazing goals and maintained successful careers.

Suicide is perhaps one of the eighth leading causes of death in the United States.

*The highest-at risk groups include young people addicted to drugs and\or alcohol or suffering from
depression, people diagnosed with schizophrenia (of whom 10% to 13% does commit suicide), and the
elderly, who suffers with depression. Although most individuals contemplating suicide generally do so in
isolation, they often provide indications and clues to their irrational thoughts. Eight out of 10 human
beings who commits suicide talk about it with someone prior to completing the act; 30% of individuals
who attempt and complete suicide and 75% of the elderly, who do commit suicide visit primary care
providers within a month beforehand; and in excess of 80% of elderly suicidal persons provides some signs
surrounding their suicidal intent, such as relative weight loss, notable isolation, or the giving away of
valuable possessions.*

The Basic Functions of the Nursing Suicide Prevention Protocol

This protocol is seen in most hospitals and it tells us that: in most health care settings, nurses
spend more time with patients than any other health care providers. But few nurses are trained to
assess suicide risk and how to intervene. In 1998, medical centers throughout the country began
establishing research-based suicide prevention nursing protocol, in order to improve the quality of
care and reduce the legal vulnerability of health care providers and their facility.

Recommended measures: the protocol should be designed as a team consisting of a psychiatric nurse practitioner, an education and training specialist, a mental health nurse specialist, a mental health staff nurse, a mental health worker, a social worker and a rehabilitation specialist. This measured should ensure that a standard is used to assess and intervene, with-all patients at risk for suicide.

Is The Patient Verbalizing, or Exhibiting Any Suicidal Ideations?

Individuals reflecting on suicide, more than often they may exhibit visible signs of self-destructive behaviors. Some might even make explicit suicide threats or engage in proceeding with the actual attempt. All self-destructive behaviors and comments surrounding suicide should be taken seriously. Distinctively, suicidal patients may often express or display feelings of hopelessness, unworthiness, lack of control over their lives, apathy about their future, self-reproach, distrust of others, fatalism, and futility. They might make veiled or indirect statements about their death. Engage in giving away personal possessions that are of great value to them.

Clients might also exhibit, or suffer from some of the following:

a) Draft up a will or make funeral arrangements.
b) Procure a weapon, or lethal doses of drugs.
c) Have a history of significant personal loss or humiliating experiences.
d) Withdraw from friends, family, and coworkers.
e) Lack a social support system.
f) Exhibit a depressed mood (sadness, melancholy, and lack of interest in life).
g) Demonstrate chronic sleep disturbances.
h) Abuse alcohol and other substances.
i) Suffer from chronic illness.
j) Have a family history of suicide.

If the nurse observes any of these factors or behaviors, or if the patient or his family reports any of them to the patients nurse, they should document them in the patient's chart. But these clues can't be viewed in isolation. For example, a patient may exhibit suicidal ideation (or contemplation) as described above; yet hold profound religious belief that would prevent him from actually committing the act. Risk factors are usually evaluated within the overall context of each individual patient background.

The nurse should conduct a mental status exam in order to observe the patient's mental functioning, while making the following notations in each of these areas.

a) Appearance, e.g. Appropriate, clean, proper hygiene, or inappropriate disheveled, poor hygiene.
b) Orientation, e.g. recognition of people, place, time and circumstance.
c) Cognition, e.g. Concentration, attentiveness.
d) Speech, e.g. Normal, slurred, pressured, loud, guarded irritated, expressive, and inexpressive.
e) Interaction during interview, e.g. Cooperative, indifferent, suspicious, seductive, vague.

f)   Mood, e.g. Stable, depressed, euphoric, anxious, sad.
g)   Congruent with mood, e.g. flat, blunted, labile, catatonic.
h)   Perceptions, e.g. Normal, hallucinations.
i)   Thought processes, e.g. focused, unfocused, tangential.
j)   Thought content, e.g. Normal, delusional, obsessive, and grandiose.
k)   Insight, e.g. self-awareness, denial.
l)   Effectiveness of coping skills: effective, somewhat effective, ineffective.

Patients should then be questioned specifically about their suicidal ideation, their intent and if they have a plan.

Ideation, the patient should be asked whether they have any thoughts of harming or killing themselves. Though it may be veiled, suicidal ideation usually occurs before the overt suicidal activity takes place. The suicidal person may make a statement such as "take care of my dog for me," etc.

Plan: The goal then is to find out if the patient has already thought of ways to kill themselves, and if so, what these methods are. This would indicate the index of danger. Any plan that is

Straight forward, easy to carry out, and has a narrow or no margin for error is highly lethal. For example, hold a gun to their head is more foolproof than a medication overdose. The plan may also provide insight into this patient's mental status.

Intent: Suicidal intent is frequently communicated before-hand by giving away personal possessions, making threats, discussing suicide methods, presenting with worsening depression or a sudden mood change, or engaging in writing suicide notes. The nurse should then try to assess the presence of these signs and to find out when the patient is thinking of carrying out his plan.

During assessment, the nurse should also use the SAD PERSONS scale to assess this tool is designed to help practitioners remember their effective plan. Here are 10 of the major suicide risk factors to remember:

Sex: Women make more suicide attempts than do men; but men commit suicide more frequently than women.

Age: Patients younger than 19 and older than 45 are at far greater risk.

Depression: Depression increases the suicide risk.

Previous attempts: Suicide rates are higher among people with a history of suicide attempts than among those with no prior attempts.

Alcohol abuse: Suicide rates are higher among alcoholics than among the general population.

Loss of rational thinking: People experiencing disorders that impair judgment such as psychoses, or bipolar affective disorder are at risk.

Social support: Those who lack supportive or meaningful relationships in their lives are at risk.

Organized plan: The more organized the plan for committing suicide, the greater the risk.

For singles or individuals without spouse: Suicide rates are higher among single, divorced, widowed, or separated people than among those who are married.

Sickness: People with chronic or debilitating illnesses are also at greater risk.

Stage 2, evaluating the patient's history ... Once an individual has been identified as a potential suicide risk, a thorough patient history must be initiated. Past suicide attempts and mental illness, physical illness, substance abuse, isolation, lack of social support, hopelessness, family history, stressful life events, anger, and impulsive behavior, should all be taken into consideration. The team should also compile information from the individual's existing medical records and from interviews conducted on the patient and their family.

STAGE 3, Intervention ... After conducting the initial assessment and history, the team must identify any risk for suicide; the patient's physician should also be identified together with any other health care team members working directly with the individual, (usually an advanced practice nurse, a social worker, and a psychologist). Together, they could implement several interventions.

Determining a treatment plan: The initial treatment plan should include counseling, medications and special observation. This should also be immediately discussed and implemented among them, their team members, and the rest of psychiatric liaison practitioners. In addition, if the individual is in an ambulatory clinic or in a community setting, they should be accompanied to an emergency room or to an inpatient psychiatric unit by a health care team member, and should never be left alone during the admitting process. If they resists treatment, but are still believed to be harmful to themselves or others, they should then be committed involuntarily. A complete evaluation should again be conducted.

These procedures, however, varies from state to state ...

Implementing the appropriate level of observation ... The patient *will* need either constant or close observation. Constant, (1:1) one-to-one observation is the universal practice in a psychiatric inpatient setting and requires a nursing staff member to watch the patient and listen to his statement for twenty-four hours, or until a psychiatrist evaluates the client. The patient's environment should be free of sharp objects, such as pencils, pens, knives and forks, as well as items that can be used for hanging like strings, electrical cords, shoe lace's belts, bathrobes, bandana's unused restraints, etc. Chemicals that they could perhaps swallow such as fingernail polish removers, bleach, medications, etc.

The one to one observation ... 1:1 is implemented on impatient units, requiring a nursing staff member to constantly watch the patient at the distant of an arm's length. This observation requires a doctor's order. On the unit, the patient's environment must be free of potentially hazardous items.

Frequent or close observation ... requires a staff member to observe the patient at least every 15 minutes during waking and sleeping hours. This level of observation can be assigned to the unit's staff on a rotating basis and can be facilitated by moving the patient to a room close to the nurses' station ... *Regardless of the level of observation, the patient's status (including mood, behavior, and location) must be documented every 15 minutes.*

Any specific treatment tactics prescribed by the patient's physician or by members of the team, should also be noted.

Development of an ongoing assessment and treatment plan:

During ongoing assessment, nurses will consider any changes in the patient's demeanor, in interaction with staff or significant others, and in interest in performing activities of daily living. The presence or absence of covert or overt suicidal ideation must be noted. Of particular concern is the patient who undergoes a sudden mood change from depressed to euphoric, e.g. this could be a covert sign of a decision to go through with the suicide plan.

Stage 4:

The Patient Is Now Stabilized: Once the patient is considered to no longer be in danger of committing suicide, they should then be referred to a mental health professional to help them explore the reasons behind their suicidal ideation and to also implement measures for stabilizing and support. The patient may receive group or individual counseling, prescription medications when appropriate and social service referrals. Best approach, could be suitable residential case-management services. These programs if functioning properly should be able to assist with obtaining financial assistance, housing, transportation, and budgeting, and medication supervision. After it is determined that the patient is stable and that their depression (if depression was present) is under control, discharge should then be considered. And if further support is necessary, mental health follow-up is to be arranged on an outpatient basis and monitored by the individual's case manager. Such protocol once implemented and reviewed, is often welcomed by most *Medical Centers*, who lean towards it, because the *Joint Commission on Accreditation of Healthcare Organizations,* has long approved of it.

Most hospitals and outpatient clinics can adapt it into their own setting, thus indoctrinating it as their most important line of defense against suicide. This is for primary-care clinics, psychiatric community clinics, emergency rooms, medical-surgical units, or even impatient psychiatric units.

The Constant or continuous observation approach ... is also implemented in most inpatient units as well, requiring one nursing staff member to constantly observe one patient visually. There should be no more than 4 to 6 feet between the patient and the nursing staff who's caring for that patient. In addition, if the patient wishes to ambulate, two staff members should accompany him at arm's length.

Fact Sheet on Suicidal Occurrences ... Although most articles published in the news media and other popular press points to a correlation between the winter holidays and suicides. However the *Annenberg Public Policy Center of the University of Pennsylvania* and other expert researchers suggest this claim is just a myth and indicated that in fact, suicide rates in the United States are lowest in the winter and highest in the spring, *according to the CDC's 1985, 1991 and 1999 reports.* CDC's later reports also indicated that suicide took the lives of 30,622 people in 2001 (CDC 2004). Suicide rates are generally higher than the national average in the Western states and lower in the Eastern and mid-Western states (CDC 1997). In 2002, approximately 132,353 individuals were hospitalized following suicide attempts; nearly 116,639 were treated in emergency departments and released (CDC 2004). In 2001, 55% of suicides were committed with a firearm.

Most at risk groups ...

Males: Suicide is the eighth leading cause of death for all U.S. men. According to the CDC's 2004 report, males are four times more likely to die from suicide than females. This same report indicates that suicide rates are highest among whites and second highest among American Indian and Native Alaskan men. Of the 24,672 suicide deaths reported among men in 2001, 60% involved the use of a firearm.

Females: The CDC's report on women attempting suicide during their lifetime remains about three times as often as men, however, these are far less unsuccessful than their male counterparts.

Youth: According to the CDC's report on youth suicide rate, the overall rate of suicide among youth has declined slowly since 1992. However, rates remain unacceptably high. Adolescents and young adults often experience stress, confusion, and depression from situations occurring in their families, schools, and communities. Such feelings can overwhelm young people and lead them to consider suicide as a solution. Few schools and communities have implemented suicide prevention plans that include screening, referral, and crisis intervention programs for youth. Suicide remains the third leading cause of death among young people ages 15 to 24. In 2001, 3, 900 suicides were reported in this group. Of the total number of suicides among ages 15 to 24 in 2001, 85% were males and 15% were females. A recent 2004 CDC report on American Indian and Alaskan Natives have indicated the highest rate of suicide in the 15 to 24 age group. In 2001, firearms were used in 60% of youth suicides.

African Americans: While non-Hispanic whites are nearly twice as likely as African Americans to commit suicide, suicide rates among young black men are as high as those of young white men and growing. It is believe that this is due in part to high and easy access to fire arms currently available in the African American communities. Research that indicates that from 1980 to 1997, the suicide rate among African Americans ages 10 to 14 increased 233%, compared to 120% of comparable non-Hispanic whites. *African Americans are over-represented in high-need populations that are particularly at risk for mental illnesses.*

The Elderly: Suicide rates increase with age and are very high among those 65 years and older. Most elderly suicide victims are seen by their primary care provider a few weeks prior to their suicide attempt and diagnosed with their first episode of mild to moderate depression, CDC's 1999 report. The later 2004 CDC report on older adults who are suicidal are also more likely to be suffering from physical illnesses and be divorced or widowed. In 2001, 5,395 Americans over age 65 committed suicide and of those, almost 90% were men and 10% were women. This report also indicated that firearms were used in more than 75% of suicides committed by adults.

Suicidalities major risk factors ... The first step in preventing suicide is to identify and understand the risk factors. A risk factor is anything that increases the likelihood that persons will harm themselves. However, risk factors are not necessarily causes. Research has identified the following risk factors for suicide (DHHS 1999): *Previous suicide attempts, history of mental disorders (particularly depression). History of alcohol and substance abuse, family history of suicide, family history of child maltreatment, feelings of hopelessness, impulsive or aggressive tendencies, barriers to accessing mental health treatment, loss (relational, social, work, or financial). Physical illness, easy access to lethal methods, unwillingness to seek help because of the stigma attached to mental health and substance abuse disorders or suicidal thoughts, cultural and religious beliefs, e.g., the belief that suicide is a noble resolution of a personal dilemma; others include local epidemics of suicide, isolation, a feeling of being cut off from other people, etc.*

The proactive and protective factors ... Protective factors buffer people from the risks associated with suicide. A number of protective factors have been identified (DHHS 1999): Effective clinical care for mental, physical, and substance abuse disorders, Easy access to a variety of clinical interventions and support for help seeking, Family and community support, Support from ongoing medical and mental health care relationships, Skills in problem solving, conflict resolution, and nonviolent handling of disputes, Cultural and religious beliefs that discourage suicide and foster tools for support and self-preservation.

Freud's Views on Suicidality.

Life instincts and death instincts... Freud saw all human behavior as being motivated by our drives or instincts; these, which he said, were the neurological representations of our physical needs. Freud then referred to these as life instincts ... *These instincts perpetuate:*

a) the life of the individual by motivating them to seek food, water and
b) *the life of the species, which motivates them to have sex.* The motivational energy of these life instincts, are the energy, the vigor, or *joie de vivre* that powers our psyches, Freud called this the libido, from the Latin word *I desire.* Freud's clinical experience led him to view sex as being much more important in the dynamics of the psyche than any other needs. My understanding to his view is that "we are, after-all, all social creatures, and sex is one of the most pursued of the social of needs." Plus, we have to remember that in his studies, Freud included much more than intercourse in the term sex. Although in actuality, libido has come to mean, not any old drive, but the sex drive. Later throughout his life, Freud began to believe that the life instincts did not tell the whole story, and he looked at libido as it being more than simply a lively thing and more as a pleasure principle, which keeps us humans in perpetual motion. And yet the goal of all this motion is to be still, to be satisfied, to be at peace, to have no more needs.

The goal of life, one might say is death. Freud began to believe that "under and beside" the life instincts, there was a death instinct. He began to believe that every person has an unconscious wish to die. *This seems like a strange idea at first and it was rejected by many of his students, but some people due tend to believe it has some basis in experience and therefore need therapy, or redirection.* Life can be a painful and exhausting process, for a great majority of people throughout the world there exist more pain than pleasure in life. However, it is something we are extremely reluctant to admit. Nevertheless, for them death promises release from life's struggles.

(Throughout my journey I've met, spoken to and even befriended many individuals who openly speak of when they die, as if it being a planned event like a concert, or an upcoming sport game). "I'm sure many of you have also met a few." Freud referred to a nirvana principle. Nirvana is a Buddhist idea, often translated as heaven, but it actually means *blowing out,* as in the blowing out of a candle. It refers to the non-existence, the nothingness, and a void. This void, which in reality, is the goal of all life in Buddhist philosophy. The day-to-day evidence of the death instinct and its nirvana principle is in our ultimate desire for peace and to escape from stimulation. Our attraction to alcohol and narcotics, our penchant for escapist activity, such as losing ourselves in books or movies, our craving for rest and sleep, which could sometimes present itself openly as suicide and suicidal wishes. Freud's theory is that sometimes we direct these feelings out and away from ourselves, in the form of aggression, cruelty, murder, and destructiveness toward others. Therefore, as individuals it is imperative that we seek and find those triggers that might make us want to give up living, hence to realize that life is difficult, but that once we've realized that life is difficult, it becomes difficult no more. It is scientifically proven that we can attain these goals by way of therapy, be it clinical, or perhaps even religious, or spiritual. Do not be afraid to talk to your minister, your reverend, or your priest.

CHAPTER VIII

Before Venturing Into the World of Prescribed Medications:
It is strongly recommended that you visit your physician, psychologist, therapist or state licensed medical
practitioner prior to taking any kind of medications
The Decision to Use Prescribed Medications as a drug
Essential Teaching Components for Taking Antipsychotic Medications.
A Simple Daily Plan All Patients Should Follow When Taking Medications
Co-Therapy = Group Therapy … and the benefits gained

Before Venturing Into the World of Prescribed Medications:

It is strongly recommended that you visit your physician, psychologist, therapist or state licensed medical practitioner prior to taking any kind of medications. Your individual participation and complete understanding of your illness is rather imperative …

*List of Antipsychotic Medications Antipsychotic medications, also called Neuroleptics have been available since the mid - 1950's. They have greatly improved the outlook for individual patients. These medications reduce the psychotic symptoms of schizophrenia and usually allow the patient to function more effectively and appropriately. Antipsychotic drugs are the best treatment now available, but they do not cure schizophrenia, nor ensure that there will be no further psychotic episodes. **Only a qualified clinician who is well trained can make the choice and dosage of medication in the medical treatment of mental disorders.** The dosage of medication is individualized for each patient; since each patient may vary a great deal in the amount of the drug needed to reduce their symptoms without producing troublesome side effects.*

Antipsychotic drugs are very effective in treating certain schizophrenic symptoms, especially *positive* symptoms. A large majority of schizophrenic patients show substantial improvement. Some patients however, are not helped very much by such medications and a few do not seem to need them. Clinicians generally divide the symptoms of schizophrenia into two types: Positive and negative symptoms. Acute schizophrenia is characterized by *positive* symptoms, such as hallucinations, delusions, excitement, and disorganized speech. Motor manifestations include agitated behavior or catatonia. Chronic schizophrenia is characterized by *negative* symptoms, such as anhedonia (inability to experience pleasure) apathy, flat affect, social isolation, and socially deviant behavior. Conspicuous thought disturbances might be present.

Sometimes patients and families become-worried about the antipsychotic medications used to treat schizophrenia. In addition to concerns about their side effects, there may be worries that such drugs may lead to addiction. Antipsychotic medications, however, do not produce a "high" (euphoria) or a strong physical dependence, as some other drugs do.

Another misconception about antipsychotic drugs is that they act as a kind of mind control. Antipsychotic drugs do not control a person's thoughts; instead they often help the patient to tell the difference between psychotic symptoms and the real world. These medications may diminish hallucinations, agitation; reduce racing thoughts, confusion, distortions and delusions. While allowing the individual with schizophrenia to make decisions more rationally, schizophrenia itself may seem to take control of the patient's mind and personality, and antipsychotic drugs can help free the person from his or her symptoms and allow the person to think more clearly and make better-informed decisions. While some patients taking these medications may experience sedation or diminished expressiveness, antipsychotic medications used in an appropriate dosage for the treatment of schizophrenia is not a chemical restraint. Frequently, with careful monitoring, the dosage of medication can be reduced to provide relief from undesirable side effects. Antipsychotic drugs, also reduces the risk of future psychotic episodes in recovered patients. With continued drug treatment, about 40% of recovered patients will suffer relapses within two years of being discharged from a hospital. Still this figure compares favorably with the 80% relapse rate when medication is discontinued. In most cases, it would not be accurate to say that continued drug treatment prevents relapses; rather, it reduces their frequency. The treatment of severe and/or acute psychotic symptoms generally requires higher doses than those used for maintenance treatment. If symptoms reappear with a lower dosage, temporary increase in dosage may prevent a full-blown relapse.

Some patients may deny that they need medication, deny that they have an illness, and may discontinue antipsychotic drugs on their own. This typically increases the risk of relapse (although symptoms may not reappear right away due to the long half-life some of the antipsychotic medications have). It can be very difficult to convince certain persons with schizophrenia that they need to continue taking medications, particularly since some may feel better at first. For patients who are unreliable in taking antipsychotic drugs, a long acting inject able form may be appropriate.

All patients with schizophrenia should not discontinue antipsychotic drugs without being clinically monitored. *Antipsychotic drugs, like most medications, have unwanted effects along with their beneficial effects. During the many phase of drug treatment, patients may be troubled by side effects such as drowsiness, restlessness, muscle spasm, tremor, dry mouth, or blurring of vision, etc. Many of these can be corrected by lowering the dosage or can be controlled by medications …* ***However, we must keep in mind that:***

Different patients have different treatment responses and side effects to various antipsychotic drugs. A patient may do better with one drug than another. Antipsychotic drugs have proven to be crucial in relieving psychotic symptoms of schizophrenia, such as hallucinations, racing thoughts, delusions, and incoherence, but do not consistently relieve all the symptoms of the disorder. Even when patients with schizophrenia are relatively free of psychotic symptoms, many still have extraordinary difficulty establishing and maintaining relationships with others. Moreover, because patients with schizophrenia frequently become ill during the critical trade learning or career forming years of life ages, 18 - 35, they are less likely to complete the training required for skilled work. As a result, many patients with schizophrenia not only suffer thinking and emotional difficulties, but they lack social and work skills as well.

The Decision to Use Prescribed Medications as a Drug

The following general principles are design to govern the anti-psychotic drug use: Drugs are prescribed or given to treat targeted symptoms of schizophrenia or other psychotic disorders.

Initial treatment may require parenteral dosages. These are changed to oral pills or concentrate forms as the behavior disturbance subsides. Total dosages are tailored to individual needs; wide variations exist among clients because of metabolic differences, e.g. weight, etc. As soon as practical with drugs having sedating effects, divided doses is changed to a single dose at HS to maximize the drug's sedative properties. Most clients with a chronic course require maintenance doses for sustained improvement.

All patients taken medications should know how do their clinicians choose among the various anti-psychotic agents? According to the number of clinicians interviewed, all agreed that *it is even more importantly for clinicians to review the patient's medication history.* That "if the patient has previously responded favorably to a given agent, then they should try that agent with the individual again. In fact, if a patient has been taking a drug for maintenance therapy and an acute exacerbation occurs during a stressful period, then raising the dose of the drug may diminish the symptoms. However, if a patient has responded unfavorably to a given drug because of either lack of efficacy or unacceptable adverse effects, avoid that agent." On the other hand, they also stated that *"if a patient has had no prior experience with anti-psychotic drugs, then the clinicians could use the experiences of a family member that has had a positive response to a particular anti-psychotic medication as a guide. Failing all of these suggestions, the clinician is then free to choose among the agents on the basis of their own experience and the spectrum of adverse effects."* In general, the high *potency anti-psychotic* drugs are less sedating, produce less hypertension, and have less effect on the seizure threshold, fewer anticholinergic effects, less cardiovascular toxicity, less weight gain and very little effect on marrow and liver. On the negative side, high potency anti-psychotic drugs have greater acute extra pyramidal effects. The converse is true with *low- potency* agents. Potency refers to the quantity of medication required to produce therapeutic effects, e.g., 100 mg. of thorazine (Chlorpromazine) produces the same anti-psychotic effect as 2mg. of Haldol (Haloperidol). The list of side effects of anti-psychotic medications that nurses must recognize can be divided into these following classes:

1. *Autonomic nervous system*
2. *Neurological and other CNS*
3. *Allergic*
4. *Blood*
5. *Skin*
6. *Eye*
7. *Endocrine*

Autonomic Nervous System: Among the antipsychotic, all possess anticholinergic side effects and antiadrenergic side effects; that is they interfere with the normal transmission of nerve impulses by acetylcholine and epinephrine. The most common side effects are the anticholinergic ones. These include *dry mouth, blurred vision, constipation, urinary hesitancy or retention, and under rare circumstances, paralytic ileus.*

2. *Neurological and other CNS*
3. *Allergic Effects:*

The principal allergic manifestation of the anti-psychotics is cholestatic jaundice. This occurs much less frequently than in the early days of psychopharmacology and it is usually a benign and self-limiting condition. Blood Skin and eyes: Among the other side effects agranulocytosis is the most serious. It is both potentially fatal, however, fortunately, it is extremely rare. Usually the individual gets an infection and deteriorates rapidly or begins to bleed spontaneously, requiring emergency medical attention. Skin eruptions, photosensitivity leading to severe sunburn, blue-gray metallic discolorations over the face and hands and pigmentation changes in the eyes, are all potential side effects. Clients are generally advised to avoid prolonged exposure to sunlight or to use high-grade sunscreen agent when outdoors. These conditions usually remit. One serious and permanent eye change is *retinitis pigmentosa,* this condition may occur in clients on Thioridazine (Mellaril) exceeding *800 mg. per day.* The condition may lead to blindness therefore doses exceeding 800-mg. X day is contraindicated.

Endocrine:

Lactation in females and gynecomastia and impotence in males lead a list of endocrine changes that can occur with anti-psychotic drug treatments. You should be alert to any changes in body functions reported by clients taking these medications. Factors that may alter plasma levels of psychopharmacologic agents are the following:

A. *Age*
B. *Renal Function*
C. *Ethnicity or race*
D. *Smoking*
E. *Alcohol*

A) Definition: The pharmacological action of a drug is altered by the co-administration of a second drug. This co-administration may increase or decrease a known effect result in a new effect not seen with either drug alone

B) Potentially harmful interactions are rarely studied in humans most of the literature involves potential interactions and case reports

C) Effects may be overlooked or attributed to one drug usage.
D) Drugs that induce or inhibit hepatic microsomal enzymes
E) Drugs with a low therapeutic index
F) Drugs with several pharmacologic actions
G) Drugs with competitive protein binding
H) High Risk Populations

1. Elderly
2. Substance Abusers

These can be reduced by choosing a medication with a favorable profile for interaction, reducing the dosage of current medication when adding an inhibitor for the same isoenzymt, e.g. beginning with a lower dosage and increase slowly.

A. Use therapeutic drug monitoring when appropriate
B. Observe the therapeutic and adverse effects
C. Maintain adequate hydration and nutrition
D. Be cautious in at risk populations
E. Include nonprescription drugs in pharmacologic assessment

It is imperative to keep in mind that knowledge of pharmaco-kinetics should be of primary concern with safe prescription and monitoring of medications at all times.

The extra-pyramidal side effect symptoms, or EPS side effects symptoms frequently comes and goes, however, they often worsen when the patient is anxious or stressed.

Akathisia: is a symptom defined as a compulsion to be in motion. Patients describe anxious restlessness and intense desire to move about, simply for the sake of moving. Akathisia is extremely uncomfortable for the patient and can often lead to noncompliance with medication. Mental health workers cannot always see the restlessness patient will report *anxiety* but may not go into full detail, which can be *anxiety inside* or akathisia.

Acute Dystonia: Jerking or spastic movements backward rolling of the eyes; sideward twisting of the neck, protrusion of the tongue; spasms of the back muscles; difficulty swallowing or breathing. Dystonias are extremely frightening and painful to the patient. Mental health workers should immediately report these signs to the nurse, or doctor and stay with the patient to offer support. Anti-EPS medication is usually effective in 10 to 30 minutes, depending upon the route of administration. Usually it's via an (IM).

Parkinsonism: Decreased movements and psychosocial withdrawal usually associated with tremors, muscle rigidity, and cog-wheeling *Akinisia*. Stooping posture, mask-like faces, shuffling gait and drooling. Cog wheeling can only be felt by examination.

Tardive Dyskinesia: May occur after both long and short-term use of high doses of anti-psychotic medications. Involuntary chewing, licking, or pursing movements of the mouth and tongue; grimacing, frowning, blinking, protrusion of the tongue, rocking movements and spastic, jerking movements of the limb. The earliest sings are usually fine "worm like" movements of the tongue and excessive blinking. Those get higher each year of use from 1 to 7 years. By 7 years, there is a 50 - 60% chance of Tardive Dyskinesia. *Tardive Dyskinesia may be irreversible.*

Tardive Dystonia: Slows sustained involuntary twisting movements of the limbs, trunks, neck or face; including involuntary eye closure (blepharospasm).

Sedation: Low potency anti-psychotic drugs tend to be more sedating. Clozapine *Clozaril,* is especially sedating. Tolerance to sedation tends to develop over a matter of days to weeks.

Seizures: Anti-psychotic drugs particular low potency, lower the seizures threshold. Clozapine *Clozaril* lowers the seizure in a dose dependent fashion. Seizures are more likely to appear in patients with marginally controlled seizures or in a state of withdrawal from drugs or alcohol. *Although there still remains a vast and significant number of unmet needs in regards to the cure and proper treatment in the field of mental health, pharmaceutical companies now appear increasingly motivated by the findings* *of recent scientific clinical researches. Therefore, pharmaceutical corporations like Bristol Myers are now encouraged to produce medications that help meet the need of patients with psychotic disorders.*

Noted throughout these, were the significant changes in the treatment of patients diagnosed with bipolar disorder that had been treated with *Aripiprazole. Aripiprazole* is a new antipsychotic medication that was still currently being investigated by the American Psychiatric Association and awaiting approval release from The FDA at the time of this research. According to their data scientific and pharmacological data, Aripiprazole is designed primarily to aid in the suffering of patients who struggle daily with schizophrenia. The new study was presented to the APA at its 155 annual meeting in May 2002. And it showed that compared to the placebo controlled study, Aripiprazole, had a much more rapid response toward reducing the symptoms of acute mania, which took merely 4 days after treatment was initiated.

The study also showed that such positive changes were tolerated and that patient's remain stable even after therapy had been discontinued. Noted also throughout the studies, was a decrease in significant differences in clinical incidence associated with drastic weight changes. Throughout the study, patient who took Aripiprazole continuously demonstrated rapid onset of symptoms improvement. Patient diagnosed with manic episodes were also treated and Aripiprazole proved to be as effective in the treatment of bipolar disorder as well as schizophrenia. Expert investigations indicated that among the 262, placebo controlled studies, patient diagnosed with acute mania showed significant change in behavior shortly after treatment was initiated. Such treatment proved to be significantly meaningful in the reduction of acute manic symptoms, such as elevated mood irritability, thought disorders, abnormal thought content and disruptive aggressive behavior.

Researchers also focused closely on differentiations among the percentages of patient treated with placebo and those that were treated with Aripiprazole. This separation increased during the three-week treatment period as measured by mean change from baseline in the total score on the Young Mania Rating Scale (Y-MRS). Week three, Y-MRS total score decreased by 8.15 and 3.35 for aripiprazole and placebo respectively. Furthermore, 40 percent of patients treated with aripiprazole responded to treatment, compared to only 19 percent of patients treated with placebo. In this study, response was defined as a decrease of > 50 percent in Y-MRS total score. The study was primarily associated with most commonly observed adverse events, such which showed that there were only headaches, nausea, (stomach) dyspepsia, (sleepy) somnolence and anxiety.

Although Aripiprazole is an investigational antipsychotic medication, it produced improvements in positive, negative and depressive symptoms of schizophrenia were carefully monitored and documented. In a 52, week study of aripiprazole versus haloperidol, according to the data collected and presented to the American Psychiatric Association (APA), the data found throughout the study showed that significantly fewer patients treated with aripiprazole discontinued therapy for lack of efficacy or adverse events than those treated with haloperidol. And in a separate 26, week study demonstrated, aripiprazole proved to be significantly better than placebo in the prevention of relapse. Although one of the most difficult challenges mental health providers face when treating patients with schizophrenia is a long-standing commitment to treatment due to their tolerance to adverse effects. However, data collected from these studies suggest the potential for significant benefits of aripiprazole in the long-term treatment of schizophrenia. Aripiprazole = Abilify, is believed to have a mechanism of action that is fundamentally different from available antipsychotics. Aripiprazole exhibits potent partial agonism of D$_2$ dopamine receptors, and is also associated with partial agonism of $_{5HT1A}$

serotonin receptors and antagonism of $_{5HT2A}$ serotonin receptors. Partial 'agonism' refers to the ability to both block a receptor if it is over-stimulated and to stimulate a receptor when activity is needed.

Moreover, the studies demonstrated maintenance of effect, safety and toleration of Aripiprazole. Throughout the 52-week study of 1,294 patients diagnosed with acute relapse of schizophrenia, a significantly larger number of patients remain on the aripiprazole treatment compared to those on the treatment of haloperidol during the full duration of the study. While both drugs showed similar improvement of positive symptoms, aripiprazole demonstrated improvement of negative and depressive symptoms from baseline to endpoint that were greater than those achieved with haloperidol. On an even more important note, aripiprazole was shown to be associated with significantly less extra pyramidal symptoms (EPS) compared to haloperidol. The most commonly reported adverse events associated with aripiprazole in this study were insomnia, psychosis, anxiety and akathisia; incidence of insomnia, psychosis and anxiety were similar to haloperidol, while incidence of akathisia appeared to be considerably less with aripiprazole than those reported with haloperidol.

A 26-week study of 310 patients with stable, chronic schizophrenia demonstrated that treatment with aripiprazole was associated with significantly fewer relapses and a two-fold increase in time to relapse compared to placebo. In this study, aripiprazole was associated with improvement in psychotic symptoms as indicated by a significantly different change from baseline to endpoint in PANSS-Total score versus placebo. Aripiprazole was well tolerated in the study, with side effects similar to placebo. However, the majority of somnolence and gastrointestinal events were noted during the first week of treatment and out of all reported events, very few appeared to have lasted longer than 7 consecutive days. Schizophrenia is a chronic mental illness that affects approximately one percent of the world's population.

The antipsychotics demonstrated improvement in symptoms and reduction in side effects. Patients with schizophrenia who were switched from olanzapine, risperidone or haloperidol to aripiprazole, the still investigational antipsychotic medication, demonstrated improvement in symptoms and a reduction in certain side effects commonly associated with those antipsychotics. In another study, involving 311 stable schizophrenia patients, three separate switching strategies were employed in the switch to aripiprazole, at full dose (without titration) from prior antipsychotic treatment; switch to aripiprazole at full dose along with tapering of prior treatment for two weeks; and switch to aripiprazole with titration to full dose while simultaneously tapering previous treatment for two weeks. The results proved to be similar across all three methods of switching strategies remain generally safe and well tolerated in all groups.

The results of all these new studies were presented to the American Psychiatric Association, APA at its 155th Annual Meeting. Experts in the field of psychiatrist and mental health providers interviewed throughout the study concluded that there is a very high rate of switching medications among patients with schizophrenia, and in many incidences the switching is driven by side effects. However, in this study, patients were successfully switched to aripiprazole from commonly used antipsychotics, and in many cases there were proven distinct benefits to the switch. Study data suggested that there were specific differences observed in parameters of safety and toleration that were dependent on prior antipsychotic treatment (results were presented as mean change from baseline).

At the end of eight weeks, patients switched to aripiprazole from olanzapine demonstrated a statistically significant weight loss of 2.03 kg and showed a decrease in prolactin levels and improvement in extrapyramidal symptoms (EPS). Patients switched from risperidone to aripiprazole showed statistically significant decreases in prolactin levels, with reductions in weight and EPS. Patients switched from haloperidol showed improvement in EPS and decrease in prolactin levels, with minimal weight change.

Overall, patients who were switched to aripiprazole from olanzapine, risperidone or haloperidol showed improvement in measures of safety and toleration, regardless of the switch strategy employed. Patients across all switch strategies demonstrated improvement in EPS as measured by the Simpson-Angus Scale (SAS), Barnes Akathisia Scale and Abnormal Involuntary Movement Scale (AIMS). In addition, a reduction in prolactin levels was seen following switch to aripiprazole regardless of switching strategy.

Variable reductions in weight were also seen in patients in all groups. Aripiprazole treatment was well tolerated in all three groups, with the majority of adverse events reported as mild to moderate in severity. The incidence of adverse events was generally comparable between the groups, with the most frequently reported adverse event being insomnia. The majority of insomnia was mild or moderate and was cited as a reason for discontinuation in only 2 of the 309 patients. There was no difference in discontinuations due to adverse events associated with the different switching methods. In addition, patients switched to aripiprazole showed statistically significant improvement on the Positive and Negative Syndrome Scale (PANS S), a commonly used scale for evaluating symptoms of schizophrenia, regardless of switching strategy or prior antipsychotic treatment (i.e. olanzapine, risperidone and haloperidol).

The pharmaceutical company that holds the patent for such, has filed the regulatory applications for Aripiprazole in the treatment of schizophrenia, bipolar disorders, depression and Tourette syndrome in the U.S. and Europe, back in October and December of the year 2001. My last inquiry in October 2002, regarding this data showed still pending; therefore a trade name was yet to be established. Nevertheless, sources recently informed me it had been approved in Mexico and the USA and a commercial area's market name had since been established, as Abilify.

Essential Teaching Components for Taking Antipsychotic Medications.

A Simple Daily Plan All Patients Should Follow, When Taking Medications

It is highly recommended that patients follow these simple, but rather imperative techniques for personal care when self-administering psychotropic drugs, in order to help decrease some expected discomfort and attain healthier daily living.

Dry mouth: Rinse mouth with water each time after taking medications. Brush teeth more frequently, chew sugarless gum, and apply lip balm to lips and nostrils as needed.

Nasal Stuffiness: Avoid using nasal spray and nasal drops.

Weight Gain: Eat more vegetables and less sugar, starch and fats. Increase protein intake, daily exercise and follow a diet that has been prescribed by your doctor, or a dietician.

Difficulty Urinating: Drink 6 to 8 glasses of fluids each day … preferably water. Notify your doctor and nurse immediately. Practice relaxation exercises, which would promote normal urination. Take showers with lukewarm water and warm baths … listen to running water.

Constipation: Immediately implement an output sheet … document and make sure to notify your doctor and nurse about any changes in your daily bowel movement. Drink 6 to 8 glasses of water each day. Incorporate green vegetables, brand, a daily green vegetable smoothie e.g. (shredded wheat), prunes, raisins and fruits into your daily diet. Take laxative medications only when recommended by your doctor.

Tips for Proper Personal Hygiene and Maintain Appropriate Body Temperature:

Decrease of normal bacteria in mouth might result in infection. Avoid foods in high sugar. Observe your tongue for signs of thick white coating. Increase mouth care, including the gargling with mouthwash.

Some medications may increase the risk for bad sunburn:

Use sunscreen and lip balm when going out in the sun. Wear clothing that protects your skin, including hat and sunglasses. Regularly take your temperature orally and document and avoid extreme high temperatures such as hot tub baths.

Vaginal Dryness: Use lubricant such as KY jelly and notify your doctor and nurse.

Keep documentation.

Menstrual Period Stoppage:

Document the length of time that each cycle has been interrupted and notify your doctor and nurse. Give specific information if you are using birth control.

Decreased moisture around eyes: Highly recommended use of caution if you are wearing contact lenses to avoid eye irritation.

If noted changes in sexual interest (increase or decrease) notify your doctor and nurse.

Rest and Activity is rather imperative: Keep proper documentation of daily activity and notify your doctor before making any changes in such. Implement proper rest schedule and practice getting up slowly when lying down. Dangle legs over edge of bed, have nurse check blood pressure if drowsiness is noted when arousing, or getting up.

Drowsiness: Use extra caution, when driving a car, or operating other vehicles, or machinery. Avoid the use of alcoholic beverages, or illicit drugs. Incorporate for extra resting time in your daily schedule. Avoid using medications that has not been approved by your doctor.

Muscle Tightness, Cramping in arms, legs, neck, or face: Notify your doctor and nurse immediately, make sure to take medications that have been prescribed for these side effects on schedule and as recommended by your doctor.

Compulsion to keep on moving, inability to sit down; restlessness: Notify your nurse and doctor right away take any medications that have been prescribed for side these effects as previously indicated.

Blurred Vision: Notify your nurse and doctor, keep and follow regular appointment with optometrist. Wear sunglasses when going out in bright sunlight. Wear prescribed eyewear.

An Imperative Discussion:

It is imperative that each individual understands the nature of their illness and that they also have a clear understanding of the reasons for which they are taking these prescribed medications. A high level of empathy is expected from all healthcare professionals in order for the individual to attain self-empowerment, self-reliance and independence. Each individual battling with mental illness's responsibility is to ask questions and participate in their own research, document and advocate. Do not just sit there as a victim waiting for your caregivers to have all of the answers, know every personal detail about the inner workings of the medications on your system and do everything for you. We are individuals and as individuals, medications act differently on everyone.

Furthermore, studies have shown that the more involved a patient become in the participation of their treatment, the faster they show improvement and therefore enable them to attain and live more productive lives in the community. Talk with your nurse, your clinician, your doctor, your pastor, social worker, your rehabilitation and vocational therapists, case manager, dietician and mental health worker. Participate and attend religious, social and cultural outings. Identify, document and communicate any symptoms that are either part of your illness, or medication side effects. Discuss these feelings with your nurse, doctor, primary care person, or clinician. It is highly imperative that you report any sore throat, fever, increased fatigue, vomiting, diarrhea, skin rash, unusual body movements, etc. If you are a woman and are pregnant, or believe to be pregnant, please discuss this in detail with your doctor. If you are an individual who drank alcoholic beverages, avoid such intake and start attending, social gatherings, the theater, church, and weekly alcoholic anonymous meetings. Prevent further drowsiness and increased side effects. Keep in mind that sudden stoppage of your medication could result in the return of psychotic, depressive, or manic symptoms and or other side effects. Make sure to first discuss with your doctor, psychiatrist, any intension, or decision that is concerned with you stopping your medications. Enjoy the long, safe, productive and fulfilled, independent life that God has entitled you to live. It is your earned birthright and not just the privilege of a chosen few.

Co-Therapy = Group Therapy and the Benefits Gained

Medication Groups, or *med group therapy,* has been implemented primarily for two reasons … 1 to monitor the psychotropic drug administration, side effects, etc., and 2 to address physiological problems encountered by those who must to take them daily to implement their quality of life, thus attain more productive lives. These groups are scheduled regularly, though there are several variations of this model type. Almost all function under the usage of co-therapy teams and most used psychiatrist-nurse pairs since the psychiatrists are trained in the prescriptive and medication evaluation functioning and nurses are trained in the observation of medication management. *Co-therapy teams* are considered advantageous in medication groups, because they allow for the rotation of resident staff while keeping continuity of permanent nursing staff. In a sense, most clinicians consider it best, due to its decreased level of verbal productivity, low disruption and frequent frustration displayed by their clients.

Co-therapy also allows for the periodic absence of a therapist without group cancellation and could function as an open-ended group, which does not terminate when one or the other therapist. In reality, its flexibility allows one therapist to become involved in therapeutic dyadic interaction, while the other monitors group process and provides mutual support, when facing a difficult situation.

Some medications groups' requirement is that patients must attend regularly and on time, and that they remain for the duration of the group, while others may accept patients who come late and even leave early, or stay for the entire session. Attendance to some might be generally monitored and non-attendees more aggressively pursued than those who might miss a traditional outpatient appointment. This occurs, since a missed appointment could result in failure to renew a medication and a prolonged loss of patient-therapist contact easily places the patient at risk for symptom exacerbation and relapse. Meetings every other week or even once per month are most frequently scheduled. This due to the belief being that it reduced frequency in addition to their weekly group psychotherapy leaves room for the patient to focus on their medications and problems of daily living. It is also believe that it reduces the transference and lessens their stimulation to a degree in which patients soon become increasingly comfortable in the groups session. There is also no interpretation of group process or encouragement of intrapsychic material. Patients are instead encouraged to review their medications and share whatever daily difficulties they presently encounter with the group, so that group leaders and other members can help them problem solve. Often times, a format is followed where the psychiatrist addresses each group member in regulating medication issues, and therefore devoting the remainder of the session to a general discussion. However, the primary focus of the group is medications management and the secondary focus, is basic group interaction and shared problem solving.

It is not unusual to see a "take turn" pattern develop in medication groups where group members interact only with the therapist and wait to have their issue address, with acknowledging the previous discussion. The major process task of a therapist in these groups is to gradually direct conversation toward the rest of group members and away from themselves as the sole possessor of information. This is usually accomplished in a step-like fashion over a period of months or even years. Initially the therapist themselves would provide the information, which is later followed by reflecting on a member of the group that might have experienced a similar particular problem. The therapist role then is to encourage that member to relate his experience to the group. Once that member is invited to reflect and share their experiences with the group, the therapists role then is to await for a group response, or to question whether a has experienced a similar situation, or if they care to contribute toward the subject.

The group process is complicated by several factors. 1, being due to the infrequency of the meetings (monthly meetings in particular), these, which make it rather difficult to maintain a sense of group history. From the clients perspective, this is however, less demanding on the patients, due to the decreased level of anxiety which is usually transferred in weekly meetings from group to group. The therapist, however, must retain a sense of group history in order to gauge their expectations concerning the level of interaction. 2, the groups where patients are allowed to come late and leave early, the natural flow of any particular meeting could be easily disrupted. Therapists must be prepared to integrate a latecomer, without losing whatever small momentum the group may have managed to pick up. From the patient's perspective, this natural disruption could become beneficial and served as to dilute the group process and therefore, reduces interaction anxiety. 3, most medication groups are open-ended. This simply means that new patients will be added as vacancies occur. Typically most medication group stabilizes as soon as they reach consensus, lending themselves to little turnovers. Nevertheless, once there exist, such a change, the therapist is then faced with the task of integrating a patient who requires a beginning medication group into group that has developed a higher level of interaction over time. Finally, the therapist must remember that the focus of the group is medication management and here and now problem solving, even though they will develop a sense of group history and process over time. Some medication groups may verge on becoming supportive group psychotherapy model, or some patients may progress to the stage of requiring such a model. Therapist must be prepared to evaluate the need to shift the focus of the group or to refer group members on for different treatment, if needed so as to not sacrifice the original goals of the medication group required by their of patients.

Medication groups are beneficial to:

1. Patients who can tolerate and benefit from interaction with others
2. Patients whose medication regimens are stable, but who require periodic evaluation.
3. Patients who because of their disability require "training" in medication group in anticipation

Guidelines and reasons to referring clients to group psychotherapy.

4. Patients who can benefit from realizing that others have similar problems and could be helpful to someone else thus experiencing a sense of worth.
5. Patients who may require "break-through" appointments.

Medication groups provide a type of interaction to individuals who might not otherwise interact with others. They do not necessarily increase social interaction within their communities, but seem to substitute for it. It is rather impossible to provide a definite listing of all the patients and clients who could greatly benefit from an individual psychotherapy relationship, but any of the patients experiencing one of the following deficits could likely be a candidate:
A lack of experience in the formation of lasting, reciprocal relationships.
A lack of insight into the here and now precipitants of problems and symptoms.
Problems of a primarily endogenous nature, i.e. internal anxiety generated as a response to external (not necessarily interpersonal events).

Evidence of recent events, or perhaps multiple, serious life events. Evidence of long-standing, inappropriate guilt and self-destructive behavior. Difficult with control due to ego deficit.
Evidence of behavior not suitable to group intervention, i.e. intolerance of stimulation, poor attention span, inappropriate interpersonal behavior and paranoid or violent ideation.
A sense of self-worth through key individual relationships formed during our childhood and adult life. The person with chronic psychiatric illness who has not had such a relationship available to them, or whose illness has prevented their benefiting from such may be well served by a supportive individual psychotherapy relationship.

CHAPTER IX

The Modern Day Seclusion and Mechanical Restraints
Guidelines for Placing Someone in Locked Seclusion
The Patient Bill of Rights = A Much Needed Global Review
A Right to Communicate = Communications Rights While hospitalized
Why Processing the Seclusion Situation Is Rather Imperative
The Universal Level System

The Modern Day Seclusion and Mechanical Restraints

Guidelines for placing someone in locked seclusion ... The procedure, which defines seclusion, is the confinement of an individual in a room alone, in a manner that prevents them from leaving. It is indicated only as a last emergency measure, or intervention to control violent aggressive behaviors that is dangerous to the individual self, or others. And should be initiated after all other less restrictive measures have been attempted and failed and is regularly assessed. Most psychiatric hospitals no longer, use seclusion as a form of punishment, nor should it be used at staff discretion to get back at an individual for punitive reasons, of unaccomplished tasks, etc.

Seclusion is to be considered inappropriate and unsafe for those individuals with recent history of self-mutilation, uncontrolled head-banging, pounding, thrashing, risk of falls, has stated fears of being alone in a locked room, or has voiced suicidal ideations. When an individual has been placed in lock seclusion, he should immediately be placed on constant or continuous observation. Lock seclusion, is a medical and therapeutic tool and the need for constant staff reassurance and monitoring is rather imperative. ***The order for placing someone in locked seclusion should be executed by a doctor, via a Registered Nurse request;*** it should not exceed three hours and must be terminated as soon as the patient's condition permits. This could be accomplished once the individual has contracted verbally, or whether, the nurse doctor, mental health worker, or clinician has spoken with the individual, noted a change in behavior, reach an agreement, or the individual has agreed to regain control. Seclusion treatments should only be permitted and conducted in designated seclusion rooms.

Guidelines for placing someone in locked seclusion ... It is the staff responsibility to:

1. Implement a less restrictive interventions, as defined in the patient's *Violence Prevention Plan,* including observation, listening, communicating, problem-solving, defusing interventions, quiet time, 1:1 or increased support, environmental-situational interventions, chemical intervention or time out as appropriate to the patient's situation and as per their individual treatment plan.

2. To document if such interventions are not effective, the Registered Nurse is to observe and assess the situation and contact the physician and any other appropriate team members to try to diffuse and resolve the situation.

3. If there is imminent physical danger to the patient or others, a physician or, in the physician's absence, an RN may order restraint or seclusion.

4. Restraint or seclusion may be used in emergency situations to manage dangerous behavior. It is understood that it is the patient's right to be free from restraints, thus they are entitled only for protection of self and or others. Whenever possible, informed consent will be obtained from the patient. However, it is understood that in an emergency or violent situation this might not be possible.

5. A physician's order must be obtained immediately upon initiation of restraint or seclusion. Each physician's order must be time limited, indicate the type of restraint, the start time and the maximum end time, which should not exceed three consecutive hours. The Registered Nurse cannot accept, or transcribe a physician's order that is not time limited. Restraint and seclusion orders should be written only on a designated physician's order sheet.

6. The Registered Nurse must assess the patient upon initiation of the procedure and at least every hour, a thorough assessment should also be conducted prior to the individual being released from seclusion. These assessments are documented on designated restraint- seclusion authorization forms. No seclusion episode is to exceed the three-hour limit.

7. The physician must sign the order for seclusion within one hour of the initiation of the restraint regardless of the time of day. *The Registered Nurse will remind the physician at 30 minute, intervals. If the order is not signed upon the 2ⁿᵈ call, the Registered Nurse must notify the Nursing Supervisor on duty, who will in turn contact the physician. If the physician is unable to come to the unit due to situations on another unit, the Registered Nurse must then have the chart brought to the physician to obtain his signature. If the order is not signed in 60 minutes, the medical supervisor should then be notified, either directly during regular working hours or through the Hospital administration on-call procedure, by following the off-hours policy.*

The physician must assess the patient within 1 hour of the initiation of the seclusion and document their findings in the ***Restraint Seclusion Authorization Form.*** Documentation for this procedure should also be written in the individuals progress note and such should include, the reason for seclusion, maximum time authorized, a psychiatric and physical status report and any issues pertaining to risk also must be addressed. The Registered Nurse, who is accountable for the patient will assess and document the physical and emotional condition of the patient and assign a staff member to the continuous observation of the patient.

The staff assigned to continuous observation will remain in the area directly outside the seclusion room door to monitor and document any change, or risk in behavior.

Clothing worn by the patient must be based on the Registered Nurse and physician's assessment of the individual's condition. Potentially harmful items should be removed from the patient at the onset of seclusion. At no time should and individual patient be secluded without clothing.

Eyeglasses worn to correct vision need to be evaluated by the Registered Nurse and should be removed only if patient's safety is jeopardized, or if they've agreed to surrender them for safety.

A physicians order for authorizing and removal of the glasses and the reason should also be obtained. The Registered Nurse will ascertain whether or not the patient has given written consent to notify a significant other of the use of seclusion and will follow the instructions in the treatment plans regarding notification.

The individual is to be offered meals at regular times if appropriate base on the registered nurse's assessment and all meals must consist of finger foods and fluids. At no time should the patient be *given utensils while in locked seclusion.* If the patient's condition does not allow for the patient to safely eat, dietary staff will be requested to hold their tray until the patient is able to eat.

Fluids must be offered at least every hour. *The patient should be taken to the restroom as needed* with at least a two staff member escort. A record of intake and output must be maintained throughout each seclusion episodes. Vital signs must be taken and recorded as necessary, though no less than hourly, and the individual should be offered a shower at the end of each seclusion episode.

The Patient's Bill of Rights = A Much Needed Global Review

A high quality of care requires collaboration between clients and their team of health care professionals. Therefore, open and honest communication, followed by respect and sensitivity to one's differences is rather imperative and essential to each individual patient progress. Hospitals, outpatient clinics, clinicians and therapist are to encourage their patient's to be active collaborators within their treatment. Hospitals, clinicians and therapist, are to respects the role each patient may take surrounding decision making; about treatment choices and the various other aspects of care ... this includes their need to seek legal counsel. The professional caregiver ought to strive toward being sensitive to each individual patient's needs, including cultural, racial, linguistic, religious, age, gender, physical and other existing differences among each individual client- consumer.

1. *Each and every individual patient – client has the right to receive considerate and respectful care, given by competent and knowledgeable staff.*
2. *Each and every individual patient has the right to and is encouraged to obtain relevant, current and understandable information concerning their diagnosis, treatment, and prognosis from their designated treaters.*
3. *Each and every patient has the right to know the identity of all health care providers involved in their care while in the hospital.*
4. *Each and every individual patient has the right to receive a high consideration of privacy while hospitalized. Including, but not limited to case discussion, consultation, examination and all treatment should be conducted so as to protect each consumer's privacy.*
5. *Each and every individual patient has the right to expect that all communications and records pertaining to their care will be treated with a high rate of confidentiality by the hospital, clinic and caregiver ... except in cases such as suspected abuse and public health hazards when reporting is permitted or required by law.* (Case in point might be of someone who has previously made threats against the President's life and the FBI must be notified at the time of their release, or a significant other and there are pending legal issues, etc.)
6. *Each and every individual patient has the right to expect that, within capacity and policies, a hospital, clinic, or clinician will make reasonable responses to the request of a patient for appropriate and medically indicated care and services.*

7. *Each and every individual patient has the right to expect reasonable continuity of care when appropriate and to be informed by health care providers of available and realistic patient care options prior to being discharged, or admitted into a hospital setting, or clinic.*

8. *Each and every individual patient has the right to have access to records pertaining to their medical care and to have the information explained or interpreted as necessary, unless otherwise clinically contraindicated.*

9. *Each and every individual patient has the right to have an advance directive such as a living will, health care proxy, or durable power of attorney for health care, in regards to their treatment.*

10. *10 Each and every individual patient has the right to be informed of hospitals, clinics and their clinician's policies and practices that relates to their individual treatment, care and responsibilities.* The patient also has the right to be informed of available resources as needed for resolving disputes, grievances, and legal conflicts. Each and every individual patient has the right to be informed of the clinics, therapists and hospitals charge for services and available payment methods prior to receiving treatment.

Additionally Each Patient has the right to:

a) Communicate by sealed mail with any individual, group or agency.

b) To be furnished with writing materials and reasonable postage.

c) To receive mail unless the hospital administration has determined it is medically harmful for the individual patient to receive mail. Then all such, said correspondence will be returned unopened to sender with explanation signed by hospital administration.

d) To make and receive phone calls and have public telephones available unless head of hospital determines patient has made threatening or obscene calls.

e) To wear their own clothing, as deemed appropriate attire.

f) To keep and use personal possessions, including toilet articles.

g) To have access to individual storage space.

h) *To* receive visitors at regular visiting hours, unless the head of hospital determines it is medically harmful for a particular patient to receive visitors and if so, to inform visitors, and to immediately notify them when a patient has recovered sufficiently to receive visitors.

i) To be visited by their clergy, lawyer, legal counsel or physician at any reasonable time.

j) To have noted in writing, signed by head of hospital and made part of the patient permanent clinical record, any restriction of their right to send and receive mail, make and receive telephone calls or receive visitors.

k) To spend a reasonable sum of their moneys for small purchases in such manner as determined by the head of the facility. *However, these rights may be denied or limited, if the treatment team and the hospital administration, or a representative determines that it could be medically harmful for the patient to exercise these rights. Such determination should be placed in the patient's clinical record.*

Each hospitalized individual and their attorney have the right to inspect the patient's records and make copies. After discharge, each individual or their attorney's may inspect and make copies of their record unless the hospital administration determines it to be rather harmful or finds that it violates another person's confidentiality. To my knowledge, psychiatric hospitals do not provide facilities for patients to receive conjugal visits. Therefore, *sexual relations on hospital grounds are prohibited. Violators could be subjected to severe police actions.* Suited to client's own personal needs, goals and aspirations, it is imperative that they be present during meetings or discussions affecting their treatment or service. That they may participate in the decision-making process and that they may help to provide input about desired outcomes. That they may exercise the right to dispute conclusions made by the treatment team, if such is found disagreeable. That they may participate in discharge planning, request for changes in treatment, services or medication regiment.

Patients may also exercise their right to refuse treatment or medications while in a facility *inpatient setting*, so long as he is not a threat to himself or others. However, this could change if noted that such patient has shown signs of decompensation. A probate judge would then determine and issue a court order. The patient does not have to be present in court. Therefore proper documentation is imperative.

A Right To Communicate = Communications Rights While Hospitalized

All patients have the right to: visit with and to have private conversations with clergy, attorney or legal counsel of their choice at any reasonable time, or during visiting hours. **To communicate** with others by telephone, to send and receive sealed correspondence and receive visitors during scheduled visiting hours. *Records or information that identifies the client, manner of treatment or diagnosis cannot be given to any unauthorized person, program or agency without a valid consent form, signed by the patients themselves.*

Each individual patient has the right to be informed of their rights and their grievance process. Each individual patient has the right to be heard concerning grievances, to discuss grievance with appropriate authorized personnel. To have the grievance investigated in a timely manner and expect a mediation to be available, in order to resolve each dispute. To expect assistance with appeal process if needed. The freedom from coercion, intimidation, discipline or any form of retaliation by staff or other clients as resulting from filing such grievance's. No patient should be deprived of any personal property or civil rights, including the right to vote and hold or convey property and contract, except in accordance with due process of law, and unless they have been declared incompetent by a court. Every patient is entitled to receive humane and dignified treatment at all times, with complete respect for his or her personal dignity and privacy.

In addition to these, it should also be noted that no employee working in the mental health field should, be mandated to work more than a reasonably schedule, or previously agreed amount of time. This does not only open the door for abuse upon a patient population, but it in tern does not guarantee the quality of service expected in the treatment geared for the mentally ill patient. My belief is that it is rather a very expensive, hence non coformative disservice to those whom we serve.

Why Processing the Seclusion Situation Is Rather Imperative

When the individual has regained control of their dangerous behavior, the staff member assigned to continuous observation, should initiate a debriefing procedure. This procedure should be based on an implemented Restraint and Seclusion Debriefing and Focus Review guidelines to discuss the situation with the patient and to perhaps collect information that could be useful in developing a plan with the patient to prevent further need for seclusion. These debriefings should be conducted within 16 hours of each seclusion episodes. The exact behavior of the patient that led up to the need or use of seclusion should be documented, all nursing observations and less restrictive interventions used prior to the use of seclusion should also be included and the patient's response to the interventions should be listed.

1.   The Treatment Team, the individual's care coordinator, or primary clinician should schedule the patient for a treatment plan review at the first scheduled treatment team meeting. This should take place following the use of seclusion, or restraints and any such recommended changes should then be incorporated into the individual's treatment plan. Most impatient hospitals function under a structured level system. Such system is geared as a treatment tool and a way of providing patient and public safety, while ensuring community protection and hospital accountability.

The Level System ... This system is primarily universal and is as follows:

Level 1) Verbalizes needs and thoughts, client may move about unit, or hospital ward.

Patients should be able to take care of their own physical needs, e.g. bathing, nutrition, etc. They may also participate in on-unit activities, community meetings, groups, etc.

Level 2) To verbalize personal needs. May go off unit to participate in desired social activities, to attend dining room and building activities with staff, e.g. off unit group activities.

Patients must be compliant with medication and treatment.

Level 3) Patients may go off unit, may attend and participates in groups, walks, in community meetings, activities, and actively participates in off-ground appointments, Rehab, Nursing, Psych, Social workers, doctor's order as needed with staff and follow all of Level 2 Goals

Level 4) Patients must achieve and follow all of Level 3 goals. They may go off unit and remain actively involved in treatment without reminders from staff. They may work toward discharge planning; attend dining room and all off unit activities unsupervised. They are required to attend at least 2 groups per day, e.g. Rehab, nursing, psych, social, work, discharge, etc. They may go to off grounds on planning activities with staff, or case manager.

It is rather imperative for patients to be open-minded and have full understanding in accepting their illness. Likewise, it is also very important that they and their family members show respect to all hospital and clinic staff, and that family members learn to respect their privacy. That they should try avoid being critical. That they refrain from putting their family member into overly stressful or unwelcome social situations, during their visits and that they do not engage in to the practice of setting their expectations too high, for recovery takes time. The most important thing a family member could do to help them while hospitalized, is to remain supportive and involved in helping their family members toward getting effective treatment. It is also helpful that they attend patient-family educational seminars and more importantly that they try to participate in discharge planning, by becoming involved in their aftercare together with their love ones.

CHAPTER X

Discharge and After Care = Outpatient and Staying Out
Two Wrongs Don't Make a Right Managed Care System Mental Health and the Marketplace.
Should people with mental illness participate in supported employment
Are African Americans, Latinos, Asians and other Minorities Still Caught?
In The Midst of A European Oriented Mental Health System?
The Need for More African American Oriented Mental Health Care
NIH New Data on Suicidal Behaviors among African Americans
Lead to Interventions
African Americans, Black Caribbean and Whites Differ in Depression Risk, Treatment
Studying High Rate Latino Incarceration In The Current Mental Health System
NIMH Recently Vows To Expand Public Health Education Effort to Reach Latino Men With
Depression
Asian Americans and the Mental Health System
Asian Americans Accessing Barriers Encountered In Mental Health Services
How Asian Americans View Stigma and Mental Illness
To Many Asian Americans Psychotherapy Is As Foreign As European Tradition
Asian Americans Face Reality About their Lack of Resources
PTSD, Depression Epidemic among Cambodian Immigrants
Bridging the Cultural Differences between Asian Americans and Our Society
Newly Implemented Mental Health Programs for Asian American Groups
Asian Americans Crossing The Cultural Bridge Programs
Alternative Treatment Among Asian Americans
New NIH Studies Shows that foreign born may not be fully protected against mental disorders
in the US
Recent Studies Shows Family-centered Intervention Effectively Reduces Risky Behavior among
Hispanic youth
Out of Many We're All but One
Availability of Mental Health Services for Minorities
Ethnic Cultural Sensitivity Training Is Now Implemented For All Clinicians

Discharge and After Care = Outpatient and Staying Out

Since early on in the decade, "the new millennium," consumers have shown concerns about the impact Medicaid and Managed Care approach and the determination the H.M.O.'s will have on their future treatment. We are now almost a quarter century into the millennium and 'The chronically ill, mentally developmentally or and physically challenged, are still hoping and praying that managed care, Medicaid and the various HMO's will have the knowledge on how to treat them and their presenting symptoms, as they embark on attempting to care for the indigent population among the mentally ill.

New strategies to old problems:

In analyzing the two important aspects of mental health delivery for those who have serious mental disorders and are indigent, we should question and compare to whether Medicaid beneficiaries, once enrolled in prepaid medical plans, would utilize mental health services to the same degree as the non-enrollee. And, also, whether plans would pay the mental health providers the amounts of dollars requested. The overdue debate in the Psychology Community Mental Health Journal still raises questions as to whether psychologists would have a place in the managed care systems as care givers. And why the HMO's places limits on the eligibility for mental health services in order to keep their costs within mandated limits. It has suggested that HMO's should manage physical health and that the community mental health centers should continue to manage mental health problems as a way to keep costs down and therefore still provide *Valuable Managed Mental Health Benefits.*

In comparing the mental health costs of 15 years ago to that of todays, the increase range is now more than (20%). Such, which ranked third only to woman's health and musculoskeletal. These statistics, showed that mental health costs, are surely to drastically increase in the next decade, while the services might continue to further decrease, or at best would remain stagnant. These comparisons were done at a local bank in Chicago several years ago. To remedy this situation the bank developed its own benefits program with some new features. They created an employee assistance program, a wellness program, a psychiatric hospital utilization review, and consulting psychiatrists and implemented also a benefit plan design for such changes. These programs succeeded in holding the line against the rising mental health costs.

One of healthcare's greatest challenges is in providing services for people with severe mental illness in managed care ... while focusing on the delivery of services to long-term persons, with chronic and severe mental illness. This population is more likely to be in poverty even when involved with a managed care group and these people require long-term care. Experts have pointed out that there is no easy solution for this growing group of people. However, they have also discussed that prepaid care for people with chronic conditions is valued over the fee for service arrangement because, (a) institutional care could and should be discouraged, (b) coordination of care could be further enhanced and preventive care should be greatly emphasized. However, clear standards of care have not yet emerged for this population. With using strict utilization review, a person may not receive the type of care needed. An enrollee may even be denied coverage. We as clinicians must be advocates for those of our clients suffering with long-term chronic mental illness and advocate for their treatment during this era of managed care.

However, we should also emphasize on the implementation and development programs geared to build and enhance skill, self-worth and occupational career training for those individuals who otherwise lose what little functioning capacity they might still possess.

Two Wrongs Don't Make a Right. Managed Care System Mental Health and The Marketplace.

Recently psychiatrists have appeared rather very skeptical, concerned and angry to some extent regarding managed care and the mental health system. Some have argued and stated to have found it wrong to turn clinicians into providers and patients into consumers; and also when fee for service was replaced by managed care, psychiatry was the first specialty to receive attention. They feel that psychiatric hospital beds went from extreme over-utilization to extreme under-utilization. They have also voiced their concerns about who profited prior to manage care and who is now profiting from such.

General hospital psychiatry and the new behavioral health care delivery system:

While focusing on the role of managed care in the general hospital psychiatric unit and reviewing the evolution of managed care in the mental health care field, some recommendations were made. These were geared toward further improving the clinical, administrative and financial aspects of general hospital and psychiatry care delivery and in preparation for continued managed care. Rather more specifically for when discussing cost constrainment and 'carve-outs.' In doing so, we should also place focus on the private sector and the middle-class insurance carriers as opposed to merely focusing solely on the indigent and seriously, persistently mentally ill individuals. And the changing landscape Managed Care is forcing and wrenching the restructuring of the behavioral health care delivery system.

Many caregivers are now joining forces and contracting with not - for - profit hospitals to create a provider network to provide services to Medicaid recipients. This is due to the fact that managed care companies and providers want the same things: cost savings and quality of service. Presently about 46% or more Americans are now enrolled in a managed care behavioral program. Experts continue to debate the issues, where managed care in psychiatry will be just as good or better than the current 'fee for services' for most seriously mentally ill individuals. Seriously we could not believe in the theory that if a "health plan artificially reduces the 'supply' of providers, behavioral health utilization will decline and cost will be reduced." They believe that all people whether through "carve-outs" or "capitation" should be eligible for managed care. This could be done through an employer, Medicare or Medicaid.

Management of Mental Health Benefits and Care:

Implemented an approach to the future of the mental health services ... HMO Behavioral Health in Worcester, Massachusetts and several other mental health centers in the nation have listed the following approach:

1. Treating the mentally ill in hospitals only when it is absolutely necessary,
2. Using outpatient clinics and clinicians whenever possible and appropriate. Suggesting that people also be treated on an inpatient basis by provide on-site utilization review with specially developed criteria to insure that high quality intensive care is provided during hospitalization.

The article goes on to also point out that therapies such as recreational, financial and social, etc, can be alleviated by talking to skilled professionals in the field. However, insurance would not provide payment for counseling of this type. The impression we focus on here is that emphasis is being placed on people with acute, short-term psychiatric difficulties.

However the interest should remain placed more on the long term persistently mentally ill. *Managed Cases, Drop-Ins, Dropouts* and other By-Products of Mental Health Care. In discussing intensive case management, assertive outreach teams and social drop-in centers for the severe and persistently mentally ill, the research concerning the above becomes almost impossible, due in part to the self-help nature of some of these very important areas, etc. Drop in centers and social clubs for the discharged mentally ill, all present a negative slant to some degree in areas where clinicians have had positive experience with i.e. self-help groups, drop-in center individuals can get help and awareness from a variety of sources.

Should People With Mental Illness Participate In Supported Employment?

During the mid-part of 2005, leading mental health organizations in several states throughout the nation began approving grants to churches and other religious organizations interested in serving their communities through outpatients, Faith Based mental health programs. In addition to prayer, many churches have since taken a renewed, therapeutic interest toward learning about the causes for mental illness, appropriate treatment and methodologies, for dealing with community mental health, etc. according to former colleagues with years of experience in the field. "If handled appropriately, in reality, this could easily be seen as the greatest change in mental and social engineering in the history of mankind." I believe it is a win, win situation for society as a whole, perhaps we could easily say that everyone in America will benefit from this new approach; the church, the individual and the community, as well as the field of mental health through applied research. Although we first caution these organizations to not stray too far away from the understanding of the individual's illness by trying to impose their beliefs, "these will come to you in due time," to work side by side with mental health professionals. To search, learn and find ways in which they could weave and apply both the religious as well as the therapeutic approach to treatment and to frequently open their doors to new workshops conducted by experts and well trained individual mental health care provider.

One of the first organizations in Connecticut to take on this approach and perhaps the only one in this state that came from behind its pulpit to reach out and seek advice from mental health professionals in the community is the *New Life Ministries*. The New Life Ministries is a faith based organization of women from various Christian denominations that now provides support services, personal development spiritual groups and implement workshops that deal with mental health issues.

This organization also provided services to other faith based organizations, such as the Personal Development Institute for Women, their clients whom are often pregnant women seeking outpatient services for alcohol and drug recovery. Their main objective, is provide mentoring services that help to develop their faith, as well as to equip them with the necessary tools toward becoming productive members of society. Another successful Christian organization set to receive a grant from the State of Connecticut under the Faith Base banner, was the *Phillips Metropolitan Church, AME.*

With a congregation of more than 600 members, a standing longevity for over 73 years in the Hartford community and a senior leading pastor, Reverend James B. Walker, whom at the time, had more than 20 years of seniority in ministry and the church. Phillips Metropolitan is also a collaborating partner with the Greater Hartford Urban League and the First Cathedral Church, to implement The African Family Connection Project (AFCP). It has also recently partnered with the State of Connecticut Department of Mental Health and Addiction Services (DMHAS). With its new purpose and targeted goal, being the Family Strengthening Program Model (FSPM), to deliver weekly educational sessions targeting at risk families and providing information and support, as well as tools and skills that includes a strong focus on the impact caused by substance abuse upon families. In addition, this church continues moving toward developing new partnerships with other community based initiatives, such as Capital Region Mental Health the SANDS and Strive Workforce, by implementing mentoring initiatives designed to recruit and train mentors toward supporting individuals in recovery, reentry into the workforce. As well as to mentor and support those individuals with a long history of previous involvement in the criminal justice system.

The church has done this through a series of teaching workshops and by assisting these individuals in how to best balance their lives and employment, while integrating faith based applications. A proposed responds to this approach has been greatly successful when measured under the Hope Strive Mentoring Program, this which has now lead to an expansion of their program in a short few years. The Phillips Metropolitan Church's mentoring program continues to focus on the integration of faith and recovery through mentoring and by paring positive role modeling, which is primarily accomplished through individual and group mentoring. According to all measured systems currently in place, Philips Metropolitan Church's approach, has been effective. Although it's only been a short time, the effects of this approach had been shown to be greatly successful, noticed and measured specifically in the black communities. Other churches since, now appeared daily to take the helm of this valuable opportunity that is as valuable to the churches, as to their individual communities, as a whole. However, just as the many religious organizations continue working hard toward accomplishing successful goals in the mental health and substance abuse treatments through development, collaborations and partnerships with local, state and other faith base institutions and community based organizations. There are still a large number of individuals who still remain in their trenches ready to defend, criticize and ridicule.

Are African Americans, Latinos, Asians and other Minorities Still Caught up,

In The Midst of A European Oriented Mental Health System?

The population growth within the Latino community remains at a fast moving pace throughout the United States. Between 1990 and the year 2000, the population increase was more than 58%. The growth in number rose from 22.4 million, to nearly 36 million, thus propelling such an increase to become the largest minority group in the land. Estimated census projections, have recently pinpointed that by the year 2050, more than 82 million individuals residing in America will be Latino or of Latino descent.

According to recent research data, there has been a phenomenal growth in the Asian American population in recent years. In early 1990's, there was nearly an 8.1 million Asian Americans in the United States, accounting for the 4.4% of the population. Since the 2000 census, the number increased by 40%, to 11 million, or nearly a 5% increase of the total US population; it is believe that such growth rate, is expected to remain steadily upward.

Regardless of the vast change in population growth in demographic, the mental health problem confronting the Latino population, still remains stagnant under-treated, ignored and understudied. Noted throughout my research and hands-on clinical experience in the field of mental health, is that the majority of the overall psychotherapeutic strategies and interventions, remains designed and implemented without much consideration of the change in demographics, or further studying the social, cultural impact of the Latino and other minority communities.

The fact that most therapeutic interventions have been designed and implemented primarily with the non-Black, or Hispanic, thus rather a sole white population in mind, has only served to further alienate minorities from seeking mental health services. Together with the fact that all available psychotherapy remains still unchanged, thus focusing solely on the treatment of a non-African American-Hispanic white population, it continues to overlook vast cultural differences, while pushing further away the minority population from an already, mismatched mental health services. The continuous oversite only manages to further fuel the negative by supplementing an already under funded and none used, support system for minorities in this country.

The Imperative Need for Mental Health Care within The African American Community

Approximately 12% of the U.S. population, 33.9 million people identify themselves as African Americans, Black Americans or Blacks. However, in order to remain politically correct I will use the political term "The African American" (sorry black folks my apologies if you disagree).

The African American population in the United States is increasing in diversity as immigrants arrive from many African, Caribbean and yes, Central and South American countries. Over half of the Nation's African American population or about 53% live in the South; 37% reside in the Northeast and Midwest combined; 10% live in the West. In 1997, nearly one-fourth of all African American earned more than $50,000 a year. Yet, as a whole, when compared to other racial and ethnic groups living in the U.S., African Americans remain relatively poor. In 1999, about 22% of African American families lived in poverty, compared to 13% for the United States as a whole and 8% for non-Hispanic white Americans.

Isn't There A Need for A More Diverse Oriented Mental Health System of Care?

Whether it being a fact that African Americans differ from whites in the rate of mental illness, cannot merely be a simple answer. For African Americans living in the community, overall rates of mental illness appear to be similar to those of non-Hispanic whites.

Differences do arise when assessing the prevalence of specific illnesses, e.g. African Americans may be less likely to suffer from major depression and more likely to suffer from phobias, than the non-Hispanic whites. Somatization, is more common among African Americans 15% more than among whites (9%). Moreover, African Americans experience culture-bound syndromes, such as isolated sleep paralysis, an inability to move while falling asleep or waking up, and falling out, a sudden collapse, sometimes preceded by dizziness. African Americans have also shown strong coping skills, in other familiar areas, strong family support has been rather an indicative fact for a shorter stays during impatient hospitalizations.

While non-Hispanic whites are nearly twice as likely as African Americans to commit suicide, suicide rates among young black men, are as high as those of young white men and growing. *It is believe that this is due in part to high and easy access to firearms currently available in the African American communities.* Research indicates that from 1980 to 1997, the suicide rate among African Americans ages 10 to 14 increased 233%, compared to 120% of comparable non-Hispanic whites. *African Americans are over-represented in high-need populations that are particularly at risk for mental illnesses.*

Among the homeless, while representing only 12% of the U.S. population, African Americans make up about 40% of the homeless population. Nearly half of all prisoners in State and Federal jurisdictions and almost 40% of juveniles in legal custody are African Americans. Research conducted in the areas of children in foster care and the child welfare system, we found that African American children and youth constitute about 45% of children in public foster care and more than half of all children waiting to be adopted. As people exposed to violence, statistics shows African Americans of all ages are more likely to be victims of serious violent crime, police brutality, than are non-Hispanic whites. One study reported that over 40% of African American youth exposed to violence, met the diagnostic criteria for post-traumatic stress disorder *PTSD.* Among Vietnam War veterans, 21% of black veterans, compared to 14% of non-Hispanic white veterans, suffer from PTSD, apparently because of the greater exposure of blacks to war-zone trauma.

On the other hand, Asian Americans, when compared to other ethnic groups have far underused the mental health resource and services. This has however resulted in a combined erosion and higher wear and tear, combined with delayed treatment rates via attrition. One of the surgeon general's recent research studies, on Asian Americans health services indicated that such underutilization is primarily connected to the shortage of bilingual services and low percentage of health care insurance coverage. *The report also noted that Asian Americans by tradition uses mental health treatment and services only as a last resort.*

New Data on Suicidal Behaviors among African Americans Lead to Interventions.

The prevalence of attempted suicide among black Americans, is higher than previously reported, but near the levels reported for the general population. However, certain risk factors for suicide in this group differ from the general U.S. population. The results of a nationally representative household survey called the National Survey of American Life (NSAL), funded by NIMH, were published in the November 1, 2006 issue of the Journal of the American Medical Association.

Suicide is the 11th leading cause of death in the United States, with older white men having the highest suicide rate. Significant increases since the mid-1980s in reported suicide and suicidal thoughts and actions among young blacks have highlighted an emerging and serious health issue. Sean Joe, M.S.W., Ph.D., of the University of Michigan, Ann Arbor and colleagues sought to identify the prevalence of suicidal thinking and attempts among black Americans in order to document the burden and advance development of interventions to prevent suicide in this population.

In reviewing data from 5,181 African Americans and Caribbean Americans ages 18 and older, the researchers found that the lifetime estimate for attempted suicide among African Americans and Caribbean Americans is 4.1 percent, higher than the 2.3 percent[1] reported previously, but similar to the 4.6 percent[2] for the general population.* In addition to prevalence, the researchers assessed risk factors for suicidal thoughts (ideation), plans, and attempts among black Americans. The presence of an anxiety disorder, was the strongest risk factor compared with other mental or substance use disorders, which differs from other studies in the general population, where depression is often the strongest predictor. Caribbean black men and young people aged 15-24 years had the highest prevalence of attempted suicide and the risk of suicide attempts was highest, during the first year following suicidal ideation. Marital status, often closely linked to suicidal behavior, was not a significant predictor of suicide planning or attempts. Of special importance to clinicians, the researchers found that the majority of blacks who attempted suicide sought treatment from a health professional. The researchers suggested that physicians and mental health professionals should be "skilled in talking with black patients about the risks for suicide, providing interventions for those at imminent risk for suicidal behavior, and referring patients for expert diagnosis and treatment." Further research on the transition from planning to attempts may provide better methods of screening for and preventing suicide in at-risk individuals.

African Americans, Black Caribbean and Whites Differ in Depression Risk Treatment.

A recent scientific update on the study of African Americans, showed that although black Americans are less likely than whites to have a major depressive disorder (MDD), when affected, it tends to be more chronic and severe. An *NIMH*-funded study of mental-health status also showed that we are much less likely to undergo treatment. Studies done by the *National Survey of American Life,* also shows striking differences among blacks. Fewer than half of African Americans with MDD undergo treatment, but the rate drops to about one-quarter in Caribbean blacks who emigrated to the U.S. or their descendants whom were born there.

The survey, included the largest black population in a study of this kind to date and provides a new picture of MDD's toll on subgroups of black Americans. It included self-reports from 3,570 African Americans, 1,621 blacks of Caribbean descent, and 891 non-Hispanic whites age 18 and older, interviewed in 2001 through 2003.

The researchers reported that 10.4 percent of African Americans, 12.9 percent of Caribbean blacks, and 17.9 percent of non-Hispanic whites had MDD at some point in life. However, among participants with depression, the rate of chronic depression, was highest in black groups: 56.5 percent in African Americans and 56 percent in Caribbean blacks, compared with 38.6 percent in whites.

Education and income, were not linked to higher or lower risk of MDD in any of the groups, but some other variables were. Older African Americans and whites, were less likely to have had MDD than were younger people. Compared to those of their male counterparts, rates of MDD, were similar in black Caribbean women, but higher in African-American women. Marriage was associated with lower rates of MDD in both black groups. For African Americans and whites, lower rates were reported by people from the South, the West, and rural areas. Higher rates were especially, noteworthy in African Americans and whites in major metropolitan areas.

Almost all of the respondents, regardless of race, said that MDD interfered with their home, work, or social lives or relationships. Among those who were severely impaired, African Americans and Caribbean blacks reported being unable to function in their daily lives for 71 days of the year; whites reported being unable to function for 63 days of the year.

Previous studies had shown that slightly more than half (57 percent) of adults, who have MDD undergo treatment. This study showed that the treatment rate is less than half (45 percent) for African Americans and less than a quarter (24.3 percent) for Caribbean blacks. The treatment rate for African Americans increases slightly, when the illness is severe, but in Caribbean blacks falls to 21.9 percent.

These findings "underscore the pressing need to understand the factors underlying racial differences in access and quality of mental health care and the urgency of implementing interventions to eliminate these disparities," the researchers write.

Results were published in the March issue of the *Archives of General Psychiatry* by David R. Williams, PhD. and colleagues from the University of Michigan and Wayne State University. With References by Williams DR, Gonzalez HM, Neighbors H, Nesse R, Abelson JM, Sweetman J, Jackson JS. Prevalence and distribution of major depressive disorder in African Americans, Caribbean Blacks, and Non-Hispanic Whites. Archives of General Psychiatry, March 5, 2007.

Studying High Rate Latino Incarceration In The Current Mental Health System

Although earlier research show us that Latinos tend to use the mental health services far less than half of that in comparison to whites, and that even when they do, use it, often times they dropout, shortly after treatment is initiated. Nevertheless, on the flipped side of the coin, Latino appears over represented throughout psychiatric hospitals and twice as likely as the non-Hispanic, white population to be locked up in a restricted psychiatric facility. This frightening pattern of treatment within the mental health disservice, should serve only to help illuminate the negative, thus create a cohesive advancement in the future of mental the health system by suggesting the urgent need to implement a more minority, friendly psycho therapeutic model, geared to each individual cultural characteristic. Although one must keep in mind the reason why I have chosen to focus on the Latino population, it is rather simple. I was born in a Latin American country, speak fluent Spanish, was raised under a primary Spanish education, but I am also a black Garifuna of West Indian descent. I therefore chose when to call myself a Latino, an Afro Latino or black. *We, Latin Americans, are the largest minority group, yet we remain underserved. To those whom might not clearly understand it, the term Latino is not much more than a label of convenience, though however, clearly it refers to a rather diverse group of people residing in the United States. Although some of us might have been born in America, and the term represent mostly those who were born in a Spanish speaking countries, one is still considered a Latino if they could trace their roots back to a Spanish speaking country. Individually, however, the Latino culture do represent many different nationalities and ethnicities … reason for which, although my being black, of African West Indian origin, with an Anglo sounding last name, and my parents being of West Indian, Garifuna descent, I'm still considered a Latino by my peers. Of course, I was born in a Spanish speaking country and I also speak fluent Spanish.*

Conveniently though am also represented by and embraced by the African American and West Indian American communities … with a large number of white, Caucasian associates, colleagues and best friends. Therefore, I am rather fortunate and very blessed for I am a proud member of God's Children, the human race. Currently, the socioeconomic, data indicate that many Latinos still live in one of the worst levels of economic hardships, compared to other groups throughout the United States. In the year 2000, the poverty rate for Latinos reached higher than 23.5 %, compared to the less than a 7.2 % for the white household. Nevertheless between 1990 and 1999, the number of middle-income Latino families grew steadily, while poverty rates diminished slightly. Keep in mind that although the average educational level for Latinos, was substantially lower than that of the general population, it too has increased slightly over the last decade. Nevertheless, there clearly exist much variability and diversity within our cultures … traditional Latino cultures, still tend to promote particular cultural values and scripts. To further grasp a deeper understanding of such, one must first keep in mind that cultural values are strong ideals geared by principles, which aspire to, or is embraced by a specific community. Nevertheless, scripts are the representational and organizational patterns by which individuals learn to follow social roles and are expected to remain within specific social norms. Each individual cultural group, tend to encourage specific scripts and values, which differ collectively from those other cultural groups. Moreover, cultural scripts and values are the essential components found in the mean system of any cultural group. It is imperative for clergy and therapists to clearly understand them and therefore employ them effectively, within their psychotherapy and pastoral sessions. My hope here is that African Americans, as well as West Indian Americans, too will indeed benefit greatly from this understanding.

Expanded Public Health Education, Geared To Reach Latino Men with Depression

The National Institute of Mental Health *NIMH* and the National Institutes of Health research shows that the majority of Latinos fail to recognize the symptoms of depression and is launching a new effort, through the *Real Men Real Depression Campaign.* This which provides Spanish-language materials to better inform the Latino community, about depression and to encourage men whom are depressed to seek help.

According to a report presented by the Surgeon General and other studies, has shown that Latinos are the largest ethnic minority group throughout the United States today, numbering over 56 million in population. With nearly a 60 percent of this group reporting Spanish as their preferred language. *The new Real Men Real Depression* materials, were created to help Spanish-speaking people across the country and from all over the world to understand more about depression and viewed it as a serious illness. As the nation's primary mental health research agency, NIMH is dedicated to reducing the burden of mental and behavioral disorders through research on mind, brain, and behavior. As part of that mission, NIMH provides mental health information to the public and, in particular, focuses on reducing disparities in health care.

National Institute on Mental Health *NIMH* director, Thomas R. Insel, M.D., stated that "*depression and other mood disorders cross all national, cultural, ethnic, and gender boundaries. NIMH developed Real Men Real Depression to inform the nation that depression can strike men just as it can strike women. Lack of awareness about depression is a serious concern in the Latino community. Through these new materials we hope to teach Latino men that depression is a medical condition that affects both the mind and the body, but there is hope.*" Dr. Insel concluded that "*Effective treatments are available and the success rate is very high for people who seek help and remain in treatment.*"

Based on the National Latino and Asian American study, 54 percent of Latino men, with at least one episode of major depression in their lifetime do not recognize having a mental health problem. Latinos also report reluctance to getting treatment for depression. And, like U.S.-born white males, Latino men are afraid that seeking treatment will endanger their jobs. However, there is no evidence to show that people do lose their jobs once they go into treatment. In fact, treatment may be essential to improve work performance.

According to Sergio Aguilar-Gaxiola M.D., Ph.D., whom indicated that new research and other clinical findings "*reveal that women and men may talk differently — or in the case of men, not talk at all about the symptoms of depression,*" Dr. Sergio Aguilar-Gaxiola M.D., Ph.D., was a visiting Professor of Clinical Internal Medicine and the Director of the Center for Reducing Health Disparities, University of California, Davis, and member of the National Advisory Mental Health Council; when he stated that "*Traditional gender roles in the Latino community may further contribute to an unwillingness to talk about feelings of depression.*"

These new materials include publications and broadcast and printed public service announcements (PSAs) in English and Spanish. The PSAs feature Rodolfo Palma-Lulión, a recent college graduate, whom shared his experience with depression in the hopes of encouraging other Latino men to talk about their depression and seek treatment.

"*It took me years to understand that what I was experiencing was depression. Getting help made such an improvement in my life,"* Palma-Lulión. *"I hope the Real Men Real Depression campaign will help other Latino men recognize depression in themselves and have the courage to ask for help."*

Men with depression, regardless of ethnic background, may be more likely to turn to alcohol or drugs, or to become frustrated, angry or irritable instead of acknowledging their feelings and asking for help. Some men may throw themselves compulsively into their work or hobbies, attempting to hide their depression from themselves, family, and friends; other men may respond to depression by engaging in reckless behavior.

Real Men Real Depression was launched in April of 2003. It is the first national public education effort to raise awareness that depression is a major public health problem affecting an estimated six million men annually. The primary message of the campaign's PSAs is that it takes courage to ask for help. *Real Men Real Depression* materials feature personal stories of real men from varied backgrounds. The campaign spokesmen are a combined groups of *Latino, African American, Asian, and American Indian* and include such professions as a firefighter, a national diving champion, a retired Air Force sergeant, a lawyer, and a writer.

The Real Men Real Depression approach, features in its brochure: *"Estos hombres son reales. La depresión también la es!"*

Are The Doors To The Mental Health System Closed To Asian Americans?

Here again, as researchers and mental health treaters, we must thread, carefully and respectfully, when treating, studying or researching the Asian population as a whole … just like the Latino culture, the Asian American group, is as vast and far more culturally diversified among the many represented nationalities, languages and cultures than their Latino counterparts. As recently as 2003, while I worked as the Lead Mental Health Worker and English Spanish Specialist translator on 1West, acute unit, a young Asian American, perhaps of Chinese origins, patient arrived to the now closed Cedar Crest Psychiatric State Hospital in Newington, Connecticut, it took us over twenty four hours, searching and awaiting to locate a competent, qualified, license translator to complete the proper admitting procedures.

This shocked me and at the same time, it reawakened a curiosity to further read, research, investigate and document a little deeper into Asian cultures and mental health system.

Although this might have change a bit since then, throughout our interviewing procedure, during this research other Asian Americans concurred that Asians generally tend to relay more on alternative medicine and seek help from families, friends, and family care physicians. They also added that Asian Americans whom seek psychiatric help, do it as a last resort, and that those that do resort to using mental health services, do it on a primarily short-term, treatment basis and their outcome, reports far lower patient satisfaction scores, than do white Americans, African Americans, Latinos and other ethnic groups.

A review of the uncovered literary research data, reveals a paucity of published data on the prevalence of mental illness among Asian Americans, both in the community and in primary care settings. A recent large-scale community-based study of depression conducted on Chinese Americans living throughout the United States, estimated the lifetime prevalence of major depressive disorder *MDD* among Chinese Americans to be 6.9%, lower than the national estimate of 18% previously documented on Asian Americans. This study was conducted via use of the *Composite International Diagnostic Interview.* Other researchers, whom examined the prevailing major depressive disorders among the Asian Americans, within the primary care settings in urban communities, found the MDD rate among this population to be around 20%. The multiple phase epidemiologic survey conducted, according to the researchers, estimate is believe to be comparable to what was found, within the nonminority low-income population throughout the United States. However, noted is that many of these urban health care centers, with wide-ranging clinical services, is primarily serving the Asian immigrant, whom also face financial, lingual and cultural barriers to health care.

Earlier studies, which examined the symptom profiles among Asian American clients, found that symptoms spontaneously reported by patients differed substantially from those reported when asked directly about the presence or absence of these mood symptoms. Many of them often mirrored earlier results found by other examiners, which led to new findings, discovering that only about 15% of patients among this new migrant group, spontaneously described symptoms from the psychological realm. Among the many symptoms described, most were viewed as depressed mood, irritability, rumination and poor memory. A higher number was proportioned at nearly an 80% among this group of patients, who presented their chief complaint, as their physical symptom, while in a primary care setting. What the study also found a bit confusing, was the fact that none of the patients, who were depressed in earlier studies, considered depressed mood as their chief problem. Nevertheless, nearly 95% of the same individuals had previously endorsed depressed mood, when asked to rate their symptoms using a depression rating scale.

Despite all of these findings, we believe that Asian Americans, who have recently immigrated to the United States, are not incapable of identifying or feeling emotions, but that in a primary care setting one tends to focus more on somatic symptoms and less or not at all, on their the psychological or mood symptoms. Overall, the clinical and public health implication, is that clinicians treating this population need to actively elicit mood symptoms from Asian American immigrants to prevent further under recognition and the under treatment of major depressive disorders.

Although a noted new trend in culture by sociologist and psychologist alike, have documented these recent changes; where in the past, Chinese patients had been brought up and culturally raised as of alexithymic character, *where the individual lacks the ability to understand their emotions or else are unwilling to report them.* Recent documented research study, now shows that the majority of Chinese patients suffering with depression today, have no problem, either identifying or reporting psychological symptoms to their care givers.

It is rather imperative to note that as recently as ten years ago, a study conducted on Chinese American immigrants at an urban primary care population, whom were depressed. A known researcher in the field wrote "When the subjects were asked to label their condition, more than half were unable to ascribe their symptoms to depression or any other psychiatric illness. Although when asked how the symptoms affected them, their responses showed awareness to both the internal, psychological state as well as the somatic, physical state. Out of the 30 patients interviewed in the study, twenty eight over 90% of them felt that the symptoms had affected their mind, nearly an equaling twenty four 80%) felt the symptoms also affected their body, with 22 remaining patients 76% feeling that the symptoms affected both their mind and their bodies.

Population Impact of mind-body relationship

Where depression is a wide a long time accepted concept among European and North American cultures as a distinct and well-accepted psychiatric syndrome, characterized by specific affective, cognitive behavioral, and somatic symptoms. Among many non-European cultures, such as Southeast Asian, Japanese, Chinese, the equivalent concepts of depressive disorders are still not found. This lack of translatability of the illness constructed from the dominant Western culture into Chinese and other Asian cultures still represents a significant and difficult barrier to the effective treatment of depression among Asian Americans today.

In Western medicine, the reporting of internal mood and anxiety states has long been considered the norm for symptom conception and presentation in depression. Somatization, which is often defined as replacing psychological needs with physical symptoms, has been considered a barrier to both the diagnosis and treatment of psychiatric disorders. The psychologizing of symptoms and the valuation of this ability to parse and analyze one's internal emotional states is particular to Westernized cultures. The separation between the body and spirit dates back to the Gnostic traditions, before the time of the early Church; this one size fits all mindset continues in the modern conception of a separate body and mind.

A psychocentric focus in the understanding of mood states is a Western practice that does not fit well with Asian cultures. In traditional Chinese medicine, illnesses are conceptualized in a framework that centers around the organ systems and elements in nature, e.g., fire, wood, earth, metal, water, etc. There is no dichotomy of the mind and body, whereby there would be physical illnesses that are distinct from illnesses of the mind. All illnesses classified as psychiatric or not in Western tradition, are explained within this system. In many Asian American traditions, *one can have anxiety over life, for example, but not an anxiety disorder.* Anxious or depressive feelings, are the natural emotional ripples in the course of life, secondary to a person's medical and interpersonal problems and not conceptualized as a disease entity.

For many Asian patients, therefore, the reporting of physical symptoms is a more familiar and culturally appropriate way to communicate their distress … It is therefore imperative for us to realize that training providers to understand the symptom presentations in different cultures, and by broadening psychiatric classification systems to incorporate the belief systems of other cultures in future psychiatric approach to treatment, we believe might be possible to begin bridging the gap between care providers and their patients.

Most Asian Americans view mental illnesses and psychiatric disorders as a highly stigmatized surrendering condition typically associated with *craziness, mental retardation, severe autism, or hereditary defects.* Many interpret these where only those persons who are unable to otherwise function in society should seek psychiatric help, thus reinforcing their cultural belief that *only crazy people seek mental health services.* Stigma also carries a heavy burden among these communities. *To the Asian American individual associated with the stigma of mental illness, are often led to a loss of face, affecting their social acceptability to them and the patient's family members. As a result, psychiatric services are typically avoided altogether.*

Caregivers should also be aware of the damaging effects often surrounding the use of literal translation of psychiatric terminologies, which can serve to further intensify and deepen the fear. An example of wide and commonly used term, such as the term 'mental disorder' according to Chinese translators, if not careful this could literally translate in Chinese as *jing shen bing,* which actually means *craziness* to most Chinese and Chinese Americans. They also cautioned us when using frequently used terms, such as depressive disorders, or '*yu zheng,*' (Chinese) it could then be perceived as a serious mental disorder leading to insanity or dementia among many Asian Americans.

While psychotherapy principles are applicable and of course, useful for treating Asian Americans, it needs to be pointed out that talk therapy provided by professionals, has not existed in traditional Asian cultures. Less acculturated Asian Americans may feel awkward or anxious, talking to a stranger about their worries and fears. In many traditional Asian societies, where privacy is almost nonexistent (and indeed, I believe there is no word for privacy in the Chinese language), disclosure of behaviors that are not sanctioned by the society, remains a risky and unfamiliar practice. During personal crises, a direct, pragmatic problem-solving approach, looking for immediate and tangible solutions to issues would be more culturally appropriate. The often non-direct role of therapists and their individualistic growth-oriented psychotherapeutic approaches may not be compatible with the needs and expectations of such patients.

Although very few studies have been published on the effectiveness of psychotherapy for Asian Americans, many questions remain about whether conventional psychotherapy principles and skills apply due to cultural differences. Recent case-study methods to analyze various psychotherapy cases of several Chinese American and Japanese American individuals, seen by Western therapists, found various forms of misunderstanding and culturally ignorant treatment practices, and these ineffective and often harmful practices, went unrecognized by the Western therapists. Such a study highlights the importance of providing ethnically sensitive psychosocial intervention. It is therefore imperative to propose that all physicians, who treat diverse cultural populations be provided with formal training in intercultural communication to improve effective quality of care. Recently the *Accreditation Council for Graduate Medical Education,* began requiring that all training programs provide supervised experience of treating patients from culturally diverse backgrounds. Many states in the nation have since established guidelines for professional development for mental health service providers to ensure culturally competency among all mental health practitioners.

Although Asian Americans have been seen as *the model minority* with household incomes higher than the national average. Behind this glamorous facade is the fact that Asian Americans are a highly heterogeneous group with 14% of the population living in poverty. In 2004, 16.8% of Asian Americans, were uninsured, which was comparable to the rate of the national uninsured population (15.7%). Approximately 62% of Asians living in the United States are foreign born, and English proficiency poses a problem for many of them in seeking health services, particularly for mental health issues that require more advanced language skills. The most recent analyzed data from the Chinese American Psychiatric Epidemiological Study, concluded that language barrier, financial resources, time constraints, and knowledge of access to treatment are factors related to the limited use of mental health services among Asian Americans.

Epidemic Levels of PTSD among Cambodian Immigrants Refugees

Recent studies sponsored by the National Institute of Health (NIH) showed that although it's been over forty years since Cambodian refugees fled from the Khmer Rouge reign of terror to the United States. These studies concluded that most Cambodians who resettled here remain traumatized. Other combined studies funded by the National Institute of Mental Health (NIMH) and National Institute on Alcohol Abuse and Alcoholism (NIAAA) found that sixty-two percent suffered from posttraumatic stress disorder (PTSD) and 51 percent from depression. This amounted to a six-to-seventeen percent when compared to the national average. The researchers conducting the study concluded that the more trauma they endured, the worse their symptoms. In the August 3, 2005 edition of the *Journal of the American Medical Association (JAMA)*, the RAND Corporation's Grant Marshall, PhD., and colleagues reported these findings in the nation's largest Cambodian community.

Their survey showed that an estimated three million out of Cambodia's seven million people died during the repression and civil wars of the 1970s and most of those who survived suffered multiple traumas. Moreover, although it has been over forty years since they've been in the U.S., the majority of the refugee community speak little or no English, they remain at income levels below poverty, and still rely on public assistance. Since previous studies of such refugee populations have been criticized for possibly overestimating rates of mental disorders, Marshall and colleagues set out to allay such concerns by employing a more conservative approach. Native Khmer speakers conducted highly structured two-hour interviews with 490 randomly-selected former refugees, ages 35-75, in their Long Beach, California homes, beginning in 2003. They used standardized questionnaires for gauging levels of violence exposure and alcohol use disorder and standardized diagnostic interviews to determine the prevalence of PTSD and depression.

On average, the refugees reported experiencing 15 of 35 types of pre-migration traumas assessed. For example, 99 percent nearly starved to death, 96 percent were enslaved, into forced labor, 90 percent had a family member or friend murdered, and 54 percent were tortured.

Even after arriving in the U.S., 34 percent said they had seen a dead body in their neighborhood, fewer than a third were spared from the psychiatric disorders assessed. Rates of PTSD and depression tended to be highest among those who were older, poorer, weaker English speakers, and unemployed. Forty-two percent had both disorders, and severity of the disorders increased with trauma exposure. The risk factors that predicted depression, were so similar to those that predicted PTSD that the researchers suggest that both disorders may, in fact, reflect "a single continuum of posttraumatic stress." The 62 percent of those surveyed who had PTSD in the past year compares to a prevalence rate of 3.6 percent in the general adult population. The 51 percent who met criteria for major depression compares to a rate of 9.5 percent of U.S. adults.

Rates of alcohol abuse among the refugees were much lower than in the general population and were not associated with PTSD, likely reflecting the influence of cultural factors. The study did not assess the extent to which participants sought treatment for their disorders, but the interviewers gave them information about local mental health clinics. Still, the study "raises questions about the adequacy of existing mental health resources in this community," noted the researchers. They also suggested that the U.S. has not succeeded in its goal of promoting the long-term health and well-being of these refugees. Also participating in the research were: Drs. Terry Schell, Marc Elliott, Megan Berthold, Rand Corporation; and Dr. Chi-Ah Chun, California State University.

Bridging the Cultural Differences between Asian Americans and Our Society

As pointed out earlier, providers treating less acculturated Asian Americans should treat somatic complaints because they are an essential and legitimate indicator of mental distress. Such complaints should not be seen as a lack of psychological sophistication. Many Asian Americans who present with physical symptoms have no difficulty in reporting and talking about their mood and anxiety symptoms when prompted by clinicians.

When Talking to Asian Americans about psychiatric illness ... In addition to understanding the characteristic profiles of symptoms presentation among less acculturated Asian Americans, clinicians should strive to use frameworks and language that resonate with their patients. Since many Asian Americans with traditional illness beliefs who are depressed may have different perceptions about psychiatric disorders, clinicians need to skillfully explore how the psychiatric terminology will be perceived and to clarify misunderstandings of the terminology that may exist. For instance, in traditional Chinese medicine, all illness is the result of imbalance in the elements and forces within the body and nature. Therefore, reframing depression as an imbalance in the body's system *i.e., monoamines* that can be helped with selective serotonin reuptake inhibitors (SSRI), would be better received than an explanation that focuses on neurotransmitter reuptake mechanisms or distorted cognitive perceptions. It is frequently helpful to use a patient's own terminology and framework to help them understand the nature of the illness and the benefits of treatment.

Newly Implemented Mental Health Programs for Asian American Groups

Several specialized mental health programs have recently been established to provide services to the Asian American populations in cities with a high concentration of ethnic groups, such as Miami, Boston, New York, Los Angeles, and San Francisco. These programs are generally staffed with bilingual, bicultural professionals and support personnel. The result has already began to show positive effects among the population whom now feels more at ease, when accessing these programs, consequently the delay between onset of symptoms and contact with the mental health system is swiftly shortened. Although, such should not come as a surprise, since studies has long shown positive results between ethnic match, therapist and client; among all, lead to better treatment outcomes.

Crossing The Cultural Bridges With Our Asian American Brothers

Investigators have documented their findings on the large numbers of less acculturated Asian Americans unfamiliar with traditional mental health services frequently present to their case to primary care physicians, herbalists, acupuncturists, or other alternative practitioners for help when suffering from psychiatric illnesses. These smart researchers have therefore, realized the need for primary care physicians to be skilled in identifying mental illness. Many studies have shown, however, that patients in primary care with mood and anxiety disorders, often go unrecognized. Improving the recognition and treatment of mental illness in primary care settings is a major public health issue, particularly among ethnic minorities. *The New York Chinatown Clinic*, lead the march in pioneering *The Bridge Program* to integrate primary care and mental health services to service the Asian American indigent population. The key elements of the Bridge Program include co-location and collaboration between mental health service providers and primary care physicians in treating mental illness and training of primary care physicians and support staff in handling patients with psychiatric disorders. This Bridge Program is now being successfully replicated at several other Asian health care centers in Boston and in Oakland, Calif. Preliminary results suggest that integrating mental health and primary care increases referrals to and treatment acceptability of mental health services by Asian Americans.

Shared Alternative Treatment among Asian Americans and Other Minorities

Asian Americans and several other minority groups often use traditional Chinese treatment for their medical and psychiatric problems, either in isolation or in combination with Western medical treatment. Common practices include meditation, tai chi, bone-setting, acupuncture, various herbal treatments, etc. While the use of alternative and complementary treatment have increased in the United States in the past decades, scientific research groups, continuously rigorous argued and try to pinpoint their inadequate evidence regarding its effectiveness and their potential side effects. Although this is a tedious and complex process, it is necessary to systematically investigate the effects of these treatment modalities on mental illness so that patients will be able to make informed decisions.

Modern Technologies Meet Modern-day Psychiatric Services:

The digital revolution, cyberspace microprocessors and videoconferencing, smart phones, etc. brings tremendous opportunities to clinical care, education, research, and administration. Due to wide access and the availability of computers and technological support, it is now possible to provide mental health services anywhere in the world. It has recently been discovered and now broadly put to use the benefit found within this rapidly evolving technology, which can address problems of disparities in mental health services caused by the shortage of bilingual and bicultural clinicians. A study conducted on immigrants and refugees in Denmark and several other European countries have documented on the positive outcome in treatment by ethnic specialists, with similar language and cultural backgrounds through videoconferencing and cell phones, compared with a face-to-face interview with a non-ethnic specialist assisted by an interpreter.

While the promises of delivering mental health services through telemedicine is great, there are still several obstacles to be overcome, before telepsychiatry can become a mainstream service. These include issues of credentialing and licensing of providers, obtaining liability coverage and health insurance reimbursement for services provided through videoconferencing. Nevertheless, this is a new tool in the treatment that still needs fine-tuning, it's here now and it is here to stay!

Foreign Born May Not Be Fully Protected Against Mental Disorders In The US.

Although most Latino immigrants tend to do overall well in mental health, when compared to their US-born counterparts, a recent NIMH-funded research study, found that the protective benefits of foreign nativity, varies widely across subgroups of this population. Factors such as, neighborhood stability, perceived discrimination, and the strength of family bonds, all combined to influence the prevalence of mental disorders across distinctive Latino ethnic groups. These findings reflects varying immigration and acculturation processes experienced by Mexicans, Cubans, Puerto Ricans and other Latino groups.

A research team, lead, by Dr. Margarita Alegria of Harvard University, placed its primary focused on the information gathered through the *National Latino and Asian-American Study (NLAAS)* to examine the effect of foreign nativity on the prevalence of mental disorders within Latino immigrant populations. The researchers initially divided the survey population into two groups; Late-Arrival Immigrants (LAI), or those whom arrived in the US after age six and those who arrived in the United States before age six, or (IUSC). The latter group also included Latinos, who were born in the United States, as native born and early-arrival immigrants, who shared similar language skills and acculturation experiences. In contrast, late arrival immigrants, may have limited English skills and closer connections to traditional customs, family structures, and religious values. Survey participants were further divided based on ethnic background and country of origin. These divisions allowed researchers to show that nativity, is only part of the larger picture, when considering susceptibility to various mental disorders. Previous studies of the "immigrant paradox," which refers to the tendency of children of immigrants to have a higher prevalence of mental disorders, than their parents, focused primarily on nativity, while overlooking other sources of risk. By dividing the Latino population into subgroups based on country of origin, as well as late (LAI) and early (IUSC) arrival to the US researchers were able to identify other factors, such as familial and cultural ties, income disparities, and perceived social standing, which interact to influence the prevalence of mental disorders. For example, Mexican LAI immigrants showed lower risk of depressive disorders, compared to their IUSC counterparts. However, when family cultural conflict and family burden were taken into account, LAI Mexicans, experienced similar levels of risk for depression as IUSC. No differences in risk for anxiety disorders were found for LAI, versus IUSC Latinos. Yet, surprisingly, results showed that immigrant families with incomes of $15,000 a year or less, seemed to experience lower levels of anxiety disorders, than those families, who made above $35,000. The researchers, proposed that the unexpected protective effect of poverty, was likely due to a higher perceived social standing, within the low income families. At the same time, thought that lower-income families may have lowered expectations for success, compared to their more affluent peers. This may help to limit some of the stressors associated with trying to improve one social standing and achievement. The study highlights the need for further investigation of the varying cultural and sociological influences that affects mental health in immigrant populations. Nativity alone may not be as protective as once thought. Rather, family harmony, marital status, and integration in employment may be key factors toward decreased risk in depression and anxiety disorders. Including comparisons of immigration arrival across subgroups, within an ethnic population in future studies could be a valuable tool in determining additional factors that may increase or decrease the risk for psychiatric disorders in,

Latino and other immigrant populations. However, as we begin to study the major impact on the most recent immigrant population in the last 13 months we shouldn't be at all surprised at the elevated numbers of MDD affecting the overall impact.

Family-centered Intervention Effectively Reduces Risky Behavior among Hispanic Youth.

A family-centered program that improves parent-child dynamics and family functioning is more effective at discouraging Hispanic youth from engaging in risky behavior than programs that target specific behaviors, according to a study published in the December 2007 issue of the *Journal of Consulting and Clinical Psychology.*

Hispanic adolescents are at higher risk for substance abuse and risky sexual behavior than other ethnic groups, according to the U.S. Centers for Disease Control and Prevention. And while they represent 14 percent of the U.S. population, they account for a disproportionate 18 percent of all HIV/AIDS cases in the nation. Several types of interventions exist that aim to reduce or prevent risky behavior like substance use and unsafe sexual behavior among non-Hispanic white youth, but no studies have been conducted to determine the relative effectiveness of similar programs targeted to Hispanic youth. Guillermo Prado, Ph.D., of the University of Miami, and colleagues randomly assigned 266 eighth-grade Hispanic youth and their primary caregivers (usually the mother) to one of three interventions: Familias Unidas plus Parent-Preadolescent Training for HIV Prevention (PATH) English for Speakers of Other Languages (ESOL) plus PATH

ESOL plus Heart Power for Hispanics, an American Heart Association program

Familias Unidas plus PATH was designed to promote positive adolescent development by increasing parental involvement and teaching more effective parental communication techniques. The program was designed to be more consistent with Hispanic cultural expectations, in which life is family-centered and vital to an individual's emotional support. PATH is designed to specifically increase parent-adolescent communication about sexual behavior and HIV risks, but it does not target family dynamics specifically.

Heart Power for Hispanics is designed to encourage healthier behaviors among Hispanic youth to reduce obesity and heart disease risks. The interventions were conducted over one year, and researchers followed up with participants at one and two years after the intervention ended. They found that the Familias Unidas plus PATH intervention was much more effective than the other two interventions in reducing cigarette use, and moderately more effective in reducing illicit drug use and unsafe sexual behavior among the adolescents. "It is noteworthy that Familias Unidas + PATH produced favorable outcomes among the youth, even though most sessions in this group were conducted only with the parents." said Dr. Prado. "The findings also suggest that targeting specific health behaviors such as cigarette smoking and risky sexual behavior within the context of strengthening the family may be the most effective approach for Hispanic adolescents."

Out of Many We're All but One

Mental Health Could Be Influenced by Culture and Immigration Status

The culturally-relevant research provided clues that may help reduce health disparities, according to the special issue of *Research in Human Development*, examined the current trends in prevalence and risk factors for mental disorders across the lifespan in diverse U.S. minority populations. Past research suggests that factors such as culture, race, ethnicity, gender and age can significantly influence overall health, as well as health care attitudes and access, and responses to treatment. A better understanding of the complex role that cultural backgrounds and diverse experiences play in mental disorders is crucial, as NIMH, researchers suggest, a stride to create personalized treatment for those with mental disorders.

The most recent presented workshops organized by NIMH and the Family Research Consortium, listed five articles providing insight into NIMH-sponsored national studies of mental health among the minority populations in the United States. These covered the potential cultural risk factors for suicide, among Native American youth, as well as one of the first major studies of mental illness among ethnically diverse teens. NIMH research scientist Cheryl Boyce, PhD, and Andrew Fuligni, PhD, of the University of California, Los Angeles, discuss in an introductory article the main themes represented in the special issue and particular cultural considerations that appear to be the most relevant at different stages of life for the mental health of U.S. minority populations. Recommendations for further research may help inform efforts to reduce health disparities. Notable findings from this special issue included:

Age at immigration appears to affect the onset of mental disorders in Asian Americans. Based on data from more than 2,095 Asian Americans collected for the National Latino and Asian American Study (NLAAS), David Takeuchi, PhD, University of Washington, and colleagues found that those who immigrated during childhood, as well as U.S. born Asians, were much more likely to have a mental disorder in their lifetimes than other immigrant generations. Asian immigrants who arrived at age 12 or younger had a greater risk for psychiatric disorders during childhood than their U.S. born counterparts; this risk, along with risk for substance abuse, increased during adolescence. Asian immigrants who arrived before age 41 also had a greater risk of onset for mood disorders during or shortly after immigration, whereas those who arrived after age 41 were more likely to have experienced onset before immigration.

Information on more than 2,554 Latinos interviewed for the NLAAS showed that age at immigration was also key in the mental health of this diverse minority population, found Margarita Alegría, PhD, Harvard University, and colleagues. In general, past age 7, the older the person at immigration, the later the onset of psychiatric disorders. Those who arrived later in life had lower lifetime prevalence rates than younger immigrants or U.S. born Latinos. However, after about age 30, the risk of depressive disorders increased among these later-arriving Latino immigrants, whereas risk tended to decrease between ages 30-40 for U.S. born Latinos and immigrants arriving before age 7. Latinos arriving between ages 0-6 had very high risks of onset shortly after immigration, but after several years, their lifetime prevalence rates approached those of Latinos born in the United States.

Researchers working with Harold Neighbors, PhD, University of Michigan, studied the interactions between culture, race, and ethnicity with depressive symptoms among a subset of participants from the National Survey of American Life, comprising 3,438 African Americans, Caribbean Americans, and white Americans. They evaluated social, group, and individual characteristics related to behavioral responses (such as coping strategies) to life stressors, group and personal identity, ideology, and beliefs about racial relations, and how these factors intersected with symptoms of depression. African Americans in this study did not show a significant relationship between depressive symptoms and high-effort coping strategies, while Caribbean Blacks and white Americans experienced increasing symptoms of depression linked to increasingly high-effort coping, in relationship to other beliefs and values.

Nearly 20 percent of Native American middle school students in a single reservation attempted suicide, double the rate for the general teenage population, according to a study led by Teresa LaFromboise, PhD, Stanford University, and funded by the Substance Abuse and Mental Health Services Administration. The researchers evaluated 122 students who belonged to the Metis or Ojibwa tribes living in the Northern Plains and found that a sense of connection or belonging to their school community appeared have a strong, protective effect against suicidal thoughts. Overall, the two strongest predictors for thinking about suicide were depression and substance abuse. Data on the mental health of diverse teens in the Houston area suggest few differences in risk for mental disorders based on ethnicity. Robert Roberts, PhD, and Catherine Ramsay Roberts, MPH, PhD, both at the University of Texas, interviewed 4,175 European American, African American, and Mexican American youth and found that, overall, teens of European American descent were at lower risk for anxiety disorders, and African American youth were at lower risk for substance use disorders and having more than one mental disorder. Unlike adults, total family income (or socioeconomic status) was not linked to increased risk for any disorder for any of the three groups; however, the *perception* of lower income was associated with increased risk for all groups.

Availability of Mental Health Services for Minorities

The current public mental health safety net of hospitals, community health centers, and local health departments are vital to many African Americans, especially to those in high-need populations. African Americans account for only 2% of psychiatrists, 2% of psychologists, and 4% of social workers in the United States.

In 2000, during the time of this research, nearly 1 in 6 African Americans remained uninsured, compared to the nearly 20% of the U.S. population. Rates of employer-based health coverage are somewhere around the 60% for employed African Americans, compared to nearly 80% for employed non-Hispanic whites. It is believe that these estimates have since grown in numbers Medicaid coverage, are at around 22% among African Americans; however, less than one-third of African Americans with a mental illness or a mental health problem get care. Yet, the percentage of African Americans receiving needed care is only half that of non-Hispanic whites. One study reported that nearly 70% of older African American adults are receiving these needed services. Although research also indicates that African Americans are more likely to use emergency services or to seek treatment from a primary care provider than from a mental health specialist. Moreover, we may use our churches and other alternative therapies more than do whites.

While African Americans of all ages are underrepresented in outpatient treatment, but rather over represented in inpatient treatment. e.g., few African American children receive treatment in privately funded psychiatric hospitals, but many receive treatment in publicly funded residential treatment centers for emotionally disturbed youth. The appropriateness and outcomes of mental health services among the African American community measures the few clinical trials evaluating the response of African Americans to evidence-based treatment, the limited data available suggest that, for the most part, African Americans respond favorably to all treatment. However, there is cause for concern about the appropriateness of some diagnostic and treatment procedures, e.g. Compared to whites, exhibiting the same symptoms, African Americans tend to be diagnosed more frequently with schizophrenia and less frequently with affective disorders.

In addition, one study found that 27% of blacks compared to 44% of whites received antidepressant medication. Moreover, it is also noted that the newer medications that have fewer side effects are often prescribed less to African Americans than to whites. Although data suggest that blacks may metabolize psychiatric medications more slowly than whites, blacks often receive higher dosages than do whites, this which in turn leads to more severe side effects. As a result, African Americans may stop taking medications at a greater rate than whites with similar diagnoses. Pharmacologic treatment among Asian Americans also focuses primarily on ethnicity as a major important factor in an individual's response to medications. The cytochrome enzymes that are important for metabolizing psychotropic medications are known to have polymorphic variations or genetic mutations that give rise to different forms of the same enzyme *isoenzymes*. Many studies have shown that higher proportions of Asians than whites have a less active form of CYP2D6 and CYP2C19 isoenzymes. These findings are consistent with other studies that show that Asians as a whole tend to metabolize antipsychotics far slower than their white counterparts. In addition to genetic differences, many environmental factors, such as diet, the use of herbal medicines and other lifestyle differences, play important roles in determining drug metabolism rates and clinical responses to medications. *All of these factors must be considered when prescribing medications to Asians and other minority patients since, thus far, most of the data on pharmacologic treatment are based primarily on white subjects.*

Ethnic Cultural Sensitivity Training a Mandate Requirement to All Clinicians?

We must keep in mind that culture plays a very important role in influencing the formation and presentation of psychiatric problems and patients' beliefs about their illness. Asian Americans, Latinos and other newly arrived ethnic groups with their characteristic and diverse cultural background and specific immigrant status, today pose a challenge to clinicians. Improvement in the recognition and treatment of mental illness in Asian Americans can be achieved by training clinicians in cultural sensitivity, redesigning the structure of service delivery in outpatient clinics, educating immigrants about mental illness, and broadening the nomenclature and practices in psychiatry to incorporate the belief systems of other cultures.

With the rapid changing demographics in the United States, it is important that all clinicians be able to provide culturally sensitive care to their clients and be fully prepared to care for Americans as a whole. These skills are especially are more important today in psychiatry than ever, where clinical judgments are invariably influenced by the ethnicity and culture of both psychiatrist and patient. In an effort to reduce and eliminate health care disparities, the *Accreditation Council for Graduate Medical Education* today requires that all training programs provide supervised experience of treating patients from culturally diverse backgrounds. Many states have also established guidelines for professional development for mental health service providers to ensure culturally competency among all mental health practitioners.

CHAPTER XI

A Face-To-Face Encounter with Pediatric Intellectual Development.

A not so sweet little story about chemical induced mental retardation, impinged on the unborn.
Andrew's first experience with mental illness concerning a child, was when he was eleven-years old. His mother had recently loss her job at the university and their home to the bank. The family had relocated to another city and moved into a tiny house owned by a family friend, on the outskirts of the city of San Pedro Sula, Honduras's industrial capitol. Their new neighborhood was miles away from where he'd spent his earlier years, grown up. Their economic status was vastly different, he now had to make new friends and start over from scratch. (Trying to be half as popular as he had previously been in his old neighborhood and readjusting proved rather difficult at his age). Nevertheless, this new neighborhood was a kind of a rural unusual town in and of itself, lots of farms, ranches, cattle, wild animals and rivers. Barrio Las Palmas, was a small blue-collar community surrounded with a largely poor, but very decent, hardworking, supportive individuals. Right away and almost instantly, he'd noticed that they were the only black family in the area. At first he believed it was going to be tough making new friends, although during such times, Honduras, was a country more class conscious and less concerned with race and the color of one's skin. His West Indian and African American heritage and his bilingual abilities, in such a case, definitely had its pluses.

This was the early part of 1970, and perhaps the main reason for his popularity, was that back then most everyone throughout the Central American region wanted to learn English. During such, less than 5% of the Honduran population spoke English, and by now most everyone dreamt of eventually moving to the United States of America, where almost everyone wanted to English. Thirty-nine years later, it appears as if we were all looking forward to a reverse migration, today everyone want to learn Spanish. As I've noticed recently, even politicians have embarked on such a systemic quest, perhaps merely to try and potentially catch a percentage of that growing Latino vote. Finding himself in this new neighborhood where no one around there looked nor sounded like him, his oldest brother, who was eleven years older, had recently moved out to live on his own. His oldest sister had recently gotten married and relocated and his second oldest sister studied at the university and stayed on campus. His mother had also recently developed a heart disease, and had been hospitalized prior to their relocating, reasons for which his grandmother had taken his other three younger brothers to live with her on the coast, leaving just him and his nine-year-old sister. The drive to where his grandmother lived was only three hours away, but it seemed to be more like a world away from the one in which he now lived. In part, this was due to his being only eleven years old at the time and not being allowed to travel unsupervised on board interstate bus lines. Months went by; however, it did not take his sister long before she'd made lots of new friends. At this time, his mother remained in and out of the hospital, following up with doctor's visits and sometimes being readmitted for overnight observations. Although she had no immediate relatives in town, she had several close friends and supportive neighbors, some of whom, even kept an eye on her each time she was re-hospitalized.

He also had a close cousin, Daliah, who although she did not live in exactly the same city, she was highly concerned about their well-being and took time to visit regularly. With all that was going on in their lives, both emotionally and financially, he had been compelled to quit school that year and spent most of his time hanging around, playing ball, wondering off in the woods and exploring the nearby outdoors, while making attempts at new friendships. Their running water at home had been shut off due to lack of payment and he now had to walk several blocks to collect water from the nearby public fountain for washing, bathing, cleaning and laundry. By now he had also befriended a couple of people in the neighborhood and was able to collect drinking and cooking water from their outdoor faucet, the nearest being about half a block away … several houses down from the Espinoza's home. The Espinoza's, was utterly a unique family. They were hard working, caring, well liked, and nevertheless, unique in a true sense of the word. They seem to live within a day, to day psychological phenomena, yet not once did they appear miserable, resentful, nor sad. Mr. Espinosa and his loving devoted wife, Chavelita, were two of the nicest people in the little community. Their unusual story, however, still is one of the saddest ones he had ever encountered.

The Espinoza's had five biological children, Stella, Nela, Fidel, Luis and Graciela. Out of their five children, four of them were mentally retarded, or developmentally disabled. However, it was due to the unusual surrounding circumstances within the Espinoza's unusual life that Andrew came to experience his first collective, psychologically challenged selective group of adults and it was through such, that he was also able to stumble upon and closely observe his first developmentally disabling pediatric case.

Although it's been many years since, their case study still puzzles and astonishes him to this day. Andrew and Luis had begun establishing a rapport; they played soccer together and oftentimes, even hiked in the woods. They also rode their bikes and together hunted birds and iguanas at times; they helped milking cows at the Pinto's farm in exchange for free cheese. However, to him it still remained a constant intrigue, as to why out of the five children, Luis was the only one who enjoyed, common intellectual, functioning abilities among his siblings? Though at the time, not much attention was paid to his state of mind. Often Luis displayed unexplainable mood swings that would sometimes turn his playing into fistfights. The active rumors around town were that his father had been a drinker, that he was an alcoholic and that as a result of his drinking; his other four children had been born intellectually handicapped. Some people throughout the small community argued about Luis being normal because Mr. Espinosa had eventually stopped the drinking for several years, but that he began to drink again around the time Graciela, their youngest daughter was conceived. Graciela was about six, or seven years old when Andrew moved into the neighborhood. He personally never saw the man drink, nor did he ever see Mr.

Espinoza appear drunk throughout the time they were neighbors. Though the particular myth was baseless and made no sense, everyone around appeared to believe it. As Andrew grew older and came to age, he automatically made it his business to familiarize himself with alcoholism in depth, its significant functions and the negative, scientific stresses it places on one's body. It was afterward when he eventually realized they were all wrong and determined that it had all been no more than false rumors. Given the fact that the fetus is formed in the mother's womb, rather than in the sperm, delivered into the woman, the father is merely the donor and not the recipient.

Said case would have had a more scientific basis if their mother had been the alcoholic, this would've revealed a more reasonable explanation for why all the children had been struck, resulting in *FAS*, or fetal alcohol syndrome. In further critical analysis of the Espinoza's situation, he recalled that Mr. Espinoza worked for the ESNEN, a fuzzy chemical environmental branch of the Honduran sanitation department. Mr. Espinoza's job consisted of being around impoverished neighbor hoods, out in the field, eradicating, or spraying for rodents, mosquitoes and other common third world pests and parasites. He remembered seeing him and his crew unknowingly mixing, spraying extremely toxic chemicals, such as DDT and other lethal chemicals with their bare hands and they wore no mask, nor any other type of protective gear. In those days most chemicals were not publicly known to be harmful to mankind as they are today and those who, perhaps knew about their dangerous and disastrous effects, made every effort to frequently keep it very quiet.

Although now DDT and other toxic chemicals have been banned throughout the United States, they were still being ship and used commonly in Honduras and many other Latin American and Caribbean countries. Anyone who lived in Honduras throughout the seventies, perhaps still thus remembers frequently seeing these men dressed in their gray uniforms, walking around in small brigades-like groups of eight, spraying this stuff around without even wearing masks over their

faces or gloves to protect their hands. It is thought, however, that those responsible for manufacturing and marketing these chemicals were knowledgeable and therefore, responsible for the failure to properly educate these men using the chemicals about the dangers encountered. Of course, it is interesting to accept that alcoholism might have also played a crucial role in this story, but it would've been a minor one by virtue of the carelessness and naive negligence of Mr. Espinoza, rather than in the immediate physical contact with his wife after working with the chemicals. Physical yes, but perhaps in the manner their father might have failed to use precautions to decisively protect his family. Realistically speaking, Mrs. Isabel (Chavelita) Espinoza and her four developmentally disable kids were merely the innocent victims to a naive and ignorant practice. Chavelita was just a common homemaker who stayed at home and who'd been dealt a bad card in life. She'd found a relatively peaceful joy and inherent spiritual comfort by staying at home taking care of her four mentally challenged children. Though poor and uneducated, she displayed the unconditional love, compassion and understanding they so needed. She implemented it in such ways, as if she'd possessed some kind of advance training in psychology.

Stella, the eldest, was about twenty-two years old; Nella, the second girl was about twenty; Fidel was about nineteen, Luis, about twelve and Graciela seven. Luis was also the only one enrolled in elementary school. They were all a selective group of poor, struggling families, who were besides very proud and supportive of each other. They all got along rather well. Andrew's new neighborhood was utterly a unique little community. It was surrounded by farms, factories, rivers, sugarcane fields, pineapple and orange walks, lots of broad open fields in which mischievous boys played cowboys and Indians and hunted, and rode horses bareback. Everyone was concerned, loving and supportive of each other. Andrew had grown to like everyone. Until one day, when Nella made a bizarre move that changed everything and turned their little, peaceful community upside down. Andrew was over by the neighbors collecting drinking and cooking water, he on most occasions carried two buckets, a plastic one for drinking and cooking, and a metal one in which he collected water for washing dishes, bathing, etc. A couple of minutes of his being there, he'd noticed that Nella had walked in to the yard and was heading straight toward him. She immediately began hitting him for no obvious reason; he moved out of her way and thought that she was trying to be playful at first. He smiled and moved out of her way, but she relentlessly continued following him around and this time making growling noises, with an angry look in her eyes, as her anger escalated into making loud, animal-like sounds, due to her inability to talk.

Nella continued making weird facial and physical gestures and definitely wished to fight him. Andrew promptly collected both of his buckets and began to walk away, but then she eventually reached into her mouth with her hand and pulled out a live green, slimy hawker from deep down her throat and flung it at him. The hawker landed on the right side of his face and at that point he lost control. He swung the plastic bucket, which he carried in his left hand at her, without immediately realizing perhaps his strength or the heaviness of the water contained in the bucket and the apparent closeness of his reach. The blow landed on her right temporal lobe, it was a hot summer day and blood immediately began to gush from her head, covering her entire face. Andrew panicked, dropped his buckets, jumped the fence and ran home to hide under his bed. He hardly remembered seeing her fall to the ground as he ran away, though he readily confesses not really looking back; "I was too scared."

A few minutes later, Mr. Espinoza, his wife, Nella, her two brothers and sisters, and it would appear that the whole town was knocking at his door. "I thought they were coming to lynch me." His mother had just been discharged from the hospital and this time she'd been diagnosed with high blood pressure and a heart condition. Andrew, however, was more concerned about his hide than that of his mother's health. "Lucky for me, Mr. Espinoza was a calm, well-mannered man who apparently was used to his children's bizarre behavior. He also understood the poor conditions of mother's health." Mr. Espinoza, clearly spoke very softly, Andrew still refused to come out from where he was hiding. "I could hear him telling my mother that he knew his children were sometimes terrors and are always getting into trouble and that some of the neighbors are pretty much fed up with them, but that she did not deserve this." He reminded her that he also punishes them whenever anyone complains to him, or his wife about them. "Just yesterday I had to take Fidel out and beat him with a wet rope, because he stole a car and crashed into a light pole." All he wanted was a couple of Lempiras toward Nella's medical bill. Of course mother was in no condition to punish Andrew. His cousin, Deliah, was up visiting them and she gladly offered her services. Deliah was about six feet tall, one hundred and eighty pounds and she went under that bed pulled Andrew outside the house and let his little behind have every ounce of her weight. She whooped his behind with a wide leather belt right in front of everyone. His mother also made him apologize and offered to effectively pay for Nella's entire medical expenses. Luckily for all, the cut on Nella's head wasn't as deep as they first thought. She required just a bottle of hydrogen peroxide, a tube of antibiotic ointment and band aids. From that day on, Nella, her two sisters, and her brothers stayed far away from Andrew and he was content by not being bothered with them ever again.

Andrew did not remain in the neighborhood much longer after the reported incident. The following trip when his cousin came to visit, he pleaded, begged and was able to convince her that if she'd taken his sister to live with her in Puerto Cortes, his mother would soon follow. His suggestion proved him right. That is how he finally got out of San Pedro Sula, Honduras' proud industrial capitol. Ever since then, he duly remained intrigued and mystified about the whole mental health affliction situation. Years later, unknowingly he entered the university and majored in psychology, but would never work as a psychologist. Puerto Cortes is situated on the North coast of Honduras and is known as being one of the largest and most significant international seaports in Central America. Hernan Cortes was its original founder, that's why it takes his name.

Hernan Cortes was also the founder and conqueror of Mexico. He is accredited with nearly and completely decimating the complete native population of that country. Ironically, he was also captured and decapitated right in Puerto Cortes. Puerto Cortes besides has one of the largest black, English and Garifuna speaking population on the Honduran mainland, second only to La Ceiba, the third largest Honduran city. Honduras is largely comprised of West Indian descents and Garinagus people who were brought to Honduras over 200 hundred years ago after being expelled by the British from Saint Vincent. These two cities are compared only to the three islands off the mainland for its African cultural heritage. The varied reasons for such a large population of African descendants having settled there is primarily due to two factors; 1) during the slave trade most blacks worked on the docks, boats, extensive waterfront warehouses and in close by towns and 2) throughout the early part of the 20th Century, the British and American banana companies also imported hundreds of thousands of Blacks from Jamaica, Barbados and other West Indian islands to work on their plantations. However, rather historically, most blacks later chose to remain settled throughout the Honduran coastline even after emancipation. The larger cities in the mountainous interior of the country became populated mainly by descendants of former enslaved Mayan Indians and other tribal natives who worked the agricultural fields, the lumber and in gold and silver mines. Of course, the meztisaje or mixture among the racial cultures in Honduras is rather vast, due to the long history of intermarriages between the European, Native Americans and descendants of black Africans.

Research Warns That Stopping Antidepressant While Pregnant May Pose Risks.

Pregnant women who discontinue antidepressant medications may significantly increase their risk of relapse during pregnancy, a new study funded by the National Institute of Health's National Institute of Mental Health found. Women in the study who stopped taking antidepressants while pregnant were five times more likely than those who continued use of these medications to experience episodes of depression during pregnancy, reported Lee Cohen, M.D. of Massachusetts General Hospital and colleagues in the February 1 issue of the *Journal of the American Medical Association*.

Depression is a disabling disorder that has been estimated to affect approximately 10 percent of pregnant women in the United States. Recently there has been concern about the use of antidepressants during pregnancy; however what has not been addressed is the risk of depression recurrence should someone discontinue antidepressant use. This study sheds light on the risk of relapse associated with discontinuing antidepressant therapy during pregnancy. In the study, Cohen and colleagues enrolled pregnant women already taking antidepressants and then noted how many of the women decided to stop taking their medications. They then assessed the risk of relapse for the women who stopped versus maintained antidepressant therapy. Contrary to the belief that hormonal changes shield pregnant women from depression, this study demonstrates that pregnancy itself is not protective. Among the pregnant women who stopped taking antidepressants, 68 percent relapsed during pregnancy compared to 26 percent who relapsed despite continuing their antidepressants. Among the women who discontinued use and relapsed, 50 percent experienced a relapse during the first trimester and 90 percent did so by the end of the second trimester.

This study demonstrates the importance of weighing the risks not only of antidepressant use, but also the risk of relapse should antidepressants be discontinued. It highlights the importance of women discussing with their physicians their own individual risks verses benefits of continuing antidepressant use during pregnancy.

Online Intervention Could Benefits College
Women at Risk for Eating Disorders

A study funded by the National Institutes of Health's (NIH) National Institute of Mental Health (NIMH), published in the August 2006 issue of *Archives of General Psychiatry* found that an Internet-based intervention program may prevent some high risk, college-age women from developing eating disorders. The researchers conducted a long-term, large-scale study via randomized, controlled trials of 480 college-age women in the San Francisco Bay area and San Diego, Calif., who were identified in preliminary interviews as being at risk for developing an eating disorder. The trial included an eight-week, Internet-based, cognitive-behavioral intervention program called "Student Bodies," which had been shown to be effective in previous small-scale short-term studies. The intervention aimed to reduce the participants' concerns about body weight and shape, enhance body image, promote healthy eating and weight maintenance, and increase knowledge about the risks associated with eating disorders.

The online program included reading and other assignments such as keeping an online body-image journal. Participants also took part in an online discussion group, moderated by clinical psychologists. Participants were interviewed immediately following the end of the online program, and annually for up to three years thereafter to determine their attitudes toward their weight and shape, and measure the onset of any eating disorders.

"Eating disorders are complex and particularly difficult to treat. In fact, they have one of the highest mortality rates among all mental disorders," said NIMH Director Thomas Insel, M.D. "This study shows that innovative intervention can work, and offers hope to those trying to overcome these illnesses." Over the course of a lifetime, about 0.5 to 3.7 percent of girls and women will develop anorexia nervosa, and about 1.1 to 4.2 percent will develop bulimia nervosa. About 0.5 percent of those with anorexia die each year as a result of their illness, making it one of the top psychiatric illnesses that lead to death.

Anorexia generally is characterized by a resistance to maintaining a healthy body weight, an intense fear of gaining weight, and other extreme behaviors that result in severe weight loss. People with anorexia see themselves as overweight even when they are dangerously thin. Bulimia generally is characterized by recurrent episodes of binge eating, followed by self-induced purging behaviors. People with bulimia often have normal weights, but like those with anorexia, they are intensely dissatisfied with their bodies. All eating disorders involve multiple biological, behavioral and social factors that are not well understood.

The intervention appeared to be most successful among overweight women who had elevated body mass indexes (BMIs) of 25 or more at the start of the program. In fact, among these women in the intervention group, none developed an eating disorder after two years, while 11.9 percent of the women with comparable baseline BMIs in the control group did develop an eating disorder during the same time frame. BMI is a reliable indicator of a person's body fat by measuring his or her weight and height.

The program also appeared to help women in the San Francisco Bay area who had some symptoms of an eating disorder at the start of the program, such as self-induced vomiting; laxative, diet pill or diuretic use; or excessive exercise. Of those in the intervention group with these characteristics, 14 percent developed an eating disorder within two years, while 30 percent of those with these characteristics in the control group developed an eating disorder during the same time frame. The authors suggest that the intervention helped these high-risk women become less concerned about their weight and shape, while also helping them understand healthier eating and nutrition practices. *"This is the first study to show that eating disorders can be prevented among high-risk groups,"* said lead author C. Barr Taylor, M.D., of Stanford University. *"The study also provides evidence that elevated weight and shape concerns are causal risk factors for developing an eating disorder,"* he added. The study suggests that relatively inexpensive options such as Internet-based interventions can have lasting effects on women at high risk of developing an eating disorder. *However, the authors note that the results cannot be generalized widely because there were differences in the women's baseline characteristics and treatment responses between the two sites used in the study.* Also, the rate at which the women stuck with the program was very high—nearly 80 percent of the online program's Web pages were read—suggesting that the participants were unusually motivated. *"Women who are less motivated may be less likely to participate in or stick with this type of long-term intervention,"* added Taylor. In addition, women with restricted or no access to computers would not be able to benefit from an online intervention program. However, the authors conclude that such Internet-based programs may be a good first step in a diligent program designed to screen women for potential eating disorder risks. Additional study authors are Susan Bryson, MS, MA of Stanford University; Kristine H. Luce, PhD of Stanford University; Darby Cunning, MA of Stanford University; Angela Celio, PhD of the University of Chicago; Liana B. Abascal, MA of San Diego State University; Roxanne Rockwell of San Diego State University; Pavarti Dev, PhD of Stanford University; Andrew J. Winzelberg, PhD of Stanford University; and Denise E. Wilfley, PhD of Washington University Medical Center.

The Fluctuation In Sex Hormone Levels, Could Affect Circuit Activity Flow In Woman's Hormonal Cycle

Recent imaging studies conducted by the National Institute of Mental Health (NIMH), has revealed that fluctuations in sex hormone levels, during women's menstrual cycles, affect the responsiveness of their brain reward circuitry. While women were winning rewards, their circuitry was more active, if they were in a menstrual phase preceding ovulation and dominated by estrogen, compared to a phase when estrogen and progesterone are present. According to Karen Berman, M.D., chief of the NIMH Section on Integrative Neuroimaging. *"These first pictures of sex hormones, influencing reward-evoked brain activity in humans, may provide insights into menstrual-related mood disorders, women's higher rates of mood and anxiety disorders, and their later onset and less severe course in schizophrenia,"* Dr. Berman added that *"these studies may also shed light on to the reasons as to why women are more vulnerable to addictive drugs during the pre-ovulation phase of the cycle."* This research was also supported by Dr. Berman and her colleagues, Drs. Jean-Claude Dreher, Peter Schmidt and other colleagues from the NIMH Intramural Research Program report on their functional magnetic resonance imaging (fMRI) study and posted in the online *Proceedings of the National Academy of Sciences* report January 29, 2007.

Philip Kohn and Daniella Furman of the NIMH, section on Integrative Neuroimaging, David Rubinow of the NIMH Behavioral Neuroendocrinology Branch and other participating colleagues also contributed to the study on the reward system circuitry which includes: the prefrontal cortex, *seat of thinking and planning*; the amygdala, *the fear center*; the hippocampus, *the learning* and the *memory hub*; and the striatum, which *relays signals* from these areas to the cortex. Reward circuit neurons harbor receptors for estrogen and progesterone. However, how these hormones influence reward circuit activity in humans, still remains unclear to science. The research is ongoing.

To pinpoint hormone effects on the reward circuit, Berman and colleagues scanned the brain activity of 13 women and 13 men while they performed a task involving simulated slot machines. Women were scanned before and after ovulation, and the MRI pictures showed that the reward system responded differently when women anticipated a reward compared with when the reward was actually delivered, depending upon their menstrual phase.

When they hit the jackpot and actually won a reward, women in the pre-ovulatory phase activated the striatum and circuit areas linked to pleasure and reward more than when in the post-ovulatory phase. Researchers also confirmed that the reward-related brain activity was directly linked to levels of sex hormones. Activity in the amygdala and hippocampus was in lockstep with estrogen levels regardless of cycle phase; activity in these areas was also triggered by progesterone levels while women were anticipating rewards during the post-ovulatory phase. Activity patterns that emerged when rewards were delivered during the post-ovulatory phase suggested that estrogen's effect on the reward circuit might be altered by the presence of progesterone during that period.

Men involved in the research showed a different activation profile than women during both anticipation and delivery of rewards, men had more activity in a striatum *signal relay station* area during anticipation compared to women. The study also showed that women had more activity in the frontal cortex *executive hub* area at the time of reward delivery compared to men.

This Study Indicates Increased Risk for Depression among Girls with Low Birth Weight

This new study shows where girls' risk for developing depression after puberty increased significantly if they had low birth weight, yet low birth weight didn't appear to be just one more risk factor for depression. Rather, it seemed to increase the risk effects of other adversities. The research study funded in part by the National Institute on Mental Health, (NIMH), indicated that among the 5.7 percent of girls involved in the study who had low birth weight, more than 38 percent developed at least one episode of depression as teens, compared to only 8.4 percent with normal birth weight. This clearly points to the fact that teenage girls with low birth weight, also have one other risk factor, i.e. such as teenage pregnancy or sexual abuse. Therefore, their odds of developing depression increases to nearly 20 percent versus 3.6 percent for normal birth weight girls. The research also shows that if these girls have two, or more risk factors, then such risk would rise to 68.5 percent versus 19.7 percent for normal birth weight girls. Nevertheless, if these girls have no other risk factors, then their low birth weight poses no additional risk. Research also pointed to no increase depression risk in low birth weight teenage boys.

Drs. Elizabeth Jane Costello, Adrian Angold, Duke University, and colleagues, suggests that *"these recent findings indicates that the adaptations in the womb that optimized survival under adverse conditions that can lead to low birth weight may later impair girls' ability to cope with stress."* Adding that *"their lower thresholds for stress-triggered illness may remain latent until they encounter adversities that strain their capacity,"* The report was published in the *Archives of General Psychiatry* of March 2007.

The researchers drew on assessing depression among 1,420 North Carolina boys and girls, ages 9-16, during the 1990s, relying on mothers' recollections of birth weights and other risk factors. "Low birth weight predicted depression, only in adolescence and only in girls," even after other depression-related adversities — such as living in a dangerous neighborhood, having single or mentally ill parents, or poor health — were factored into the analysis, report the researchers. Even though boys are more prone to low birth weight, fewer than five percent of low birth weight teenage boys became depressed — about the same rate as other boys. The researchers note that boys appear to be more prone to early developmental insults and have higher rates of early-onset disorders like ADHD and autism, while girls seem more prone to later-onset disorders like depression. Social phobia, post-traumatic stress disorder and generalized anxiety disorders were three times higher in girls with low birth weight than in boys or girls with normal birth weight. However, evidence suggested that this was likely a reflection of the fact that these disorders co-occurred with depression. These latest findings strongly encourages *"pediatricians and parents of girls who were of low birth weight should pay close attention to their mental health as they enter puberty."*

Links to Depression Found In Bone-Thinning Among Premenopausal Women

A recent study funded in part by the National Institute of Mental Health (NIMH) and the National Institutes of Health (NIH), shows us that premenopausal women with even mild depression have less bone mass than do their non-depressed peers. The research study conducted on the level of bone loss is at least as high as that associated with recognized risk factors for osteoporosis, including smoking, low calcium intake, and lack of physical activity. Hip bones, the site of frequent fractures among older people, were among those showing the most thinning in depressed premenopausal women. The reduced bone mass puts them at higher risk of these costly, sometimes fatal fractures and others as they age, the researchers note in the November 26 issue of the *Archives of Internal Medicine*.

The report was submitted by Giovanni Cizza, MD, PhD, MHSc, of NIMH and the NIH National Institute of Diabetes and Digestive and Kidney Diseases (NIDDK); Farideh Eskandari, MD, MHSc, and NIMH Deputy Director Richard Nakamura, PhD. Who indicated in their report that *"Osteoporosis is a silent disease, often times the first symptom a clinician sees is when a patient shows up with a broken bone. Now we know that depression can also serve as a red flag – that depressed women are more likely than other women to approach menopause already at higher risk of fractures."*

Researchers also concluded that after bone mass reaches its peak in youth, bone-thinning continues throughout life, accelerating after menopause. Preliminary studies had suggested that depression may be a risk factor for lower-than-average bone mass even in young, premenopausal women. Results of the current study lend considerable weight to those earlier findings. The study's design reduced the possibility that the lower bone mass was linked to factors other than depression.

The study included 89 depressed women and 44 nondepressed women, all participants in the research were between 21 and 45 years old and all were premenopausal. Except for depression, the two groups were similar in risk factors, including calcium, caffeine, and alcohol intake; smoking; level of physical fitness; use of oral contraceptives; and age of first menstrual period. Both groups were of relatively high socioeconomic status and were well nourished. The single difference between them was that the depressed women was currently taking antidepressant medications. Although earlier studies suggested that older adults taking antidepressants called selective serotonin reuptake inhibitors had more bone fractures than others, nevertheless, the latest study showed that medications showed no direct link to low bone mass in premenopausal women. The researcher study also found that 17 percent of the depressed women had thinner bone in a vulnerable part of the hip called the femoral neck, compared with 2 percent of those who were not depressed. Low bone mass in the lumbar spine, in the lower back, was found in 20 percent of depressed women, but in only 9 percent of nondepressed women. Bone mass was measured via an X-ray technique called DXA scanning. There was also no significant link between the degree of bone loss and the severity of depression or the cumulative number of depressive episodes, the researchers found. The depressed women had been diagnosed with mild depression and were having or recently had depressive episodes. Other NIH and NIMH contributors to the study, such as the NIDDK, the NIH Clinical Center and the National Center for Complementary and Alternative Medicine, concluded that *"Depression generally isn't on clinicians' radar screens as a major risk factor for osteoporosis, particularly for premenopausal women, but it should be,"* Blood and urine samples also showed that depressed women have imbalances in immune-system substances, including those that produce inflammation, compared to their healthy peers. This additional finding strengthens the case for a suspected link between depression-induced imbalances in the immune system and accelerated bone loss. The blood and urine samples were taken every hour for a full day, providing a truer picture than does less frequent testing, as had been done in previous studies. The immune-system imbalances may be tied to excess adrenalin, since the part of the nervous system that produces adrenalin is over-active in depressed people. Increased adrenalin can over-stimulate the immune system. Compared to the others, the depressed women in this study had higher levels of immune-system proteins that promote inflammation, and lower levels of those that prevent it. The study also showed that one of these inflammation-promoting proteins, IL-6, is known to promote bone loss. And that at the molecular level, bones routinely break down, and their minerals, notably calcium, are reabsorbed into the blood, where they travel throughout the body to perform crucial functions in cells. At the same time, the body builds the bone back up. Researchers concluded that the imbalances found in this normal loop of bone re-absorption and build-up, such as high levels of IL-6, could promote bone loss, the researchers suggest.

The National Institute of Mental Health's *NIMH* mission is to reduce the burden of mental and behavioral disorders through research on mind, brain, and behavior. The National Institutes of Health *NIH*, is *the nation's top medical research agency*, it spearheads 27 Institutes and centers and is a component of the *U.S. Department of Health and Human Services*. Which is the primary federal agency for conducting and supporting basic, clinical and translational medical research, and it investigates the causes, treatments, and cures for both common and rare diseases. For more information about NIH and its programs, visit the NIH and NIMH website.

These Recent Studies Is Believe To Show Proven Results In Medication and Psychotherapy Treatment for Depression Among Low-Income Minority Women

A recent press released in combined treatment with medication and psychotherapy, show reduced depressive symptoms in women from minority populations, according to a recent research funded by the National Institute of Mental Health (NIMH). Participants in this study were mostly low-income, African-American and Latino women, whom are at high risk for depression. All of the participants in the controlled trials, were clients of county health and welfare services. Participants, were randomly assigned an antidepressant, psychotherapy, or referral to a community mental health service provider. The lead author of the study, Jeanne Miranda, Ph.D. of the University of California at Los Angeles Neuropsychiatric Institute, concluded that *"structured care reduces major depression in these diverse and impoverished patients."* Also adding that *"this study broadens the knowledge base by evaluating depression treatments among young, predominantly minority women. It is the first study to let providers know that treating depression in this population, can significantly improve the ability of these women to feel and function."*

The results show that low-income women, in minority populations benefit from depression treatment, when it is paired with intensive outreach and encouragement to support the interventions. Not only did women achieve lower levels of depressive symptoms, but they also gained higher levels of functioning in daily life.

Outreach support, also included transportation, child care, and spending considerable time to gain the trust of each of the participants, which was an essential part of the study. Miranda and colleagues screened thousands of women for ethnicity, major depression, and exclusionary factors, while they attended Women, Infants, and Children food subsidy programs and family planning clinics, in four suburban counties near Washington, D.C.

Three cultural groups were recruited. Of the 276 women who met criteria, consented to treatment, and were randomized in the trial, 117 were black, 134 were Hispanics, and 16 were white. The median age was 29.3 years, 60 percent lived at or below the federal guidelines for poverty, and 37.1 percent had not graduated from high school. The women had experienced extremely high rates of trauma exposure, including rape, child abuse, and domestic violence. High rates of post-traumatic stress disorder were also found. Each month for 6 months, participants completed a version of a standard psychiatric measuring tool to compare depression symptom and functioning scores over time.

Women assigned to medication, were treated with paroxetine for 6 months. If a patient did not tolerate the antidepressant or show a significant response, bupropion, an antidepressant with a different medical profile, was prescribed. Women assigned to psychotherapy, were treated by experienced psychotherapists in 8 weekly, cognitive behavioral therapy (CBT) sessions. The treatments were most often provided in or near the county clinic where the women, were identified. CBT taught participants techniques to manage mood, disprove thinking that may keep them depressed, engage in pleasant activities, reverse self-defeating beliefs, and get social support from others. Medications and psychotherapy, were both significantly more effective in decreasing depressive symptoms than the community referral sample, which received little treatment. With community referral, researchers made appointments for care, but very few women attended the sessions. Medications were more effective than no treatment at 6 months for reducing patients' depressive symptoms, improving home and work life, and increasing their ability to get along with others and engage in social activities. Psychotherapy was more effective than no treatment at 6 months for decreasing depressive symptoms and relating to others, but it did not improve home and work life.

The 88 women in the medication group were twice as likely as those referred to community care to achieve a significant reduction on depression rating scale scores.

Researchers believe that without outreach involving education, encouragement to comply with treatment, transportation, and child care, few poor women are likely to receive appropriate depression treatment. The results ultimately suggested that treating depression in this population improves the functioning of these young women if they have the tools to overcome barriers to care and receive treatment services. The research findings appear in the July 2 issue of the *Journal of the American Medical Association.*

The Search for The Gene That Causes Schizophrenia Remains Alive and Well.

Despite promising evidence that a gene closely linked to schizophrenia could be found on human chromosome number 1, an international team of scientists who scoured the chromosome in more than 2, 900 patients, concluded that it wasn't there. In conclusion, members of the scientific research team sponsored by the National Institute of Health stated that "the bad news is that we couldn't find it, however, the good news is that we could now fully concentrate our efforts on other regions of the genome, such as chromosomes 6, 8 and 13." The result of the findings was published in the Gene Hunters 'April 26, 2002 issue of Science.

Fast forward (The Scientist 20/16), Schizophrenia and the Synapse: "compared to the brains of healthy individuals, those of people with schizophrenia have higher expression of a gene called 'C4,' according to a paper published in NATURE 1/27/16 "The gene encodes an immune protein that moonlights in the brain as an eradicator of unwanted neural connections 'synapses.' These findings, which suggest increased synaptic pruning, is a feature of the disease, are a direct extension of 'genome-wide association studies' that pointed to the 'major histocompatibility' locus, as a key region associated with schizophrenia risk.

The research remains alive and well! According to a recent NIH funded research, (suspect runaway synaptic pruning during adolescence ... schizophrenia strongest known genetic risk, has now been deconstructed). Schizophrenia's genomic skyline ... the site in chromosome 6 harboring, the gene C4 towers, far above other risk associated areas on schizophrenic genomic skyline, marking its strongest known genetic influence. This new study is the first to explain how specific gene versions works biologically to confer schizophrenic risk "I awaited over thirty years to write this valuable piece!"

This article here highlights the arduous scientific searches during the earlier part of the millennium. Such articles were already highlighting the challenges of identifying the genetic roots of complex diseases. "Schizophrenia being such a complex psychiatric disorder, it just can't be explained by either a single altered gene or a single environmental cause. There are clearly genetic components, but they are likely to be varied and to interact in many ways with non-genetic factors." The scientist concluded in their statement. Although recent studies has suggested that genes associated with susceptibility to schizophrenia would be found on the 'q' or long arm of chromosome 1, a region separated from the short arm, known as "p." In their study, researchers laboriously searched for associations between genetic markers on chromosome 1 and schizophrenia in families that had more than one member diagnosed with the disease. This approach, called genetic linkage analysis, is used to detect the location on the chromosome where disease genes reside. Nevertheless, by pooling their resources and data, and agreeing on how to attack the problem in a large sample of affected families, the scientist have been able to quickly use this type of genetic linkage analysis to tell if they were on the right track. Such which resulted in a conclusion that it is still possible that genes on chromosome 1 q contribute to the disease, but these would influence only a small proportion of patients. "Biology is complicated, and the search for genes that contribute to large numbers of cases is endless." "Although a variety of genetic and environmental factors are at play in cancer, cardiovascular disorders and diabetes, nevertheless, despite the difficulties, we are getting closer to understanding the molecular causes of schizophrenia." Said the leading scientist, while they praised and hinted at the advances in imaging, neuro-anatomy, genetic analysis and psychopharmacology being daily implemented and brought forth in the fight against the debilitating disease. The estimated population of Connecticut as of July 23, 1868, was 521, 965; by 1880, the population had increased by more than 19 percent to 622,700. As of July 1900, the population showed an increase of more than 47 percent and was estimated as 908,420. During the thirty two year period that the Connecticut Hospital for the Insane had been opened, the number of inpatients had increased in 1900 to 2, O78 with an admission rate of 228 per 100,000 population. Thereafter, associated with the steady increase of the population of Connecticut, was an obvious increase in the number of persons who needed psychiatric services.

This trend influenced the construction and opening of the Norwich State hospital in 1904 and, of Fairfield State Hospital in 1933. At the close of the 1940 fiscal year, 7,532 patients were hospitalized in the three state psychiatric hospitals, with an admission rate of 412 per 100,000. Such which showed an increase of more than 80 percent since, 1900. Meanwhile, the population of Connecticut had increased during the same forty-year period to 1,711,800; or by more than 88 percent. On June 30, 1940, the reported population was of 7,532, within the three state hospitals; comprised more female patients, 51.56 percent than male patients 48. 44 of these, or almost 66 percent, were first admission and slightly more than 34 percent, had two or more admissions. More than 53 percent of the patients were over 50 years old and almost 29 percent of this group was over 60 years old; more than 36 percent were between 30 and 50 years of age; and almost 11 percent was under 30 years of age. Up until in the 1950's, throughout most of America very little written statistical data were available on the number of mental patients and the incidence of mental illness. Most of the information was obtained from the individual's institutional records and from reports done by the various Special Commissions, appointed by the Governors of each state. According to an annual report done by the Department of Mental Health for the period ending on June 30, 1958, readmission has played an increasingly significant part in the volume of total admissions. In 1948 they represented 30% of admissions (excluding transfers), whereas in 1957-58 they constituted some 40%. The degree of influence of readmission has been continually enlarged since 1938. In that year they constituted 20% of total admissions. For each ten-year period there has been a 10% increase in the proportion of readmission has. During fiscal year 1962 the readmission has exceeded the first admissions by 844 and comprised almost 56 percent of all the patients admitted to the three state hospitals; and the male patients exceeded the female patients by more than 11 percent. Almost 69 percent of the patients had been admitted on the 30 day physician's certificate; more than 26 percent, on a voluntary status;

slightly more than 2 percent, as transfers from penal institutions; and less than one percent, by order of the circuit, probate and superior courts.

In 1967 the readmission has to the three hospitals comprised 63 percent of all admissions compared to 37 percent in 1955; the admission rate was 361 per 100,000, population. Since 1955 the length of hospitalization has shown a steady decline; 56 percent of the patients in the state mental hospitals that year, remained for less than three months; whereas in 1967, 78 percent, remained less than three months and 91 percent, less than one year. "During such time, more than 25 percent of all patients had been charges of the hospitals for 20 years or more." During the 1967 fiscal year 10,300 persons were admitted to the three State hospitals. 3,792, or almost 37 percent, were first admissions and 6,508, or more than 63 percent, readmission has; male admissions and readmission has continued to exceed female admissions and they accounted for more than 58 percent of the first admissions and almost 67 percent of all readmission has. Although almost 54 percent of all admissions were by 30 day physician's certificates, a marked shift to informal admissions was noted at Fairfield Hills Hospital, which accounted for more than 45 percent of its total admissions; whereas, only 3 percent of the admissions to Connecticut

Valley Hospital and less than one-half percent, to Norwich Hospital, were on an informal basis. More than 40 percent of the admissions to Connecticut Valley Hospital and 37.5 percent, to Norwich Hospital, were on a voluntary basis.

During the fiscal year of 1972, 14,181 patients were admitted to the three State hospitals. 4,309, or more than 30 percent, were first admissions and 9,872, or almost 70 percent were readmission has; male admissions and readmission has continued to exceed all female admissions and they accounted for almost 70 percent of the first admissions and slightly more than 70 percent of all readmission has. Almost 49 percent of the admissions were by a 15 day, physician's certificate; almost 38 percent, were on a voluntary basis; less than 5 percent, by court order; and less than 1 percent, on an informal basis. Fairfield Hills had reversed the trend back to voluntary admissions and the informal method was used by less than 2 percent of their patients. The admission rate for Connecticut during this period was 520 per 100,000, population. During a period covering 103 years (1869-1972), the average daily census at Connecticut Valley Hospital, formerly (Connecticut State Hospital), computed on a 12 month, basis at intervals of ten-year increase from 225 patients in 1869 to 3,206 in 1939 and decreased thereafter to 1.037 patients in 1972 (FY). During the first 70 years there was an increase in the number of patients hospitalized at Connecticut State hospital of almost 1,325 percent. From 1939 to 1959 (before unitization), there was a decrease of more than 10 percent in the hospital population. During the next thirteen years (including the period of decentralization), the decrease was more than 61 percent.

Throughout Connecticut and the rest of the country, admissions consistently exceeded the discharges through the mid 1960's. At a ten-year interval, the number of admissions ranged from a high of 54.7 percent above the number of patients discharged in 1899 of 4.2 percent above, in 1969. During a three-year period, from Jul 1, 1964 to June 30, 1967, the number of discharges consistently exceeded the number of admissions by more than 12.6 percent during (FY) 1964-

1965 by more than 28 percent during FY 1965-1966; and by more than 12 percent during FY 1966-1967. During the next three years, the trend was reversed and the number of admissions exceeded the number of discharge by less than 1 percent to more than 4 percent. During the fiscal year ending on June 30, 1971, discharges exceeded admissions by less than one half of a percent and during the year ending June 30, 1972, by more than 2 percent.

Highlights of the Past, Could Lead Us On The Present ... Our Future!

Punishment before Treatment ... the treatment for the mentally ill of today's roots, was planted in the seventeenth-century American Colonial mind set. Prior to that era, mental illness was viewed not as a treatable illness, rather as a form of a *cursed, demonic possession and a state of being suitable, only for destruction.* During such times several methods for treating and dealing with the mentally ill emerged in the United States of America and throughout the rest of the world. These two major trends were the institutional care, in the form of state and county mental hospitals and then deinstitutionalization. This latter resulted in a form of community mental health movements of the 1960's. This transition created a new form of institutionalization based in the community, and was predicated on the two-thirds reduction in resident population of large public institutions. In the early part of the seventeenth century, beliefs in demonical possession and witchcraft were the most prevalent attitude toward this type of illness in America. Neither mental illness nor its proper treatment were cared for, or understood. The Salem Witch Trials of the mid 1600's represented the culmination of an exorcist, abusive approach to the mentally ill. In the latter half of the century this approach gave way to milder forms of incarceration designed to protect the general public from those afflicted with mental illness without causing unnecessary harm to the patient.

There were essentially two classes of mentally ill persons back then, (a) the propertied and (b) the poor. Propertied families were expected to build cell-like outbuildings to house their afflicted members, as well as to absorb the cost of care, such as feeding, treatment, clothing, as well as to providing the bare essentials. Several solutions to the care of the poor insane developed over the latter half of the century and these were the predecessors of community mental health system as we know it today ... foster home placement, and hospitals for the mentally ill. The poor insane presented problems for the whole community. Their behavior, often in the public eye, caused people to worry about the real or imagined harm the afflicted persons might do to themselves or others. Laws were developed to prohibit the insane from wandering from one community to another, forcing communities to assume responsibility for their own ill members. A tax system was levied to provide financial assistance to families who could not afford to build proper outbuildings for their mentally ill. Town officials were charged with the responsibility of housing and caring for the mildly insane individual who had no families or whose families could not care for them. The population and concentration of mentally ill individuals residing in the communities increased toward the end of the seventeenth century. This brought about the concept of workhouses and almshouses as a way to provide shelter for the poor and the mentally ill. Though this period was characterized, at worst, by punitive, abusive treatment of the mentally ill and, at best, by benign community neglect, it gave birth to many concepts central to the understanding of psychiatric chronicity today. However, it was during that time that the stigma of mental illness in this country was established and from it we can still recognize the early development of contemporary concept of care, "public vs. private treatment," boarding out or foster placement community responsibility for care of the mentally ill, and the need for special institutions for the care of the mentally ill.

By the end of the seventeenth century, institutionalization had been replaced witch-hunting; yet, the basic objective was still to protect society, not to care for the individual. By the early half of the eighteenth century, however, treatment of the mentally ill actually regressed to include repressive confinement and mental and physical torture in the form of isolation and neglect. It wasn't until the latter half of the eighteenth century that changed gradually appear on the horizon.

At that time, Philadelphia became the center of humanitarian and rational reform under the influence of the Quakers, most notably, Benjamin Rush. The first general hospital in America, the Pennsylvania Hospital, was founded to treat mental as well as physical illness. It offered the first attempts at curative treatment for the insane. Though treatment by present standards was still somewhat barbaric, it represented the first signs of humanitarian, rational views of mental illness and a focus on the care and cure of the individual, rather than solely on the protection of society. Fourteen years later, the Eastern Lunatic Hospital opened its doors in Williamsburg, Virginia. It was the first hospital in America built exclusively for the mentally ill, and it remains the only state hospital of its kind for more than 50 years.

Treatment methods of the time included bloodletting, water immersion, spinning, and excessive use of restraint. The rational humanitarian treatment reform in America is credited to Benjamin Rush, similar movements in Paris, France and York, England, undoubtedly influenced Dr. Rush. Philippe Pinel, at the Hospital Salpetriere, in Paris instituted "moral treatment" throughout Europe by taking mental patients out of chains, removing them as public spectacles, and applying concepts of human trust and interaction as treatment. Similarly, William Tuke instituted The Retreat in 1786 in York, England as a reaction against the abusive medical treatments of the times. The Retreat, based on principles of non-stigmatization and the maintenance of a family-like environment, kindness, and consideration, is mostly noted for its role in eliminating the practice of bloodletting as an accepted form of treatment for insanity. Against this background, Rush instituted major reforms in the physical conditions of asylums and hospitals; the introduction of work and recreational activity as therapeutic; the separation of the seriously insane from the mildly insane; the separation of the violently insane from other inmates; the separation of male and female patient units into different units; the hiring of intelligent and compassionate male and female attendants to interact with patients, participate in activities, and engage in normal social discourse; and the restriction visitors who might be disturbing to the patients.

Before the establishment of the State of Connecticut Department of Mental Health in 1953, each of the three state hospitals were autonomous and there existed very little to no communication among them. *The Joint Committee of State Mental Hospitals,* (JCOH) which originally served in 1940 as an informal, unofficial forum for the three superintendents and selected members of their respective Boards of Trustees (would later become an official agency in 1945). It had little impact on the hospitals, their staffs and their patients. The three Boards continued to set their own policies and to operate independently ... Department heads of the three hospitals had little, if any, contact with each other, no collaboration, cooperation or consultation existed and the resources of one hospital were not extended to the other hospitals. Each of these state hospitals operated within their own isolated communities and was largely self-sufficient. The implementation of the concept of a central authority, implicit in the creation of the new Department elicited considerable suspicion and defensive behavior on the part of the Boards of Trustees and the superintendents. Political resources and community loyalties were mobilized to protect the vested interests and the existing territorial boundaries.

Doctor Blasko, became the first appointed Commissioner of Connecticut's Department of Mental Health, he was perceived as an-outsider, who threatened the *status quo*. His visits to these hospitals created considerable anxiety. This was reinforced by his attempts to upgrade the services being rendered to patients and to implement innovative and modern psychiatric therapies, as well, as to establish training and research programs. His efforts to improve conditions, led to the appointment of a Coordinator of Research and Training, as a member of his senior staff. It would be the first time representatives of psychiatry and nursing from each of the three state operated hospitals were brought together to discuss existing training programs, and to help plan new ones. Unfortunately, these contacts were limited and did not improve relationships between the hospitals and their staffs. Dr. Blasko served as Commissioner for three years until

June 1957. Shortly thereafter the Legislature enacted a law, which invested, departmental authority in the person of the Commissioner, thus converting the Boards of Trustees to an advisory status.

The next decade might be viewed as a period of transition from decentralized, toward centralized authority. The senior staff of the Commissioner of Mental Health, contributed unwittingly to the unspoken, but obvious struggle of the administrative staffs of each of the three hospitals to remain autonomous and resist changes from outside their respective institutions. The coordinating multidisciplinary staff appointed by the Commissioner, was in the untenable position of being "plenipotentiaries, without portfolios," while at the same time, being classified as technical supervisors of their counterpart in the facilities operated by the Department of Mental Health. Although without line-authority, they represented the Commissioner and often by implication, were vested with his authority.

The daily operation of each facility would again become the responsibility of the Superintendent and rarely were his decisions challenged. At times, communications between these three facilities and the Office of the Commissioner were guarded and restricted. The administrator of one of the hospitals once gave explicit orders to his nursing leaders (that they were to listen to the Chief of Nursing Services, but not give any information that would reflect negatively on the hospital). This same superintendent, with the support of his Board, was able to submit the implementation of certain standard nursing practices, regarding the preparation and administration of medications, etc. The institution created weekly psychiatric nursing workshops around special problems and programs in the early 1960s and had considerable impact on nursing in the three state hospitals. Representatives from the three hospitals began meeting with their Chief of Nursing Services on a scheduled basis. Problems were discussed and solved, training programs were developed, supervision in individual and process-oriented interactions was provided and programs were designed and implemented. Selection criteria and evaluation in practices were standardized and individual nursing care plans developed for all patients. Participants in these workshops increased in knowledge and skill and utilized every opportunity to work with other nursing personnel in the development of their skills.

Peter Bryce (1834-1892) laid the groundwork for the care of the mentally ill in Alabama, not by the mere holding of a position, but by his own sensitive, patient nature and by the inauguration of treatment methods that marked him as a pioneer in psychiatry. Bryce, a native of South Carolina, was elected superintendent of the newly created, not yet completed, Alabama Insane Hospital in 1860, when he was only 26 years old. He gave the remaining 32 years of his life to the hospital that now bears his name. He strongly encouraged the idea of "moral treatment" toward the insane, discarding the use of shackles, jackets and other medical restraints. Although such was now almost seventy years old, it was still virtually unknown in this country. When the first person was admitted into Bryce Hospital back in 1861, the young physician enforced strict discipline among his attendants, requiring nothing short of absolute courtesy, kindness and respect toward the patients. This conscientious nursing practice unheard of at the time bore fruit in the form of warm relationships and by 1882 a policy of absolute non-restraint was fully implemented. Doctor Bryce also set up working programs, farming, sewing, maintenance, and amusement programs for his patients; such programs were valuable both as therapy and as a means of making ends meet. The very survival of the hospital during its early years, when the state's interest and finances were directed to other needs, could be listed as one of the superintendent's greatest accomplishments. Doctor Bryce created a mental institution recognized as one of the best managed in the country. An understatement, but nonetheless true, is Bryce's own assessment, which was written prior to his passing: "I feel that I have done my work and I hope, hence without self praise, rather a hope that I'd be permitted to say… I have done it well!"

American Historic Asylums

The following is a list of America's Vanishing Historic Asylums, State Hospitals, Sanitariums, County Homes, Retreats and Other Mental Institutions.

This list, focuses on the historical and architectural preservation and is not intended in any way to be used when compiling factual data, nor taken as support for institutionalization. Although several groups of preservationists are currently working to preserve some of these specific places, many of these historic state hospital sites are in danger of demolition, destruction, or some other sort of serious negative alteration: Kansas State Hospital is due for demolition in the near future and the Buffalo State Psychiatric Hospital in Buffalo, New York, was torn down in September, 2002.

The listed sites here, has been catalogued in an attempt to present America's historic state hospitals and insane asylums, which were founded before and in the latter half of the 19th century. The listing focuses on the facilities built on the "Kirkbride plan," but it is not necessarily limited to the Kirkbride hospitals. The asylums of the 19th century represent to many a darker period in mental health care, with their involuntary incarceration, barbaric and ineffective treatments, and number of reported cases of abuse toward patients. However, there is also a legacy of progressive institutional treatment left by Dorothea Dix, Thomas Story Kirkbride, John Galt, and others represented by these buildings and sites. Treatments and philosophies, which seem rather outdated today, at the time, however, represented great improvement in the treatment of the mentally ill. A large proportion of these historic institutions are no longer mental hospitals, what remains of them, are rather the magnificent castle-like buildings, wrought of brick and stone in incredible detail, a legacy of an attention to detail in architecture which seems to have been long forgotten. The scope of this list presented here are of some hospitals which are still in operation, hospitals which are still standing, but are now closed, hospitals that are still standing but are no longer used as hospitals, and hospitals that have been long since or recently been demolished. Although this list focuses primarily on mental institutions run by state governments, which were most commonly called "state hospitals," however, some city and county asylums have been included as well. In addition, there are some medical hospitals and sanitariums included, although these are not the primary focus of the list. These include certain Pennsylvania state hospitals, which in some cases are actually medical hospitals and not mental health institutions at all. These are probably in actuality more numerous than the state hospitals, but information on them seems to be far more, scarce than for the state institutions. Institutions, which are similar to, or have overlapping functionality with insane asylums, include prisons, medical hospitals, sanatoriums, and poor farms. Although a few of these might be included in this list (especially where they share locations with insane asylums), the focus of this list is not on these types of facilities. *Readers should keep in mind that this list is not quite complete, there are a numbers of asylums that have not yet been added at the time of the research publication.*

The Architects

The primary architects of many of these buildings included H.H. Richardson, George Kessler, Gordon W. Lloyd, Stephen Vaughn Shipman (who designed several), state capitol architect Elijah E. Myers, Ward P. Delano, Isaac Perry, John Notman, Frederick Law Olmsted (landscapes and grounds), A.J. Davis, H.W.S. Cleveland, Edward O. Fallis, Warren Dunnell, Charles C Rittenhouse, Richard Karl August Kletting, John A. Fox, and others. Thomas Story Kirkbride, while not an architect, devised the basic floor plan many of these architects used in the design of their main asylum buildings.

Sanitariums

To most people, the word "sanitarium" currently has identical meaning to the disgusting words 'insane asylum.' However, a century ago, the typical sanitarium was most likely a hospital or residential health spa. Some historic sanitariums were state-run tuberculosis hospitals, and a few were actually insane asylums. The most famous historic sanitarium was (The SAN) the *Kellogg Sanitarium* in Battle Creek, Michigan. This sanitarium was a hospital/health spa variety, and was depicted in the film and book "The Road to Wellsville," Kellogg's corn flakes were invented at this institution. Several historic sanitariums are included at the end of the listings for each state. Many of these hospitals with their imposing main buildings are quickly vanishing from the American landscape.

The Famous Kirkbride Plan for the Building of State Hospital

This excerpt is based on annual reports written by Dr. Thomas Story Kirkbride himself, Doctor Kirkbride served as superintendent at the Pennsylvania Hospital from 1841-1883. Dr. Kirkbride's progressive therapies and innovative writings on hospital design and management became known as the "Kirkbride Plan," these, which influenced, in one form or another, almost every American state hospital built by the turn of the century.

Dr. Kirkbride created a humane and compassionate environment for his patients and he believed that the beautiful setting described below restored patients to a more natural balance of the senses. Dr. Kirkbride spoke of his plan as linear. Buildings were arranged *enéchelons*. The center building was more imposing than the others and had a dome, in agreement with the classical tastes of the time …

The center buildings were used for administration offices, extended wings right and left for patients. From the ends of the wings short cross sections dropped back to connect with more buildings, for patients, which were parallel to the original wings.

The Kirkbride plan ... included a large building with a tall central wing and wings attached on either side in a symmetric fashion were known as the Kirkbride hospitals. Asylums based on a plan of scattered cottages. Hospitals, which started as Kirkbride, but later, added cottages are included under the Kirkbride category above instead of this cottage category. Preserved hospitals can still be in use as psychiatric hospitals, used for other purposes, or abandoned. Many of these are in danger of demolition at this time, although few are currently undergoing some sort of remodeling or renovation. Many of these former institutions are also found under *Asylum Tourist* listing and are now historic museums and some are still in operation, there is also a large number of these former institutions which have been converted and used for other purpose including residential use, others as prisons and some have also now became colleges.

"Each ward was enough out of line so that fresh air could reach it from all four sides and it was not under observation from the other wards." *Dr. Thomas Story Kirkbride*

Previous Names Commonly Given To Psychiatric Hospitals

Over the years, factors such as changes in the mission of the state hospital, changes in philosophy, and even changes in terminology have left these facilities with many names. Some state hospitals have had several names, and it seems like any institution that lasted from the 19th century into the 20th century had at least one name change.

Examples of Names (tending from earlier to recent)

- Lunatic Hospital
- Lunatic Asylum
- Asylum for the Insane
- Insane Asylum
- State Hospital
- Mental Health Center
- Psychiatric Hospital
- Regional Center
- Retreat
- Developmental Center
- Center

List of Historic Psychiatric Hospitals

Many are now demolished, closed, exchange to prisons, condos and even colleges

Alabama *Asylums* –
Bryce Hospital for the Insane, Tuscaloosa *Sanitariums* –
Belle Aire Sanitarium (Mobile)
Alaska
No listings at this time.
Arizona *Asylums*
Phoenix Insane Asylum
Arkansas
Arkansas State Hospital (Arkansas Insane Asylum), Little Rock, 1883. No historic structures remaining (?)
Arkansas Training School for Girls, Alexander
California Asylums –
Atascadero State Hospital
Agnews State Hospital 1885
Camarillo State Hospital Ventura County
Highland State Hospital
Stockton State Hospital, 1853
Metropolitan State Hospital near Los Angeles
Modesto State Hospital
Napa State Hospital
Norwalk State Hospital
Pacific State Hospital
Patton State Hospital
Colorado Asylums
Fort Logan Mental Health Center
Colorado State Hospital (Colorado Insane Asylum)
Pueblo, 1879 *Sanitariums*
Mount Airy Sanitarium
Connecticut
Norwich State Hospital
Fairfield State hospital
Connecticut Valley Hospital
Institute of Living
Cedar Crest Hospital
Delaware *Asylums*
Delaware State Hospital for the Insane, Wilmington
District of Columbia, Washington, D.C. Asylums
St Elizabeth *Sanitariums*
Washington Sanitarium and Hospital
Florida
Asylums
North East State Hospital, MacClenny
Georgia Asylums

Central State Hospital, Milledgeville 1837
Georgia Retardation Center
Sanitariums
Blackman-Walton (Atlanta)
Hawaii
No listings at this time.
Idaho
No listings at this time.
Illinois Asylums
Alton State Hospital
Anna State Hospital (Southern Illinois)
Bartonville State Hospital, Peoria, 1885 (aka Peoria State Hospital)
Chester State Hospital
Chicago State Hospital
Elgin State Hospital
Kankakee State Hospital (Eastern Illinois)
Manteno State Hospital Watertown Asylum
East Moline State Hospital
MR & DD, State Homes
Institute for the Feeble Minded, Lincoln
Indiana Asylums
Evansville State Hospital (Woodmere)
Madison State Hospital (Southeastern Insane Hospital)
Madison Richmond State Hospital
State Homes
Home for Feeble-Minded Youth, Fort Wayne
Sanitariums
Dillsboro Sanitarium
Iowa Asylums
Mt Pleasant State Hospital
Cherokee State Hospital
Des Moines County Infirmary and Asylum for the Insane Hospital for the Insane, Dubuque
Woodward State Hospital (in Woodward) Independence *State Homes*
Institute for Feeble-Minded Children, Glenwood
Kansas Asylums
Kansas State Imbecile Asylum Winfield State Hospital
Winfield Larned State Hospital Parsons State Hospital, Parsons Wells Asylum, Atchison
Menniger Clinic (1925)
Kentucky Asylums
(Western Kentucky Asylum), Hopkinsville, 1848 Eastern State Hospital, 1824
MR. & DD, Disabled, State Homes
Waverly Hills Tuberculosis Sanitarium
Louisiana Asylums

Jackson State Hospital (East Louisiana State Hospital) Central Louisiana State Hospital (Pineville)
Sanitariums - Fenwick Sanitarium (Covington)

Maine *Asylums*
Bangor Insane Hospital
MR & DD, Disabled, State Homes
Valley Farm (Maine School for Feeble-Minded), West Ponwal

Maryland Asylums
Bay View Asylum.
Highlandtown Eastern Shore State Hospital,
Cambridge Sheppard-Enoch Pratt Hospital, Towson
Spring Grove State Hospital, Catonsville
Springfield State Hospital (and Warfield Complex Development Project) *Sanitariums*
Laurel Sanitarium (Laurel)
Solomon Sanitarium

Massachusetts *Asylums*
McLean Hospital, Waverly
Metropolitan State Hospital for the Insane Sanitariums:
Essex Sanitarium, (Middleton)

Michigan *Asylums*
Ardmore Center, Livonia Caro State Hospital
Pontiac State Hospital (Clinton Valley Center)
Kalamazoo State Hospital (I) at Asylum Lake
Kalamazoo State Hospital (ii) Newberry State Hospital
University of Michigan in Ann Arbor Lapeer School
St Joseph's Retreat, Dearborn
Eloise Hospital (Westland, Wayne County)
Sault Sainte Marie State Hospital

Minnesota *Asylums*
Anoka State Hospital
Brainerd State Hospital
Cambridge State Hospital
Hastings State Hospital, 1888
Moose Lake State Hospital
Rochester State Hospital
St Peter Regional Treatment Center, 1866 Willmar State Hospital
Wabasha Sanitarium
State Sanitarium at Walker Medical Hospitals:

Missouri *Asylums*
St. Vincent's Insane Asylum, St. Louis.
Marshall State Hospital or State Home (Marshall, Missouri) St Louis County Insane Asylum
East State Hospital (Meridian)
East Mississippi State Hospital (Meridian), 1885
Mississippi State Hospital (Whitfield)

North Mississippi Regional Center (Oxford)
South Mississippi State Hospital (Laurel)
Kuhn Memorial State Hospital (Vicksburg)
Montana *Asylums*
Montana State Hospital (at Anaconda)
Nebraska *Asylums*
Norfolk Hospital for the Insane, 1885
Nevada *Asylums*
Nevada Mental Health Institute, 1882
New Hampshire *Asylums*
New Jersey *Asylums*
Ancora State Hospital
Hudson County Asylum, New Jersey
New York *Asylums*
Newville State Hospital Creedmore State Hospital
Harlem Valley State Hospital
Hudson River State Hospital (Poughkeepsie)
Utica State Hospital
Dannemora State Hospital
Matteawan State Hospital (now Fishkill Correctional Facility)
Rochester State Hospital
Willowbrook State School (Staten Island)
Western New York Institution for the Deaf-Mute (New York)
St. Lawrence State Hospital in Ogdensburg, 1890
Rockland Asylum on Blackwell's Island, 1839
Bloomington Lunatic Asylum, 1808
New York Asylum for Idiots, at Syracuse
Sanitariums:
Loomis Sanitarium, (Liberty)

North Carolina *Asylums*
Appalachian Hall, Asheville
Broughton Hospital, 1874 (Morganton)
Cherry Hospital, 1880
Dorothea Dix Hospital
State Hospital at Raleigh
Sanitariums:
North Dakota *Asylums*
Grafton State Hospital Jamestown State Hospital
Ohio *Asylums*
Fairhill Psychiatric Hospital
Mt Vernon State Hospital
Toledo State Hospital, 1888
Dayton State Hospital

Columbus Hospital for the Insane
Cleveland State Hospital, 1855
Athens State Hospital
Southeast Longview Asylum
Massillon State Hospital
Lima State Hospital

State Homes
Dayton Ohio Soldiers and Sailors Home

Oklahoma Asylums
Central State Hospital, Norman
Eastern State Hospital, Vinita
Western State Psychiatric Center, Fort Supply

Oregon Asylums
Dammasch State Hospital, Wilsonville
Eastern Oregon State Hospital at Pendleton
State Insane Asylum at Salem

Pennsylvania Asylums
Allentown State Hospital
Blossburg State Hospital
Byberry Hospital
Danville State Hospital
Friends Hospital
Harrisburg State Hospital
Mayview State Hospital, 1818
Nanticoke State Hospital
Norristown State Hospital (near Philadelphia)
Pennhurst State Hospital, Spring City
Pennsylvania Hospital (Philadelphia)
Scranton State Hospital
Warren State Hospital
Woodville State Hospital
Schuylkill County Almshouse and Hospital for the Insane
Farview State Hospital
Western Pennsylvania Hospital for the Insane at Dixmont
Pennsylvania State Hospital general/medical hospitals Philipsburg State Hospital
Shamokin State Hospital Hamburg State Hospital

Puerto Rico Asylums

Rhode Island Asylums
Butler Hospital for the Insane, 1847
Dexter Hospital for the Insane
Asylum for the Incurable Insane at Howard, 1870

South Carolina Asylums
Columbia State Hospital

South Dakota *Asylums*

Yankton State Hospital

Hiawatha Insane Asylum for American Indians, 1902.

Tennessee *Asylums*

Bolivar State Hospital

Texas *Asylums*

San Antonio State Hospital Rusk State Hospital

Terrell State Hospital

Wichita Falls State Hospital

La Lomita Mission

Tropical Texas Center,

Mission Utah Asylums - Utah State Hospital

Vermont *Asylums*

Brattleboro Retreat, 1838

Waterbury State Hospital

Eastern State Hospital, Williamsburg (Original) Eastern State Hospital, Williamsburg (Current)

Western State Hospital, Staunton

Central State Hospital, Petersburg

Augusta County Asylum

Washington State *Asylums*

State Insane Asylum near Tacoma (Steilacoom)

Eastern State Hospital at Medical Lake

West Virginia *Asylums*

Fairmont State Hospital

Weston Asylum 1858

Lakin State Hospital (Colored Insane), near Point Pleasant

Huntington State Hospital

Wisconsin State *Asylums*

Mendota State Hospital

Winnebago State Hospital, aka Northern Asylum for the Insane

Winnebago Mental Health Institute, 1873 (Oshkosh)

County Asylums

Sauk County Poor Farm and Insane Asylum, 1871

Rock County Insane Asylum

Dunn County Insane Asylum

Richland Center Asylum

County Asylum, Lancaster

Monroe County Asylum, Sparta

County Asylum, Sheboygan

County Asylum, Marinette Medical Hospitals

Wisconsin State General Hospital (Madison)

Wyoming *Asylums*

Casper State Hospital

Evanston State Hospital
Sheridan State Hospital
Canada *Asylums*
Asylum, Hamilton, Ontario, Canada
Asylum, Kingston, Ontario, Canada
Asylum for the Insane, London
Ontario, Canada Asylum, Orillia, Ontario, Canada
Asylum, Toronto, Ontario, Canada
Other Asylums
St Agnes Hospital for the Chronically Insane (US)

Historic Review behind the American Psychiatric Hospital Deinstitutionalization

From Jails to Prisons … The Emergent Need for The Church's Intervention

Researchers involved in closely following this study, have concluded that deinstitutionalization doesn't work and that "we simply just switched the mentally ill from one place to another." Meaning that instead of sending sick people to the hospitals for treatment where they could actually benefit or deal with their hopes of getting better, sick people are now being put into jails. This lack of treatment in the system does not serve the mentally ill person or the community in a positive form. It is however, rather costly to taxpayers who will continue pouring money into a bottomless well … while further confusing those whose lives is already raveled and confused.

Confining Michael X, to the Hartford County Jail could be another indicator of the growing mental illness crisis. Throughout the United States persons with mental illness are now being jailed repeatedly instead of treated in psychiatric hospitals. Often times for creating disturbances in their communities. Although many of these men and women have long been diagnosed with schizophrenia, they are again released to the streets and each time they're back to using alcohol, sniffing glue or paint fumes, smoking marihuana, crack and even other stronger illicit drugs, thus exacerbating their schizophrenia and other illnesses which lead to their disorderly behavior. According to recent newspaper accounts, "many of these individuals have been locked up so often they have admitted to liking their jailers and it even being a place they now call home."

As early as ten years ago, when police officers encountered someone on the streets suspected of suffering from a mental illness they would have taken them to a hospital emergency room, a psychiatric hospital, a community mental health center or a better suited facility that would supposedly help the chronically mentally ill deal with their illness. Now they don't even bother …

Many police departments have instead become cynical, untrained and rather frustrated about the whole approach. Police officer appear rather frustrated while responding to a call, thus causing increased stressors upon these individual, resulting in death. Additionally too often rooky cops quickly learn that two hours later, individuals previously detained are right back out on the streets. "The circle of sending the person with mental illness to jail instead of health care facilities really doesn't work." Additionally, police departments throughout the country and their officers, has long been denied opportunity to specialize in proper approach toward deescalating the mental ill individuals, during psychotic episodes, due to bad political maneuvers. Their mobile crisis intervention failed them miserably, or are totally none existent.

Nevertheless, this practice has become almost nonexistent. The odyssey of repeated incarceration for severely ill people, was previously common in the United States throughout the 18th and 19th centuries although back then many Americans found such practices inhumane and uncivilized. Their sentiments found organized expression in the *Boston Prison Discipline Society*, which was founded in 1825 by *Reverend Louis Dwight, a Yale graduate and Congregationalist minister*. Shocked by what he saw when he began taking Bibles to inmates in jails, established the society to publicly advocate improved prison and jail conditions in general and hospitals for mentally ill prisoners in particular. According to the medical historian, Gerald Grob, Dwight's insistence that mentally ill persons belonged in hospitals, aroused a responsive chord, especially since his investigations demonstrated that large numbers of such persons were confined in degrading circumstances.

Dwight's arduous campaign led the Massachusetts legislature to appoint a committee in 1827 to investigate conditions in the state's jails. The committee's investigations report directed to the State General Court concluded in its documentation that in fact many lunatics and persons suffering from mental illness were being confined, often in inhumane and degrading conditions. The report showed that in one jail, a man had been kept for almost ten years. "He had a wreath of rags around his body and another round his neck. He had no bed, chair or bench, a heap of filthy straw, like the nest of a swine, was in the corner. "The wretched lunatic was indulging in some delusive expectations of being soon released from such wretched dwellings." He then wrote in its report and the committee concluded that *the situation of these wretched beings calls very loudly for some redress*. They seem to have been considered as out of the protection of laws. Less attention is paid to their cleanliness and comfort than to the wild beasts in their cages, which are kept for show."

Among the specific recommendations of the committee was that all mentally ill inmates of jails and prisons should be transferred to the Massachusetts General Hospital and that confinement of mentally ill persons in the state's jails should be made illegal. Three years later, the Massachusetts General Court overwhelmingly approved a bill providing in its budget monies to build a state psychiatric hospital for 120 patients. It opened in 1833 as the State Lunatic Asylum at Worcester. When the hospital opened, more than half of the 164 patients received during that year came from large work houses, almshouses, and prisons. One-third of these patients had been confined in these institutions for longer than 10 years.

Dorothea Dix, the most famous and successful psychiatric reformer in American history, came to pick up where Dwight had left off. In 1841, with the *American asylum-building movement* under way, Dix began a campaign that would focus national attention on the sad plight of the mentally ill in jails and prisons and would be directly responsible for the opening of at least 30 more state psychiatric hospitals. At the time she began her crusade, Dix was a 39-year-old teacher who had been left a bequest by her grandmother, allowing her to give up teaching. Her father had been shiftless, poverty stricken and irresponsible … fanatically religious, with a penchant for writing theological tracts in fits of inspiration, and her childhood had therefore been very difficult. Her father may in fact have been mentally ill, which would account in part for her zeal to improve conditions for such sufferers. Dix's crusade began in early 1841, when she agreed to teach a Sunday school class at the East Cambridge Jail outside Boston.

While there, she noticed not only that there were insane prisoners among the inmates, but also that the insane prisoners had no heat in their cells. When she inquired about this, she was told by the jailer that it was because "the insane need no heat." Horrified, Dix reported her findings to her friends and set out to investigate other jails in Massachusetts to ascertain whether similar conditions prevailed. Over the next year, she visited dozens of jails and almshouses and then presented a report to the state legislature. This reform sat the tone for Dorothea Dix's life's work. I come to present the strong claims of suffering humanity. *"I come to place before the Legislature of Massachusetts the condition of the miserable, the desolate, and the outcast. I come as the advocate of helpless, forgotten, insane and idiotic men and women ... of beings wretched in our prisons, and more wretched in our Alms-Houses. I proceed gentleman, briefly to call your attention to the state of Insane Persons confined within this Commonwealth, in cages, closets, cellars, stalls, pens: Chained, naked, beaten with rods, and lashed into obedience."* After finishing her report in Massachusetts, Dix moved on to New Jersey, where she proceeded in the same fashion to visit jails and almshouses, then report to the state legislature and urge the building of public psychiatric hospitals in which insane persons could be treated humanely and receive treatment. By 1847, she had taken her crusade to many eastern states and visited 300 county jails, 18 prisons, and 500 almshouses. Her success in persuading state legislatures to build psychiatric hospitals was impressive, and she provided a major impetus to the reform movement.

The Reverend Louis Dwight and Dorothea Dix were remarkably successful in leading the effort to place mentally ill persons in public psychiatric hospitals rather than in jails and almshouses. By 1880, there were 75 public psychiatric hospitals in the United States for the total population of 50 million people. In 1880, the first complete census of *insane persons* throughout the United States was conducted. It is in fact, believed to have been the most accurate and complete census that has ever been carried out since. The census also included letters to all physicians, asking them to enumerate all "insane persons" in their community, a question about "insanity" on the census form that went to every household, and a canvassing of all hospitals, jails, and almshouses.

A total of 91,959 mentally ill persons were identified at this time. Out of these, 41,083 were living at home, 40,942 were in hospitals and asylums for the insane, 9,302 were in almshouses, and only 397 were in jails. The total number of prisoners in all jails and prisons was 58,609, bringing the number of severely mentally ill inmates down to only 0.7 percent of the population of jails and prisons ... That was the situation back in the 1880's.

The Reverse Act

The Policy Geared To Putting Mentally Ill Individuals Back Into Jails

A study of five California county jails carried out in 1975 by Arthur Bolton and Associates found that 6.7 percent of the inmates were severely mentally ill at the time of examination. Gary Whitmer's 1980 study of 500 mentally ill people who had been charged with crimes emphasized the causal relationship between the person's mental illness and his or her crime, and he cited examples such as a man who had "smashed the plate-glass window of a retail store because he saw a dinosaur jumping out at him"; a woman who refused to pay her restaurant bill because she believed that "she was the reincarnation of Jesus Christ"; a man who harassed two other men whom he believed to be "CIA agents who had kidnapped his benefactress"; and a woman with paranoid delusions who went up to a man on the street and "struck the victim in the right buttocks" with a hat pin. At the time of their arrests, only 6 percent of the mentally ill studied by Whitmer were involved in any treatment program, leading him to conclude that the reforms brought about by deinstitutionalization had "forced a large number of those deinstitutionalized patients into the criminal justice system." By the early 1980s, interest in the problem of the mentally ill in jails and prisons was growing, increasing as their numbers increased, and two methodologically sound studies of the problem were carried out. In Chicago, Linda Teplin, spurred by the observation that mental health professionals speculate that the jails have become a repository for the severely mentally ill. Out of the nearly 750 interviewed jail admissions using a structured psychiatric interview found that 6.4 percent of them met diagnostic criteria for schizophrenia, mania, or major depression. In Philadelphia, Edward Guy and his colleagues interviewed 96 randomly selected admissions to the jail and reported that 4.6 percent had schizophrenia or manic-depressive illness and they labeled such as an alarmingly high incidence of mental illness among inmates of a city jail.

A more inclusive but methodologically less rigorous study of mentally ill people in the nation's jails was carried out in 1992 by the Public Citizen Health Research Group and the National Alliance for the Mentally Ill. Questionnaires were mailed to the directors of all 3,353 county and city jails in the United States asking them to estimate the percentage of inmates who on any given day "appeared to have a serious mental illness." This was further defined to include only inmates with schizophrenia or manic-depressive illness who were exhibiting symptoms such as auditory hallucinations, delusions, confused or illogical thinking, bizarre behavior, or marked mood swings. The jail directors were instructed not to include as mentally ill anyone who exhibited "suicidal thoughts or behavior" or "alcohol and drug abuse" unless the person also had other symptoms as previously described. No attempt was made to identify mentally ill inmates with more subtle symptoms of mental illness (e.g., an inmate with paranoid schizophrenia who did not discuss his delusional beliefs); the survey sought to count only those who were the most severely and overtly mentally ill. Replies were received from 41 percent of the jails, which represented 62 percent of all jail inmates in the United States. Overall, the jail directors estimated that 7.2 percent of inmates appeared to have a serious mental illness, ranging from less than 3 percent in jails in Wyoming, Nevada, Idaho, and South Carolina to almost 11 percent in jails in Connecticut, Hawaii, and Colorado.

Studies of inmates with psychiatric disorders in state prisons have also been carried out, and the results agree with the results from the studies done in jails. In general, jails keep prisoners sentenced for one year or less, whereas prisons keep prisoners with longer sentences. Ron Jemelka and his colleagues reported that many such studies "used a field survey approach in which one or more key administrators in each prison system was asked to respond to a series of questions about the mentally ill in their facilities. These surveys have suggested that 6 to 8 percent of state prison populations have a serious psychiatric illness," but for a variety of reasons "facility surveys are likely to substantially underestimate the number of mentally ill offenders."

When prison inmates have been actually interviewed a high percentage of them have been found to be severely mentally ill, or suffering from some type of mental illness. A research conducted during the 1980's, reported findings from interviews of 246 prisoners in Oklahoma; 10 percent of them were found to be acutely and severely disturbed. In 1987, Henry Steadman and his colleagues published the results of interviews with 3,332 prison inmates in New York State; 8 percent of them were said to have very substantial psychiatric and functional disabilities which clearly warranted some type of mental health treatment.

A 1988 sociological and psychological study of 109 new admissions to the Washington State prison system, which used a structured diagnostic interview, also reported that 8.4 percent had schizophrenia, manic-depressive illness, or mania, while 1.9 percent more had schizophreniform disorder, and 10 percent met diagnostic criteria for depression. A similar study conducted on 1,070 prison inmates in Michigan found that 6.6 percent had schizophrenia or manic-depressive illness and 5.1 percent had major depression. Considering all these studies, researchers concluded that 10 to 15 percent of prisoners had major thought disorders or mood disorders and where in need the services usually associated with severe or chronic mental illness. Other studies have also been used to ascertain how frequently people with severe mental illnesses are put into jails and prisons. In 1991, a telephone survey was carried out of 1,401 randomly selected members of the National Alliance for the Mentally Ill, an advocacy and support group composed mostly of family members of persons with schizophrenia and manic-depressive illness. It was found that 40 percent of the mentally ill in this group had been arrested at some time in their lives and, at any given time, 1 percent of them were in jail or prison. Studies have also been done to ascertain arrest and incarceration rates for the homeless who are mentally ill. A 1985 study in Los Angeles of 232 people living in shelters and on the streets who had previously been psychiatrically hospitalized found that 76 percent of them had been arrested as adults. This is similar to the 74 percent previous arrest rate reported for severely mentally ill inmates examined in the Los Angeles County Jail. Such studies demonstrate a large overlap between mentally ill persons who are homeless and those who are in jail.

How many people with severe mental illnesses are in jails and prisons on any given day? If such illnesses are defined to include only schizophrenia, manic-depressive illness, and severe depression, then approximately 10 percent of all jail and prison inmates appear to meet these diagnostic criteria. The most recent data available in 1995 indicated there were 483,717 inmates in jails and 1,104,074 inmates in state and federal prisons in the United States, a total of 1,587,791 prisoners. If 10 percent of them are severely mentally ill, that would be approximately 159,000 people. It is also likely that the mentally ill often rotate back and forth between being homeless and being in jails or prisons. The term *deinstitutionalization* is the name given to the policy of moving chronically mentally ill individuals out of large state hospitals and then closing part or all of these institutions; it has been a major contributing factor to the mental illness crisis. This term was also used to describe the similar process for mentally retarded. The process of deinstitutionalization began in 1955 with the widespread introduction of Thorazine or chlorpromazine, which was the first effective antipsychotic medication, and received grand momentum, thus spearheading the federal Medicaid and Medicare enactment. By the following ten years, the two part deinstitutionalization immediately began moving the severely mentally ill out of the state institutions, and the closing of part or all of those institutions. This would not only affected people who were already suffering with mental illness, but would latter affect those who became ill after the policy had gone into effect and for the indefinite future because large number of hospital beds had now been permanently eliminated. The magnitude of deinstitutionalization of the chronically and severely mentally ill could easily be catalogue as being one of the largest social experiments in American history. In 1955, there were 558,239 severely mentally ill patients in America's public psychiatric hospitals. By the 1994, the same year the Connecticut CBI programs opened this number had been reduced by 486,620 patients, to 71,619 and counting. One must note the importance of these numbers, when compared to the census of 558,239 patients in public psychiatric hospitals in 1955, which is in relationship to the nation's total population of 164 million at the time.

By mid 1994, America's population had increased to 260 million. If there had been the same proportion of patients per population in public mental hospitals in 1994 as they were in 1955, the number of patients would have totaled 885,010. According to researchers, the severe impact on deinstitutionalization differed in magnitude between 885,010 and 71,619. In effect, approximately 92 percent of the people who would have been living in public psychiatric hospitals in 1955 were not living there in 1994. Their estimate indicates that even allowing for the approximately 40,000 patients who occupied psychiatric beds in general hospitals or the approximately 10,000 patients who occupied psychiatric beds in community mental health centers on any given day in 1994, this the means that approximately 763,391 severe and chronically ill individuals or over three-quarter of a million are living in the community today who would have been hospitalized 40 years ago. Such conclusive evidence shows this number being higher than either the population of Baltimore or San Francisco. The deinstitutionalization of the mentally ill however varies by state. Therefore, research geared toward assessing these differences in census for public mental hospitals, it is not sufficient to merely subtract the 1994 number of patients from the 1955 number, because state populations shifted in the various states during those 40 years. In Iowa, West Virginia, and the District of Columbia, the total populations actually decreased during that period, whereas in California, Florida, and Arizona, the population increased dramatically; and in Nevada, it increased more than sevenfold, from 0.2 million to 1.5 million. Nevertheless we could assume that the ratio of hospitalized patients to population would have remained constant over the 40 years.

Rhode Island, Massachusetts, New Hampshire, Vermont, West Virginia, Arkansas, Wisconsin, and California all have effective deinstitutionalization rates of over 95 percent. Rhode Island's rate is over 98 percent, meaning that for every 100 state residents in public mental hospitals in 1955 perhaps less than 2 patients are currently there today. Nevada, Delaware, and the District of Columbia have effective deinstitutionalization rates below 80 percent. Most of those who were deinstitutionalized from the nation's public psychiatric hospitals were severely mentally ill. The expert estimates indicate that more than 60 percent of those individuals discharged were diagnosed with schizophrenia. Almost 20 percent were suffered with manic-depressive illness and severe depression and the additional number were diagnosed with some form of organic brain disease such as epilepsy, stroke, Alzheimer's disease, and brain damage secondary to trauma. The remaining individuals residing in public psychiatric hospitals had conditions such as mental retardation with psychosis, autism and other psychiatric disorders of childhood, and alcoholism and drug addiction with concurrent brain damage. The fact that most deinstitutionalized people suffer from various forms of brain dysfunction was rather far from being understood prior to the policy of deinstitutionalization going into effect.

Through these and other documented factors, deinstitutionalization created a national mental illness crisis by discharging people from public psychiatric hospitals without ensuring that they received the medication and rehabilitation services necessary for them to live successfully in the community. Deinstitutionalization further exacerbated the situation hence once the public psychiatric beds were closed they were not available for people who later became mentally ill. This situation at present remains alive and well.

As a result, this well intended social experimentation has managed to create an epidemic that is of approximately 2.2 million severely mentally ill individuals in America who do not receive any type of psychiatric treatment what so ever. Although deinstitutionalization was based on the principles that the severe mentally ill individual should be treated in the least restrictive and humane setting ... this was further defined by President Jimmy Carter's Commission on Mental Health. The then First Lady, Roselyn Carter's ideology rested on "the objective of maintaining the greatest degree of freedom, self-determination, autonomy, dignity, and integrity of body, mind, and spirit for the individual as they participates in treatment and received services." Though this is a praise deserving goal for many in society and perhaps for a large number of those deinstitutionalized, the dream was at least partially realized. However for a substantial number of chronically mentally ill individuals, deinstitutionalization has been a colossal psychiatric nightmare. *Considering the fact that their lives are now virtually devoid of either, dignity or the integrity of body, mind and spirit.*

The popular terms *self-determination,* widely used and coined to help spearhead the march back then, today it simply means that the person has a choice of soup kitchen or garbage can. And "least restrictive setting" often turns out to be a under a bridge in a cardboard box, a jail cell, or a terror-filled existence on the streets plagued by both real and imaginary enemies.

Mental Imprisonment Deinstitutionalization
Mental Illness and Incarcerations

Throughout 1980 and 1995, the total number of individuals incarcerated in American jails and prisons increased from 501,886 to 1,587,791, an increase of 216 percent, compared to the general population which increased by only 16 percent. This however, could be a clear indication that the vast majority of this increase has been fueled by changing demographics, more stringent mandatory sentencing laws and the increasing availability of cocaine and other street drugs. It is however with little doubt that the mentally ill contributed more than their expected share to the increasing population throughout our jails and prisons.

Evidence to previous studies suggests that the relationship between mental disease and crime in Europe and other countries, indicates that prison and psychiatric hospital populations were inversely correlated. Sociologist have in fact coined this term as the *balloon theory,* due to the fact that as one rose, the other usually falls. Balloon theory as in if we "push in one part of a balloon and another part will bulge out." This theory was found to substantiate the George Palermo's 1991 conclusive analysis by researching and studying the extensive data collected from American mental hospitals, jails, and prisons between 1904 and 1987.

Experts in the sociological and psychological arena also believed that the increase number of mentally ill individuals in American jails and prisons also supports the thesis of progressive transinstitutionalism. And it is believed that these authors statistical evidence derived from the national census data, such which corroborates their clinical observation indicating that jails are in fact now a warehouse for the chronically and mentally ill. The recent data collected on psychiatrists and corrections officials observations also support the tangible increase between the numbers of psychiatric patients from hospitals to jails and prisons, thus concluded that such relationship is due in part through mass deinstitutionalization.

California was one of the first states to aggressively embark on the implementing deinstitutionalization through the Lanterman Petris Short Act of 1969 (LPS). This, Act which was primarily implemented to make it more difficult to involuntarily hospitalize an individual, or keep them in a hospital against their will, though perhaps still suffering with acute psychosis of the illness. The first published data showing that the number of mentally ill persons entering the criminal justice system was in fact beginning to double appear as early as 1972, little over a year after the Lanterman-Petris-Short Act went into effect. It was published by Marc Abramson, who was then a practicing psychiatrist in the San Mateo County. Throughout by which Abramson stated that "as a result of the newly implemented LPS, the mentally disordered individuals are now being increasingly subjected to arrest and criminal prosecution, thus exacerbating their illness and their stigma." Abramson also went on to coin the term "criminalization of mentally disordered behavior" through his writings and warned sociologist in an almost remarkably prophetic statement that "If the mental health system remains continuously pressured into forcing the release of mentally disordered individuals into a community prematurely, there will be an increase in demand on the criminal justice system to reinstitutionalize them." And affirmed that "those who castigate institutional psychiatry for its present and past deficiencies may be quite ignorant of what occurs when mentally disordered patients are forced into the criminal justice system." similar observations have been made throughout California. An early 1970's study on the Santa Clara County indicated the jail population had risen by almost 300 percent in less than four years, following the closing of Agnew State Psychiatric Hospital. Later in 1975, a study conducted on five of California jails, reported the number of severely mentally ill prisoners growing by 300 percent in little over 10 years. The number of mentally ill inmates throughout the California's state prison system grew at an alarming rate during the 1970s. Prison psychiatrists have concluded and though painfully they now easily summarized the situation as they "being literally drowning in patients, running around trying to put our fingers in the bursting dikes, while hundreds of men continue to deteriorate psychiatrically before our eyes into serious psychoses." While acknowledging that this crisis stems primarily from the recent changes in mental health laws that now allows more mentally sick patients to be shifted away from the mental health department to the department of corrections. By which today many more men and women with serious mental illness are now being sent to prisons instead of hospitals for treatment.

The second noted approach to assessing the situation between deinstitutionalization and the increasing number of chronic mentally ill individuals sent to jail and prisons is to further reexamine and understand the reasons for many causes for incarceration. A public citizen study conducted in 1992 indicated that almost 30 percent of these jails often times incarcerated the mentally ill persons who might perhaps have no charges against them, but rather are merely awaiting psychiatric evaluation, for a psychiatric hospital bed to become available, or perhaps even a simple case of someone just waiting transportation to a psychiatric hospital. These types of incarceration are conducted under state laws which permits emergency detentions of individuals suspected of being mentally ill. These are thus far now legal and primarily common in many rural states such as Kentucky, Mississippi, Alaska, Montana, Wyoming, and New Mexico.

In Idaho, innocent mentally ill persons who had broken no laws were continuously incarcerated as a standard practice until late 1991, when the legislature changed the laws and made it illegal. However, any persons requiring involuntary commitment are still first being taken to the local jail rather than to a hospital emergency room until they could be examined by a state-appointed psychologist. Until the psychologist advised hospitalization, these people would remain in jail awaiting a psychiatric hospital bed becomes available. Idaho state officials estimated that approximately 300 persons who had not been charged with any crime had been jailed in 1990 for an average of fifteen days ... each while awaiting psychiatric referral or hospital beds. However, such practice was not reserved only for the rural communities, but also for Boise, the state capital. The Ada County jail had also detained 85 persons without charges even though there were two private hospitals with available psychiatric beds just a few blocks from the jail. Recent studies conducted by the psychological and sociological communities clearly indicated though private, these hospitals are often built with federal and Community Mental Health Center grant. Their studies conducted especially in communities with poorly developed public psychiatric services, such practice remains alive and well. They have also documented testimonies given by sheriff's and other rural and inner cities law enforcement officers, whom have in fact observed, mentally ill inmates often being given paper gowns and kept in holding cells for observation up to eight weeks prior their finding a hospital bed.

According to several experts reports and my research it is known that most of the severely mentally ill individuals placed in jails are there because they have been charged with a misdemeanor. Mentally ill people are four to five times more likely to windup incarcerated for far lesser and serious charges such as disorderly conduct and threats, when compared with sane inmates. By these same definitions the mentally ill inmates is also four times more likely

than those not mentally ill to have been charged with disorderly conduct, 6 times more likely to have been charged with trespassing, and 10 times more likely to have been charged with harassment. A more recent study at the Mental Health Unit of the King County Correctional Facility in Seattle found that 60 percent of the inmates had been jailed for misdemeanors and had been arrested on the average of six times in the previous three years. 51 similar findings have been reported from other parts of the United States. In Madison, Wisconsin, the most common charges brought against the mentally ill who end up in jail are "lewd and lascivious behavior, e.g. urinating on a street corner, defrauding an innkeeper and eating a meal, then not paying for it. The label disorderly conduct on the mentally ill is seen as being too loud, menacing panhandling, criminal damage to property, loitering or petty theft. Many of these arrests records were later reexamined and researchers immediately found direct correlations between the person's mental illness and the behavior that led to repeat offences, apprehension, incarceration and ultimately prison. i.e. An elderly woman diagnosed with schizophrenia in Florida was arrested for assaulting employees and resisting arrest when she walked into a shoe store and began attempting to give away pairs of shoes and other products to customers because of being delusional, believed that she owned the store and her voices were telling her that she needed to share her wealth.

When she was asked to leave, she physically attacked the employees she then attempted a physical confrontation with police when they arrived. None of these officers on the scene had any prior experience in dealing a psychotic episode ... guns were drawn and she was finally maze with gas, cuffed and arrested. A young man with schizophrenia in New Mexico was acting bizarre in a restaurant and was arrested and later sued for assaulting a cook who came from the restaurant's kitchen and began making fun of him. Society remains uneducated, crewel and ill prepared to deal with mental illness ... yet community mental health treatment centers continue to close. Meanwhile police officers, fire and emergency personnel, and other public officials remain blind to the understanding of chronic or acute mental illness's approach. Although it has long been known and largely documented that people who suffer from paranoid schizophrenia, in particular, are likely to be arrested for assault because they may mistakenly believe someone is following them or trying to hurt them and will strike out at a person whom they might deem threatening to their safety. Yet the training to police officers and emergency personnel remains unknown or minimum at best.

Petty thievery among this homeless population on the streets could involve anything from empty soda cans, to supermarket shopping carts, to cardboard boxes, to cigarettes, food, a yacht and even a plane. Several months ago I read in a local Arizona newspaper about a man with mental illness who'd been arrested for stealing empty beer bottles to turn them in and buy cigarettes with the refund. Several years ago a Connecticut man with manic-depressive illness stole a yacht from a dock in the Connecticut River and drove it up and down the until it ran it a gown. Although one of the most common forms of theft among homeless mentally ill individuals involves the "dine and dash," this entails going into a restaurant and running out at the end of the meal because they have no money to pay. I have also been involved with cases as drastic as the stealing of a seaplane in the Virgin Islands. This man diagnosed with schizophrenia that had been discharged from Saint Elizabeth hospital in Washington D.C. sat for a period of time observing the seaplane's captain and where he kept the keys to the plane until one day he decided to steal the plane and run it aground destroying the plane and several other expensive boats in the process. Fortunately no one was killed the man was then recommitted to a long term inpatient treatment center for life. However, it is a known fact that police frequently use disorderly conduct charges to arrest a mentally ill individual when no other charges are available.

Examples of these could easily be noted when the parent of a man in Minnesota who had been diagnosed with schizophrenia told us that their son was often arrested simply for wanting to have a normal conversation with people he encountered in malls or on the streets.

Said he would follow them around and kept talking trying to get their attention and wouldn't go away until when they became afraid and asked him to leave. Of course his looks were often unkempt, which added to their fear. They would then call the police and he would again be arrested. I also read in Texan newspaper about an individual diagnosed with manic-depressive illness being arrested for disorderly conduct simply because they played loud music on their home stereo and their neighbors had complained.

Again this shows a lack of community and police understanding about the mentally ill. Most whom have perhaps studied behaviors and mental illness, would have some knowledge about people with acute psychosis, using music to block out their voices and delusions. Perhaps we have also read about people with schizophrenia being arrested for throwing out their television set to the streets because either their voices told them, or their hallucinations lead them to believe it to be talking to them. Unfortunately this happens, it is part of their illness. However, if these individuals were properly monitored, perhaps their case managers and therapist would realize that their medications needed a bit of adjustment, intense group or individual therapy, etc. Given the fact that each person suffering with mental illness, is an individual and that not all might be able to have radio or a television set in their home for it feeds their paranoia. Another problem affecting these individuals in the community is the easy and unlimited access to drug and alcohol. Alcohol- and drug-related charges are common simply because alcohol and drug use among this population frequently occurs as a secondary problem among the mentally ill. They also used it in place of their medications, or self-med. I recently heard about a woman in Washington State diagnosed with manic-depressive illness, whom was arrested for being drunk and disorderly on the street. There have been numerous arrests for driving while under the influence of alcohol or drugs; in some cases the person did not used either, but because of their bizarre behavior and perhaps even the medication's side effect and the ill trained arresting officer automatically assumes they are drunk.

Another common known charge used by law enforcement officers to arrest and remove mentally ill individuals from the street is trespassing. Researchers investigating this issue has shown persons with schizophrenia and alcohol abuse being arrested repeatedly mostly on trespassing charges throughout the country. Family members have also reported about their schizophrenia diagnosed relatives being arrested and put in jail simply for holding up signs that says *Will Work for Food* and panhandling in public areas, others have reported about their relatives arrested for sleeping in cemeteries. Trespassing arrests on mentally ill persons has also been for their delusions of owning a building, a bridge, a street, etc. recently it was reported on a man in Kansas who was arrested for refusing to leave a federal building because he thought that God had given it to him. Another man in Florida entered a bus depot and went to sleep in the bathroom because he believed he had won it in a prize from a tobacco company. Local law enforcement personnel also reported about local businesses constantly exerting pressure and demanding the police to get rid of these "undesirables" and the mentally ill loitering around their place of business. This situation worsens in areas highly dependent on tourism, where the police reputation is well-known reputation for stepping back in time and using prehistoric 18 century tactics, arresting all vagrants and homeless persons in what they consider as "cleaning the streets." Police official confide that their problems usually stem through complaints received from local business operators, demanding these people be removed from their business.

Atlanta officials have also described how mentally ill homeless persons at the city's airport are routinely arrested. Sympathy and mercy bookings are also commonly used by police officers trying to protect mentally ill individuals. This situation is particularly common among mentally ill women who are often victimized and raped, on the streets. Police officers throughout the country have admitted off the record that *they will trump up charges if they can't find something to charge them with and bring them to jail.* This at times must be done reported jail official, after noting that local state psychiatric hospitals routinely discharged severely disabled female patients to the streets. Asserting that if the mental institutions are not able to protect them by holding them until safely discharged, they will continue to arrest them for their own protection. The police arrested a mentally ill woman in Texas because she was psychotic and yelling on the streets and charged her with disorderly conduct. A Madison Wisconsin police department spokesperson told us that people often called the police because they are afraid these women may be assaulted. Although sometimes these women may not be exhibiting dangerous behaviors necessary for commitment to the State Hospital and may not want to go to the shelters and since forced medications is illegal … they remain vulnerable to sexual assaults. So the police are force to arrest and jail them for their own protection. This same theme is sounded by police captains throughout the country, who claim to arrest someone with mental illness for petty crimes because they know that at least they will be put in some kind of facility where they will receive food, shelter and perhaps even treatment. Stating that they do not invent a crime, but it's a discretionary decision by which they know that these individuals will be safe and fed.

The Los Angeles police officers has admitted it being a crisis intervention, where they frequently arrests severely mentally ill homeless persons are conducted because they are suffering from malnutrition, disheveled with dirt-encrusted skin and hair, and often bleeding from open wounds.

That it is a rather real pitiful situation to encounter these individuals who are hallucinating and haven't eaten for days. Considered more as a massive cleanup effort, because the goal is to get them shelter, food and perhaps even back on their medications. Mercy bookings are often initiated by mentally ill individuals themselves in order to get into jail for shelter or food. Some of these individuals have admitted to commit crimes near police stations and turn themselves in because once in jail they'll put them to work cleaning floors and get fed. Family members have also found the practice of jailing their relatives as being the most expedient means of getting help for the person in need of treatment.

As the public psychiatric system throughout the United States progressively deteriorates, common practice of giving priority to psychiatrically ill persons with criminal charges becomes rather apparent. Therefore mentally ill is jailed by families seeking treatment for a family member; so having the person arrested becomes the most efficient way to accomplish this goal.

This method is now crucial for getting treatment particularly in states where psychiatric services throughout hospital's priority is for people who are a danger to themselves or others. Family members encouraged either by the police or mental health officials have continuously pressed charges against their mentally ill relatives in order to access psychiatric care for them. The Public Citizen Act survey has recently released mountains of documents in which family members have admitted doing such.

Throughout the United States parent and other close relatives of individuals diagnosed with schizophrenia and other psychiatric illnesses, have began to complain about the inability of these patients getting into state hospital, even if willing, without being dangerous to self or others. And have openly concluded that rather than sitting around waiting for their relatives to become too psychotic and disaster occur, they now bring charges against them for making simple threats or damaging property. This is done similarly, in suburbia were several cases are now being documented. An example of this is the case of the parents of a severely ill young man who had no insight into his illness, he had refused treatment and psychiatrists refused to involuntarily commit him to a hospital because they claimed he was not a danger to himself or others. The young man was finally hospitalized after his parents called the police and obtained a court order barring him from their home, and when he violated the order, they had him arrested. The same judge, in fact had suggested his parents to use this mechanism in order to get treatment for their son. The judge then offered the young man a choice between jail and going to a hospital for treatment. Ironically these same jails have now become a transitional tool used in the system as vehicle by which to obtain psychiatric care from the same health treatment system that has proven to us all as a failure to treat. To ascertain the frequency in which patients are arrested after discharged from psychiatric hospitals, has become one of the most effective measures toward direct approach when assessing the entangled relationship between deinstitutionalization and the increasing number of mentally ill persons in jails and prisons. However, similar studies conducted on the general population show no major increase … included those done prior to the beginning of deinstitutionalization did not show a higher arrest rate than for the general population. Virtually every study done on the mentally ill since deinstitutionalization has shown a major increase.

A Brief Study Examining the Increased Rate of Psychiatric Patient's Imprisonment

A series of studies regarding the increased arrest rates of discharged psychiatric patients throughout American. The most accurate and are more concerned studies on this epidemic have been done between the years 1965 and 1978, which were analyzed by Judith Rabkin. These individual studies found that the arrest and conviction rates of recent discharged and former mental patients far exceeded those of the general population in at least some crime categories when patients and if these are considered as a homogeneous group. The expert noted a pronounced relative as well as absolute increase in arrests of mental patients. Especially impressive was Larry Sosowsky's study of arrest rates of patients discharged from California's Napa State Hospital between 1972 and 1975, after the Lanterman-Petris-Short Act had taken effect. Compared with the general population, discharged patients with no previous arrest prior to hospitalization were arrested 2.9 times more frequently. For the category of crimes against property e.g., shoplifting, the discharged patients were arrested 4.3 times more frequently. Discharged patients who had been arrested prior to their psychiatric hospitalization were arrested approximately 8 times more frequently than the general population.

The John Belcher's study of 132 discharged patients from Columbus State Hospital in Ohio during a 4 month period in 1985 is particularly most interesting. His studies have reported similar trends on patients who were followed up at 1, 3, and 6 months to determine what happens to them. The result of the study showed that at the of 6 months end, 18 % of the 132 patients had been arrested. However, only 65 of the 132 discharged patients had diagnoses of schizophrenia, manic-depressive illness, or severe depression, and 21 of these 32 % were among those arrested and jailed. According to Belcher, these 21 respondents were often threatening in their behaviors and exhibited bizarre behaviors as stripping and walking naked on the streets while talking to themselves. He also noted that they also did not take the prescribed medications needed to control their psychiatric symptoms and that they frequently abused alcohol or drugs. Each 21 individual former patients became homeless within the 6-month follow-up period, thus reaffirming the correlation between jail or prison, chronic mental illnesses and homelessness.

It could be easily assumed by many that jails and prisons have rapidly become surrogate mental hospitals for many people with severe mental illnesses. The estimated 10,000 mentally ill inmate population throughout the New York state's prison system now surpasses that of the number of patients in the state's psychiatric hospitals.

The Travis County Jail officials of Austin, Texas have admitted so many prisoners with mental disabilities that its psychiatric population rivaled and surpassed that of Austin State Hospital. Jail officials in Dallas County have openly admitted that on any given day one could find between 900 to a 1000 chronically mentally inmates … this is more than twice the number of patients being treated in the nearest state mental hospital.

The Seattle King County jail has become one of the largest institutions for the mentally ill. Meanwhile the San Diego County Jail reported that more than 15% of the men and 30 % of the women inmates are on psychiatric medications. According to County officials, jails are now the bottom-line mental health provider in many counties. Congressional members and other national politicians has openly admitted the Los Angeles County Jail, where approximately 3,300 of the 21,000 inmates require mental health services on a daily basis, is now dubbed as being the largest mental institution in the world. This I believe should be nothing to boast and be proud of, but rather ashamed and embarrassed as humans beings with dignity.

Is The American Impact On Deinstitutionalization A Blessing or A Curse?

The magnitude of deinstitutionalization throughout the 50 states and the District of Columbia, although Alaska and Hawaii became states after deinstitutionalization was implemented though not included. The practice s still absorbed within and affected these including the US. Virgin Islands ... Since the total population of the United States increased from 164 million in 1955 to 260 million in 1994 and since the rate of population change varied markedly for different states, 1994 state population figures can be used to calculate the number of patients who theoretically would have been in public mental hospitals in 1994 if the hospitalization rate had been the same as that which existed in 1955. The effective deinstitutionalization rate, then, is the actual number of patients in public mental hospitals in 1994 subtracted from the theoretical number with the difference expressed as a percentage of the theoretical number. The importance of looking at population change when assessing the magnitude of deinstitutionalization can be illustrated by looking at Nevada, which is especially anomalous because it actually had 760 patients in public psychiatric hospitals in 1994 than the 440 it had in 1955. Its actual deinstitutionalization rate is therefore plus 72.7 percent. However, because Nevada's total population increased more than sevenfold during the 40-year period, its effective deinstitutionalization rate, based on the population, was minus 71.4 percent.

Deinstitutionalization is the name given to the policy of moving severely mentally ill people out of large state institutions and then closing part or all of those institutions. By all de experts account it could easily be said that deinstitutionalization has played a major contributing factor to the mental illness crisis. Deinstitutionalization throughout the United States began in 1955 with the widespread introduction of chlorpromazine, a medication commonly known as Thorazine. Thorazine is considered one of first effective antipsychotic medication, and received national and international momentum 10 years later with the enactment of federal Medicaid and Medicare. However, due to its toxicity and debilitating physical side effects, chronic psychiatric patients have been known to cringe simply at the mentioning of this medication.

Updating Our Faith: A Global Theological View on Spiritual Psychiatric

Throughout the last one hundred years American psychiatry has shifted its field of activity from being primarily concerned with the custodial care of the client with mental illness to an emphasis on the treatment of ambulatory patients, and, in our time, to a concern for the family, the home, the school, the job, marriages, juvenile delinquency and narcotic addictions. At the same time, institutional patterns of psychiatric care have undergone a gradual change, leading to an open door policy in many hospitals throughout the country.

When we think of the word faith, we must also think of the meaning of anguish, pain and confusion, which exist in the hearts and minds of those individuals suffering with mental illness. We must also think of their redemption and about the loneliness, despair and depression that plagues their daily lives and weights them down. When we look at faith, we must first remember that we all want to be loved. Each of us want to know and to believe that God loves us, and faith tells us that … while it indicates that we must teach others to love God. Though it's been over a hundred and forty years, since the church had been removed from the mental health field, we pray for 'the powers that be' opens their hearts and pushes their doors wide open once again, thus allowing individual suffering with mental illness to benefit from Christian counseling by allowing a little more of God back into the field of mental health as needed. Throughout the centuries we have treated, investigated and document, what conditions and what special features have lead people to fall into the traps of mental illness. The core of this book, is to attempt to grapple with the issues raised by those questions, as we remember that even today, we poses very little rational concept upon the nature of mental illness. And about what it is, what causes it and what will actually cure it, although this is true even among world renown, psychiatrists, psychologist and the mental health and psychiatric communities as a whole. This admission of ignorance does frustrate and color our attitudes in the field, toward the large amount of competing explanations held throughout the centuries, about insanity and reasons for their causes and treatments. Insanity, mental illness, madness, or whatever other name the psychiatrists, psychologists and sociologists societies may find hip at the time, including the consumers themselves, have managed to label it up upon themselves throughout the years, it still remains an elusive phenomena … although a lifelong institutionalization today, is rather a rarity.

Today, most patients recover enough to be cared for in their own homes and their own communities. Community help for the mentally ill, has progressed enormously in the past two decades, though much work is still required to complete the job. Although we still do not know the exact causes for the major mental illnesses, schizophrenia, bipolar affective disorder (manic depression) or clinical depression, treatment is available. Researchers continue to look at genetics in an attempt to identify the causes. Though a cure may not come in our time, perhaps it will there for our children and their children. The stigma of mental illness, have not yet been fully eradicated. However, the move to equate mental illness with physical illness, has resulted in greater understanding on some fronts as to the course of the disease. Sad, though truthfully so, we still have a long way left to go, but we'll keep on working on it. This body of work, indicate that we're on the right path.

Getting Into The Business of Mental Health …
How Did I Got Into the Business?

I honestly don't know how … perhaps, it was after seeing countless individuals suffering with mental illness, wandering the streets and being pelted with rocks and bottles by the local people, growing up as a five, six, seven year-old boy, throughout various Honduran towns and cities. Perhaps triggered as I recalled walking through the streets of downtown Kingston, Jamaica, as a as a fifteen year old mariner, during Jamaica's economic downturn, political wars, as a young sailor from 1976 through 1979 ... and losing count on how many individuals we'd seeing hallucinating in public, after being kicked out of hospitals into the streets, without appropriate treatment, medicines, nor any kind of follow up care. Who knows, perhaps it was because, somewhere along the way I had lost count of how many were suffering that puzzled my mind and shock me to the core as a human? Though I had noticed less suffering in Canada and Europe, as my classmates became anesthetized. Perhaps, because I'd completely grown tired of seeing so much pain, during the 1980's and early 1990's, on the streets of New York, during our monthly trips, as we arrived and walk the streets, to observed and learn empathy and grow closer in touch with my own humanity, as I studied and conduct field research. Perhaps it was after learning about my good buddy and former shipmate, Francisco's death, who's body had been first ravaged by addictions that I wanted to really know the why and how?

The practical reality my reasons, were all of the above, although I sincerely believe that this career came to me more as a spiritual calling, rather than as a permanent occupation. A calling, which in turn generously and gradually helped me to get to know myself, grow as myself and strive toward becoming a better human being. One that might better learn to love my fellowman, thus further, deeper and better, comprehensively understand my limitations, become a better father, and a better person, in pursuit of a spiritual growth that would later, also help to theoretically preserve my life as a therapist, a philosopher, a sociologist, theologian and a child of God, with a full purpose in life to follow, study, learn and hopefully better understand.

A Mental Meltdown Upon The High Seas ...

From The Decks of Cruise Ships To The Halls of Psych 101

After practically eight years of daily struggles at sea, while dealings with drunken, drugged up staff members and countless irritating passengers on board the exclusive cruise liners, I had initially started researching their behaviors. This particular incident happened shortly after we had sailed out of the port of Miami a few days earlier my ship was full to its maximum capacity. We had automatically made a quick stop in Samana, Dominican Republic, as part of our weekly rout and we were on our way down to Puerto Rico. The tropical sun shinned nicely bright, the ambient temperature, was about seventy formidable degrees, the seas were as calm as the melodious music being played. The limbo show had just finished and the forged steel-band, still performed smooth calypso and reggae tunes, near the upper deck pool. Everyone notably appeared relaxed and all seemed to be having a good time. The upper deck was almost at capacity, some of the ship's passengers were sitting back enjoying the music and taking in fresh the sea-breeze compliment of their cruise vacation. Others soaked in the pools and checked on their tan, meanwhile some swam and others even danced. I was on duty as a security patrol officer, in great spirits, since I'd been advised I'd be promoted to chief that same week; everything that day, appear to be in perfect harmony. I had just finished making my rounds and checking all the decks, life boats, watertight doors, and fire stations, muster stations. As usual during rounds, I would stop by the pool bar, listen to some music, report the officer on the navigation bridge, calibrate my beeper and punch my clock. It was my official 3:00 to 4:00 P.M. routine. The steel band eventually took a break and I spent a couple of minutes chatting and exchanging pleasantries with several of the band members, greeted a couple of passengers and was about to proceeds doing my rounds. The steel band impressively began playing and I elected to momentarily stay for a while and listen to their new tunes, they'd been practicing on, before moving on. Shortly after reinitiating their set, I witnessed the lead steel drum player abandoning his instrument, stepping off the stage and into the crowd. I thought it was strange, but guessed it might just be a relevant part of their new act. He was boldly insisting on trying to take a female passenger out on the dance floor, she was with her loving husband and of course, she declined. I thought it rather strange, but paid little attention. He then rushed back to his instrument and as I started to walk away, I heard him promote over his P.A. "we are going to take another break and meanwhile we take a pause, I am going to preach to you the word of Jah!" The rest of the group kept on playing ... music still in the background. All of this unsurprisingly appeared rather odd, but I kept on believing that perhaps it was really a part of their act. Several minutes passed and he kept sermonizing to the mostly, all white passengers in a bizarre, militant unusual Rastafarian flair. As he continued to address the crowd, he got louder by the moment and sounded even more bizarre and threatening tone of voice. Although he wasn't a Rasta or a militant, his accent and voice had changed and he began to look more intimidating and threatening, almost as if he been possessed. The guitarist and band leader subsequently began signaling to me with his head, while rolling his eyes, indicating that I tried getting him off the stage. I slowly walked up to him and asked him calmly to him and suggested "we leave the deck and come grab a cup of coffee, or a cup of tea, while we sat and talk about what was going on."

My calm approach and my easy plea, merely served to further infuriate and extremely frustrate him. He subsequently picked up his instrument (a heavy steel drum) then threw it into the crowd and his preaching grew even louder and more bizarre. This time he became much more divisive, his remarks were now racist and discriminatory, vulgar and demeaning, in an almost threatening manner to the white passengers, as well as offensive to myself, his fellow black bandmates and other African Americans out on the deck. As each minute passed by, he got louder and extremely irrational, delusional. He proceeded to use derogatory and racist slurs toward the Italian officers and the white passengers, while strongly claiming to have been preaching the word of Jah. I had tried calling the navigation bridge and the Staff Captain's office for help, but got no immediate reply. Subsequently I then noticed that he was now foaming at the mouth, it was a sort of thick white froth. After realizing this, I calmly walked up to him and gently placed my hand on his right shoulder, (while ordering that he had to cut it out before someone got hurt.) I incessantly persisted calling the bridge on my hand-held 'Walkie-talkie and had tried in vain to reach some of the other officers on the bridge by telephone and via radio to seek their assistance, minutes earlier. It was about an hour before the captain's cocktail party started, I assumed the captain, staff captain and most other officers were perhaps, in the process of getting dressed up and ready for their traditional weekly awaited party. A few minutes later, after several more attempts, the staff captain finally came down, but by now I had already almost gotten the obnoxious and dangerous situation under control. The captain then began demanding that we took him down in the hatches and chained him up in the holding cell. Together with two other security officers I escorted him down, but declined to put the handcuffs on him to prevent from further infuriating him. I had instinctively realized that he was actively undergoing some emotional and psychological painful distress and did not want to impose further unnecessary stressors. I did not attempted to search him before locking the cell's door. This was a sensible oversight and a huge mistake that could've certainly cost me my life. Since once inside the cell, he requested that I sent someone to get his Bible, I immediately sent for it and once it was delivered to me, I passed it to him, he then handed me over an eight-inch long switchblade. He afterward told me that the only reason he did not stab me or anyone else with this knife, was because I had treated him with considerable, inherent dignity and marked respect. He repeatedly continued thanking me for having treated him like a man and like a human being. He also thanked me for saving the Staff Captains life, while telling me that he was ready to take him down today. A man, who's name I've safeguard and kept his confidentiality since 1982, stood six feet four, inches tall, weighing about two hundred and thirty five pounds of solid muscle. That was perhaps not my first, albeit my worse face to face encounter with religious madness. It wasn't hard to note that he regularly lifted weights and I was barely a six feet and half inch tall, and weight about a hundred and sixty pound at the present time. I was an athlete in my prime, a runner, Scuba diver and a soccer player, but certainly no match for his physical strength, his psychosis and a sharp switchblade knife. It was perhaps due to the fast lifestyle most musicians and other entertainers experienced aboard the cruise ships at the time, they tend to medicate themselves with drug and alcohol. Although he wasn't a known heavy drinker he frequently smoked marijuana to self-medicate. My particular opinion then was that he had probably felt his psychosis approaching became paranoid and had gotten himself prepared for an outright ferocious assault with hisww pocket knife. God was guiding me that day at sea. I later found out he also had previous hospitalizations in mental hospitals throughout the Caribbean. Although I had never in the past seen him taking any medications, nor talking about his mental illness, but I had occasionally witnessed and spoken to him about drinking and about his excessive pot smoking, several times in the past. Like many other individuals we stumbled upon throughout our communities, whom regularly experience such horrifying fears due to their mental illness perhaps, they merely try to medicate themselves, the only way they understand how to. Usually it's the wrong way … they engage in the unlimited use of illicit drugs. Through such ways, in which often times they wind up hurting themselves, getting killed, unfortunately hurting, or killing someone else.

Establishing Our Core Values. Aid to Recovering From The Illness

Putting people first is not only the humane thing to do, for it is the right thing to do. It is also the most effective way to help people with serious mental illnesses … and it is not a hand out, it is rather a hand's up. The values that underlie development of community-based services for people with serious mental illnesses and/or co-occurring substance use disorders who are trying to get back on their feet. Housing and spirituality are as important to the individual as all other traditional service components. Each of these values has at its center an abiding belief in the dignity and worth of the individual.

Financing housing and support services for people with serious mental illnesses and/or co-occurring substance use disorders who are homeless is a challenge for local providers. The public mental health and substance abuse treatment systems, as well as the system of services for people who are homeless, have multiple players. These include public and private mental health and substance abuse treatment providers, and general and specialty health care providers, as well as the social welfare, housing, criminal justice, employment, and education systems, among others. The funding streams that finance these systems and services are complex and sometimes contradictory, with competing incentives among funding sources.

Planning is the first critical step in developing an integrated, comprehensive system of care for people with serious mental illnesses and/or co-occurring substance use disorders. When the planning is done, the real work begins. Putting people first is our duty ... it is the humane thing to do; but also it is the most effective way to help people with serious mental illnesses or co-occurring disorders escape homelessness.

Recent research reveals that service providers who respect the individual's right to self-determination are more likely to result in residential and psychiatric stability and sobriety. The following chapter examines the concept and practice of recovery, person-centered values, and system-level values that form the foundation for effective services to prevent and help to end homelessness among people with serious mental illnesses or co-occurring disorders.

The Concept and Practice of Recovery

The good news is that we now know that *people with serious mental illnesses and/or co-occurring substance use disorders can and do recover.* Understanding the concept and practice of recovery is fundamental to the development of effective services for people with serious mental illnesses and/or co-occurring disorders who are homeless.

Our Definition Versus Consumer's Definition of Recovery

There are as many different definitions of recovery as there are individuals who recover. However, as mental health and substance abuse treatment systems move toward recovery-based systems of care, many have developed working definitions to guide their efforts. The Connecticut Department of Mental Health and Addiction Services has endorsed a broad vision of recovery as: a process of restoring or developing a positive and meaningful sense of identity apart from one's condition and then rebuilding a life despite or within the limitations imposed by that condition (Evans et al., 2002). *For many, if not most, homeless individuals who have mental illnesses and substance use disorders, recovery will involve some type of professional intervention, including the use of medication, where appropriate.*

Recovery from Substance Use Disorders

The term *recovery* has been used extensively in the field of substance use, where it refers to a return to sobriety (Ralph, 2000). For many individuals, spirituality and peer support are critical to their recovery from addictions. Thus, for example, individuals in 12-step groups for recovery from addictions express their belief in a power greater than themselves. Secular substance use recovery groups, such as Women for Sobriety and Self-Management and Recovery Training (SMART), focus on individual empowerment and emotional growth. They share with the 12-step tradition a belief in the importance of self-help as a way to obtain and maintain sobriety. People with both a mental illness and a co-occurring substance use disorder face the daunting task of recovering from both disorders. Self-help groups specifically designed to meet the needs of people with co-occurring disorders, such as Double Trouble in Recovery, provide individuals the opportunity to share common problems and to help others in their recovery from both mental illnesses and substance use.

Recovery from Mental Illness

Use of the term "recovery" only recently has been applied to people with mental illnesses, in part because of the mistaken belief that having a serious mental illness is a lifelong condition. The most frequently cited study that disproves this notion is a longitudinal study of severely disabled individuals in Vermont. Investigators found that 34 percent of former hospital inpatients who received mental health services, including psychiatric rehabilitation, in the community achieved full recovery in both psychiatric status and social functioning, and an additional 34 percent improved significantly in both areas (Harding et al., 1987). Twenty-seven studies (including Harding's) published between 1960 and 1991 show equally promising rates of recovery from serious mental illnesses (Ralph, 2000). More recent research examines the relationship between illness self-management, an evidence-based practice in the mental health field, and recovery from serious mental illnesses. Researchers found that illness self-management skills, including greater knowledge of mental illnesses, coping skills, and relapse prevention strategies play a critical role in people's recovery from mental illnesses (Mueser et al., 2002).

However, much of what is known about mental health recovery comes from the writings of mental health consumers themselves and supports what has been called the "simple yet powerful vision" (Anthony, 1993) of mental health recovery. Ultimately, recovery from a serious mental illness is a very personal process that involves the recovery of hope, of meaningful activities and relationships, and of self-esteem and self-worth. Many consumer advocates believe that recovery involves the development of both key relationships with supportive individuals and core beliefs about mental illnesses (Ahern and Fisher, 1999). Accordingly, they believe an individual can recover regardless of whether he or she takes medication.

Recovery from Homelessness
Recovering from homelessness also is a process, according to a study conducted by SRI Gallup, Inc. the researchers defined recovery from homelessness as being sober, employed, and housed; they identified six themes that support this process: spirituality, self-insight, security, self-awareness, support, and suppression of poor self-concepts and negative attitudes

Person-centered values are at the heart of a system that empowers people with mental illnesses and substance use disorders to recover. Lack of support or connection to others may be the single most important reason why people are homeless, according to the SRI Gallup survey. For many homeless people, outreach workers are the first to break through the isolation and begin to move people toward a life of greater health and personal stability. Outreach is about *"compassion translated into concrete action. It is about regarding all human beings as intrinsically valuable."* (Kraybill, 2002).

Person-Centered Values
The key values that support recovery can be described in a number of ways. For example, people with mental illnesses and substance use disorders who have survived trauma (defined as physical or sexual abuse) speak of "safety, voice, and choice" as the values that must guide services designed by and for them (NASMHPD, 1998). Researchers trying to quantify recovery to make it measurable use the terms "hope, taking personal responsibility, and getting on with life" (Noordsy et al., 2002). Spirituality and self-help are key tenets of the 12-step approach to addictions. While these values are described similarly, some important points stand out.

Their Choice.
People with serious mental illnesses and/or co-occurring substance use disorders who are homeless should be given *real* choices in housing, treatment, and support services. They should be informed of the full array of options available to them. Services cannot be "one size fits all"; they should be tailored to the individual's needs.

Their Voice.

A well-known tenet of the mental health consumer movement says, *"Nothing about us without us."* People who have serious mental illnesses or co-occurring disorders, should have a say in the programs, policies, and services designed to serve them.

Their Empowerment.

Many people with serious mental illnesses or co-occurring disorders, especially those who are or have been homeless, are disillusioned with services they have received in the past and are disenfranchised from the service system. They should be *educated* and *empowered* to make choices in matters affecting their lives and to accept *responsibility* for those choices (Federal Task Force on Homelessness and Severe Mental Illness, 1992). For most, this should include participation in developing their treatment goals and recovery plan.

Their Dignity and Self Respect.

The use of *people first* language (e.g., *people* who have serious mental illnesses, *people* who are homeless) is more than an exercise in semantics. Language shapes thought, and treatment service providers must recognize that the people they serve deserve the same respect that providers expect from them.

Their Hope.

Hopelessness breeds helplessness and despair. For many, *recovery of hope is essential for recovery from serious mental illnesses or co-occurring disorders.* Recovery from these disorders is an achievable goal that makes all other goals possible.

System-Level Values

A recovery-oriented system of care, according to the Connecticut Department of Mental Health and Addiction Services, "identifies and builds upon each individual's assets, strengths, and areas of health and competence to support achieving a sense of mastery over his or her condition while regaining a meaningful, constructive sense of membership in the broader community" (Evans et al., 2002). Specific system-level values that can help achieve this vision include:

Belief in Recovery.

Optimism is essential. Osher (1996) notes: *"Consumers, families, and practitioners who maintain a hopeful attitude toward recovery are associated with effective [co-occurring disorders] treatment programs."*

Any Door Is the Right Door For Services ... is geared for people who are homeless and have serious mental illnesses and/or co-occurring substance use disorders should be able to enter the service system through any service "door" (e.g., mental health services, substance abuse treatment, welfare office, jail), should be assessed, and should have access to the full range of comprehensive services and supports they want and need (National Technical Assistance Center for State Mental Health Planning *NTAC*, 2000).

Use Mainstream Resources to Serve People Who Are Homeless ... People with serious mental illnesses or co-occurring disorders who are homeless should be educated and empowered to gain access to mainstream resources (e.g., housing, mental health, and income support) for which they are eligible (Federal Task Force on Homelessness and Severe Mental Illness, 1992). Many people who become homeless are or have been clients of public systems of care and assistance, but they have been ill-served. Homeless assistance providers should help connect or reconnect individuals to mainstream programs, which is the only way to provide the long-term housing and services individuals require to break the cycle of homelessness (NAEH, 2000).

We Recommend A Flexible Approach ... Offer Low-Demand Services ...

Services should be flexible enough to be delivered in sufficient amounts, duration, and scope to support recovery, based on an individual's changing needs and preferences. Participation in treatment and receipt of services should not be required to gain access to housing. Individuals reluctant to enter treatment may require some type of low-demand service, such as a Safe Haven, to help engage them in more intensive interventions. These strategies can provide safety and help meet immediate survival needs while providing an opportunity to engage individuals in more intensive interventions.

Tailor Services to Meet The Individual's Needs ...

Each individual's preferences, treatment history, strengths, needs, and motivations must be recognized and addressed in plans designed to help him or her avoid or exit homelessness (Federal Task Force on Homelessness and Severe Mental Illness, 1992).

Develop Culturally Competent Services ...

Race, ethnicity, and culture influence everything, from how individuals express problems to whether or not they seek help and the type of services they will accept. At its core, cultural competence involves improved access to services and cultural adaptations that make services appropriate in cross-cultural settings (PATH Cultural Competence Workgroup, 2001). At a minimum, providers should be multilingual and multicultural (Federal Task Force on Homelessness and Severe Mental Illness, 1992; HHS, 2001).

Involve Consumers and Recovering Persons ...

Mental health consumers and individuals in recovery from substance use disorders play an important role in helping to empower their peers to recover from serious mental illnesses or co-occurring disorders. They make valuable contributions as agency staff and as active members of planning councils and advisory boards. Many consumers and recovering persons operate programs and services designed to help their peers recover.

Offer Long-Term Follow-up Support ...

Recovery from mental illnesses and co-occurring substance use disorders is neither a linear nor a short-term process. Relapse is to be expected, and individuals may require long-term follow-up support, especially after they move into housing or gain employment. Short-term fixes are neither cost-effective nor humane.

People with serious mental illnesses and/or co-occurring substance use disorders who are homeless have significant, complex needs ... they must be addressed i-f care is to be effective and recovery is to be achieved. The many state, spiritual and community agencies that serve people with serious mental illnesses or co-occurring disorders who are homeless must work together to plan a comprehensive, coordinated system of care that supports their clients' individual needs for recovery from these multiple conditions.

The Right Move toward Fair Housing

Decent, safe, affordable housing is everyone's goal, but it's often barred to people with mental disabilities. There are two main reasons: too little low-income housing and too much discrimination against those who want to live in it. Here's some information about both.

The public mental health system increasingly rations care in such a way that people with serious mental illnesses tend to first *"hit bottom"* before receiving the services and supports they need to live successfully in the community. In many communities, jails and prisons have become the largest providers of mental health services, and homeless shelters and nursing homes have become housing of last resort for people with mental illnesses. While not appearing on the mental health department's budget line, the costs of care for people with mental illnesses are borne by these other systems--and by taxpayers. Clearly, it is fiscally more prudent, as well as more humane, to address mental health needs before they reach the point of crisis.

The Bazelon Center for Mental Health Law has set out to reshape the debate about mental health system reform by developing and disseminating a model law for adaptation by states and localities. The purpose here, is to bring fort and make aware every individual involved with the process that there exists *(An Act Providing a Right to Mental Health Services and Supports that seeks to transcend the recurring debate about inadequate funding by providing a legally enforceable entitlement to recovery-oriented mental health services and supports, in sufficient amount, duration, scope and quality to support recovery, community integration and economic self-sufficiency).* Under a statute based on this template, states or counties may define eligibility broadly or narrowly, but may not turn away any eligible person.

The United States Supreme Court held in *Olmstead* that it is against the law to segregate people with disabilities in large institutions and recognized that it would be wrong to place people with serious mental illnesses into community settings *"devoid of the services and attention necessary for their condition."* The model law seeks to prohibit such neglect by the mental health system and to empower people with mental illnesses to be full partners in their treatment and recovery.

Supportive Housing, Combating Homelessness in Connecticut and the USA

The Reaching Home Hosts Supportive Housing Summit held in December 2006 was with a primary objective of the reaching home steering committee was to invite key leaders in the movement to end homelessness during a supportive housing summit scheduled to be held at a later date in 2007. A chief objective of the summit would be to address pertinent questions, such as:

What is supportive housing and is it effective to our society?

Supportive housing is a proven, effective means of re-integrating families and individuals with mental illness, chemical dependency or chronic health challenges into the community by addressing their basic needs for housing and offers on-going support. Supportive housing is a solution to homelessness and other mental health issues because it addresses its root causes. It is a positive alternate to more expensive and far less effective institutional settings.

Supportive housing has two major components:
(a) Safe and secure rental housing that is affordable to people with low incomes.
(b) Supportive housing ought to be independent … that is, all tenants should live in their own permanent apartments and occupancy to be provided so long as the tenant pay their rent and complies with the terms specified on their lease.

Defining Targeted Support

Support services are provided by qualified staff trained in working with people who are homeless and people with disabilities.

Targeted support services are in the following categories.
a) flexible and responsive to the needs of the individual.
b) available as needed by the tenant.
c) accessible where the tenant lives.

Supportive housing combines affordable housing with individualized health, support and employment services. Supportive housing looks like every other type of housing because it is like other housing. People living in supportive housing have their own apartments, enter into rental agreements and pay their own rent, just as in other rental housing.

Special differences is that they can access, at their option, support services such as the help of a case manager, help in building independent living skills, and connections to community treatment and employment services designed to address their individual needs.

The following is a comprehensive listed varieties on future housing models

Supportive housing comes in all shapes and sizes, and is designed to meet the needs of both the people and the communities served … albeit a refurbished hotel offering furnished single room occupancy apartments, a multi-family development where tenants with disabilities live alongside other families with low incomes, smaller or more service-oriented building, a renovated YMCA or scattered-site apartments.

Theoretically the primary focus of supportive housing is targeted to people with imperative risk factors such as homelessness, or health challenges such as mental illness or substance addiction. Whatever the configuration maybe, all of the housing allows tenants to access support services that enable them to live as independently as possible.

a) Supportive housing is designed to break the cycle of homelessness.

b) Supportive Housing Ought to Create Stability.

Unlike in-patient care, supportive housing does not force the individual to pick up and move as soon as they achieve stability. This stability is designed to give tenants the foundation on which to rebuild their lives and reduce their use of inpatient services.

Supportive Housing fosters self-sufficiency toward support services, including mental health care, job training and creation, addiction counseling, education, and training in basic life skills, which are designed to help the individual help themselves and minimize long-term dependency on government safety-nets.

Although modeled in part by the failed CBI's of the early 1990's, Supportive Housing facilitates the process of securing and retaining employment. Support staff, help tenants who are able to work make connections to vocational training, job placement, adult education and develop the necessary skills to find and retain jobs.

Supportive Housing prevents unnecessary use of emergency health care.
Tenants are helped in making connections to primary health care, to maintain good health and quell the need of using local emergency rooms as a primary source of care.

Supportive Housing promotes preventive care. Through daily contact with tenants where they live, service staff can see and respond to signs of poor health, depression, relapse into addiction, and other problem conditions. This early intervention can help a tenant secure appropriate treatment before a slight setback becomes a crisis.

Supportive Housing also promotes Socialization and reintegration through peer to peer support. Notable is the fact that many people who have previously been homeless lack social network of family and friends on which to rely for support. Supportive housing helps tenants build new social supports by fostering tenant interaction, tenants' associations and peer support groups.

Supportive housing also helps to prevent stigmatization;
Since supportive housing often combines apartments for people with disabilities with other market-rate or affordable apartments, and because it looks like the buildings around it, tenants do not experience the stigma often associated with residences serving people with special needs.

Noted is the unique combination of stable, safe housing with the presence of service personnel trained in handling substance abuse issues, which makes supportive housing the most effective environment for helping tenants in recovery maintain their sobriety ... Supportive housing is therefore prevents recidivism.

Point in Time Count

In January, 2007 for the first time in the history of the state of Connecticut, there will be a coordinated state-wide count of the homeless through the local continuums of care in Connecticut. The purpose of this coordinated effort is to collect data that can be used to update the state-wide homeless numbers and used in advocacy efforts to show the need for the creation of new units of supportive housing across the state.

HOME Connecticut effort takes shape with reports in from researchers and other consultants, HOME Connecticut's analysis and proposals for solutions to the state's affordable housing supply shortage are being drafted for consideration by executive and legislative state leaders.

The CHFA Board Set Goals for 2007

According to our sources in a recent meeting held in early November, the Connecticut Housing Finance Authority's Board of Directors affirmed that they will approve goals for 2007 in six areas pertinent to addressing the mission of CHFA … this documentation is now available on the net.

Department of Economic and Community Development (DECD) has issued the **RFP** for the third round of funding available under the *Housing Trust Fund*. This round of funding is open to both programs and projects that preserve or develop affordable housing and applications are due on December 14th, 2006. DECD will also hold a general information session and application workshop on November 8, 2006 from 9am to 12pm at the Legislative Office Building. You may research the *RFP* and related information on line, which is available http://www.ct.gov/ecd/cwp/view. asp?Q=310704&A=1098

The Corporation for Supportive Housing CSH 07 invitation to participate in their Consultation Days, which provides technical assistance in getting started on New Supportive Housing Projects.

The Community Loan Funds in Connecticut provides valuable financing and technical assistance to help nonprofit developers create affordable and supportive housing.

As part of their new directory of supportive housing programs in Connecticut and Rhode Island, the Corporation for Supportive Housing has compiled a comprehensive productive glossary, which is geared to teaching about affordable housing.

Reaching Home … Supportive Housing Summit

The Reaching Home Steering Committee has invited key leaders in the movement to end homelessness. Their goal is to turn to a supportive housing summit with the event scheduled to be held on the second anniversary of the kick-off *Reaching Home Campaign*, to consider the successes and lessons learned as we move toward our goal of 10,000 units for permanent supportive housing.

First Time State-wide Point in Time Count Scheduled for January 2007

For the first time ever, through the local continuums of care, there will be a coordinated state-wide count of the homeless in Connecticut. The purpose of this coordinated effort, in addition to the numbers that continuums are required to submit to HUD, is to collect data that can be used to update the state-wide homeless numbers and used in advocacy efforts to show the need for the creation of new units of supportive housing across the state. Continuums participating in the count will be offered assistance in the form of volunteer recruitment for conducting the count and nominal funding for incidentals involved in the count from the organizations co-sponsoring this effort. We urge you stay tuned for communication about how you can get involved in the volunteer efforts.

The 2007 state-wide point in time count was co-sponsored by the CT Coalition to End

Homelessness *CCEH*, Corporation for Supportive Housing *CSH* and the Partnership for Strong Communities.

The Lyceum host's a January CT Health Initiative Conference with HUD. The HUD's Partnership for Strong Communities *PSC* and the Stamford Housing Authority are also partnering to hold a CT Health Initiative Conference. This conference is a long awaited opportunity for the *Reaching Home Campaign* to engage at the local level with key housing authority officials and at the federal level with the Dept. of Public Health, Dept. of Health and Human Services; Social Security Administration; Dept. of Education; Dept. of Housing and Urban Development; Centers for Medicaid and Medicare Services; and the Dept. of Labor.

Summary ... Statistical Impact of Mental Illness In Our Society

The burden of mental illness upon our health and the overall productivity of individuals in the United States and throughout the world has long been underestimated and in many cases often ignored. Until recently, the data system developed and collected by the massive Global Burden of Disease *GBD* study conducted by the World Health Organization, the World Bank, and Harvard University, revealed that mental illness, including suicide, accounts for over 16 percent of the burden of diseases in established market economies, such as the United States and Canada. Which is considered far higher than the disease burden caused by all combined cancer cases.

Mental disorders are common in the United States and throughout the world. It is estimated that 26.2 percent of Americans ages 18 years of age and older, does suffer from some type of diagnosable mental disorder in a given year. This is roughly about one in four adults, according to the 2004 U.S. Census residential population, which figure translated to about 57.7 million people. Even though mental disorders are widespread in the population, the main burden of illness is concentrated in a much smaller proportion about 6 percent, or 1 in 17 of individuals who suffer from a chronic or serious mental illness.

Mental professionals estimates suggests that mental disorders are one of the leading causes for disability in the U.S. and Canada for people ages 16 to 44 ... and have concluded that often times many of them suffer from more than one type of mental disorder at a given time. And that nearly half, 46 percent of people with mental disorders may meet criteria for 2 or more disorders, with severity strongly related to comorbidity.

REFERENCES

Scriptures obtained from The King James Bible or translated from several Spanish Bibles

1,A. Adams, Jay. E Competent To Counsel. Presbyterian Reformed Publishing Company 1970

1. Bowers, M. JR., Retreat from Sanity. New York: Human Sciences Press 1974.

2. 2,A.:Brogan John C. In-depth Discipleship Manual. Biblical Counseling Foundation 1991.

3. University of San Lorenzo's Theological Seminary's PhD dissertation on theology and social engineering, 2005.

4. Away From The Field (thesis) by Sabas Whittaker IUniverse 2003

5. BROWN, G. and Birley, J. Crisis and life changes and the onset of schizophrenia. J. Health Society Behavior 9:203, 1968.

6. BROWN, G. Influence of family life on the course of schizophrenia disorders: A replication. 4. Britain's. Journal of Psychiatry 121:241, 1972.

5. BROWN, G. Life events and psychiatric disorders. Part I: Some methodological issues. Psychology. Med. 3:74, 1973.

6. Erikson, E. Childhood and Society (2nd ed.). New York: Norton, 1963.

7. Henderson, V. and Nite, G. Principles and Practice of Nursing (6th edition) New York: Macmillan, 1978.

8. Iinkeles, A. Social structure and socialization of competence. Harvard Educational Rev. 36:265, 1966.

9. Kantor R. and Herron, W.: Reactive and Process Schizophrenia. Palo Alto, CA: Science and Behavior Books, 1966.

10. Koranyl, E. Morbidity and rate of undiagnosed physical illnesses in a psychiatric clinic population. Arch. Gen. Psychiatry 36:4 14, April

11. Laing, R. The Politics of Experience. New York: Pantheon Books, 1967.

12. Lamb, H. Roots of neglect of the long term mentally ill. Psychiatry 42:20 1, August 1979.

13. Levison, D. The Seasons of a Man's Life. New York: Knopf, 1978

13A.. Narramore Clyde M. Psychology of Counseling: Zondervan Publishing, 1961

14A. Studies on Asian Americans In The Mental Health, Professor Janes Cheu Mai

14 B. University of San Lorenzo's Social Engineering Research Studies, 2000

14. Pasamanick, B. Schizophrenics in the Community: An Experimental Study in the Prevention of Hospitalization. New York: Appleton Century-Crofts, 1967.

15. President's Commission on Mental Health, Vol.II. Task Panel Report Appendix. Washington, D.C.: Government Printing Office, 1978.

16. Rabkin J. Criminal behavior of discharged mental patients: a critical appraisal of the research. Psychology Bulletin 86 (1):1, January 1979.

17. Robins, F. Unwelcomed patients: Where can they find asylum? Hospital Community Psychiatry, January 1978.

18. Sheehey, G. Passages. New York: Dutton, 1976.

19. Slavinsky, A. Risk in a Chronic Psychiatric Outpatient Population. NU 00370, U.S.P.H.S. Division of Nursing, December 1975.

20. Nursing with Chronically Ill Psychiatric Outpatient 00370, U.S.P.H.S. Division of Nursing, December 1975.

21. Strauss, A. Chronic Illness and the Quality of Life. St. Louis: Mosby, 1975

22. Szasz, T. The Myth of Mental Illness. New York: Hoeber-Harper, 1969

23. Talbut, J and LINN, L. Reactions of schizophrenics to life-threatening disease. Psychiatric. Q., October, 1978.

24. Vaillant, G. Adaptation to Life. Boston: Little, Brown, 1977.

25. Vance, E. Social disability. American Psychology. June 1973.

26. Walters, P. When to treat and not to treat adolescent depression. Medical Insight. February 1971.

27. White, R. Motivation reconsidered: The concept of a competency. Psychological Review, 1975.

28. Wing, J. Who becomes chronic? Psychiatric, Q. November 1978.

29. Zigler, E and Philips, L. Social competence and the process-reactive distinction in psychopathology. Journal of Abnormal Social Psychology, 1962.

30. Armstrong, B. St. Elizabeth's Hospital: case study of a court order. Hospital Community Psychiatry, 1979.

31. Arnhoff, F. Social consequences of policy toward mental illness. Science, 1975.

32. Bassuk, E and Gerson, S. Deinstitutionalization and mental health services. Science,1978.

33. Deutsch A. The Mentally Ill in America (1st edition.). Garden City: Dauble Day, 1938.

34. Evans, J. Premorbid adjustment, paranoid diagnosis, and remission, acute schizophrenics treated in a community mental health center. Arch. General Psychiatry, 1973.

35. Gormann, F. Asylums. Garden City: Doubleday, 1961.

36. Greenblatt, M. and Glazier, E. The phasing out of mental hospitals in the United States. American Journal of Psychiatry, 1975.

37. Joint Commission on Mental Illness and Health. Action for Mental Health. New York: Basic Books, 1961.

38. Jones, M. Toward a clarification of the therapeutic community concept; The Therapeutic Community. New York Behavioral Publication, 1973.

39. Kirk, S and Therrlin, M. Community mental health myths and the fate of former hospitalized patients. Psychiatry 1975.

40. Kleimann, G,. Better but not well: social and ethical issues in the deinstitutionalization problems and solutions of the mentally ill. Schizophrenia Bulletin, 1977.

41. Ozarin and Sharfstein, S. The aftermaths of deinstitutionalization. Psychiatric Q. 1978.

42. Rachlin, S. When schizophrenia comes marching home. Psychiatric Q. 1978.

44. Reigh, R and Segal, L. The emergence of the Bowery as a psychiatric Dumping Ground. Psychiatry Q. 50:191, 1978.

45. Reider, R. Hospitals, patients and politics. Schizophrenia Bulletin 11:9, 1974.

46. Report on the President's Commission on Mental Health, Volume I-IV. Washington, DC: Government Printing Office, 1978.

47. Ahmed M. and Young E.: The process of establishing a collaborative program between a mental health center and a public health nursing division. AJPH 64: 680, 1974.

48. Batey S. Using a resource group to coordinate services in discharge planning. Hospital and Community Psychiatry 31: 417, 1980.

49. Freeman, S. An agency model for developing and coordinating psychiatric after care. Hospital and Community Psychiatry 31: 768, 1960. Psychiatry 31: 200, 1960.

51. Kraus J. The chronic psychiatric patient in the community a model of care. Nursing Outlook 28:308, 1980.

52. Manthey M. Primary Nursing. Boston: Blackwell Scientific, 1980.

53. President's Commission on Mental Health, Task Panel Reports. Vol. 11. Washington, DC: Government Printing Office, 1978.

54. President's Commission on Mental Health, Final Report, Vol.,1. Washing-ton, DC: Government Printing Office, 1978.

55. Sarason S. and Lorentz E. The Challenge of the Resource Network. San Francisco: Jossey-Bass, 1979.

56. Slavinsky A. Nursing with chronically ill psychiatric outpatients. A published research report, NU 00370, U.S.P.H.S. Division of Nursing. December, 1975.

57. Steering Committee on the Chronically Mentally Ill Toward a National Plan for the Chronically ill. (DHHS Publication No.[ADM] 81-1077, printed 1981.) Washington, D.C.: Department of Health and Human Services, December 1960.

58. Clapis, Joseph A.: Connecticut's State Mental Hospitals, statistical Tables for year ending June 30, 1962, Connecticut State Department of Mental Health, 1962. Hartford. Table 9,

59. Joint Commission on Mental Illness and Health: Action for Mental Health, Basic Books, Inc. 1961. New York.

60. Cohen, Elaine: Mental health teaching in school health, School of Public Health and Administrative Medicine, Columbia University, 1961, New York.

61. Scherl, Donald J.: Changing influences on delivery of Mental Health services and the role of the State Mental Hospital and community Psychiatry. 25: 375-378. June 1974.

62. Conference Reports: The future role of the State Hospitals. Legal considerations, Hospitals and Community Psychiatry. 25: 383-385, June 1974.

63. State of Connecticut's Alcohol Advisory Council: The Directory of Alcoholism Services, State of Conn., 1974, Hartford.

64. Connecticut Drug Council: Inventory of Drug Services and Programs,, State of Conn., 1972, Hartford.

65. Public Act 74-306: An Act concerning custody, treatment and referral of accused persons who appeared to be insane or mentally ill, passed by the Connecticut General Assembly and signed on May 30, 1974 by Governor Thomas J. Meskill, Hartford, p1.

66. Public Act 74-280: An Act adopting an alcoholism and intoxication treatment Act, Passed by the Connecticut General Assembly and signed on May 29, 1974 by Governor Thomas J. Meskill, Hartford, Connecticut.

67. Public Act 74-224: An Act adopting the Connecticut mental health services Act of 1974, passed by the Connecticut General Assembly and signed on May 24, 1974 by Governor Thomas J-Meskill, Hartford.

68. Special Act 74-52: An Act establishing a Commission to further study and report on the transfer of psychiatric and other related services for children under the age of 18 from the Department o f Mental Health to the Department of Children and Youth Services, passed by the Conn. General Assembly and signed on May 14,, 1974 by Governor Thomas J. Meskill, Hartford.

69. Trespacz, Karen and Lang, Rosalie: Triage. Coordinated delivery of health and social life support services to the aged, Department on Aging and of Finance and Control, November 13, 1973 Hartford.

70. Joint Commission on Accreditation of Hospitals: Accreditation Manual for Psychiatric facilities 1972, JCAH, 1972, Chicago.

71. Diagnosis and Treatment of Mental Disorders (Allen Frances. MD) 72.The Fate of Borderline Patients: Success, Full Outcome and Psychiatric Practice. (Michael H. Stone)

73. Supportive Therapy for Borderline Patients: A Psychodynamic Approach. (Lawrence H. Rockland).

74. Cognitive Behavioral Treatment of Borderline Personality Disorder. (Marsha Linehan).

75. Skills Training Manual For Treating BPD. (Marsha Linehan).

76. DSM-IV Made Easy. James Morrison

77. The Chronically Ill Psychiatric Patient and the Community. (Judith B. Krauss. Ann T. Slovansky).

78. WING, J. The social context of schizophrenia. American Journal of Psychiatry, 1978. WING, J. Who becomes Chronic. Psychiatry, Q. 50:178, 1978.

79. WULFORO, J. The effect on state hospitalization of a community mental health/mental retardation center. American Journal of Psychiatry 1972.

80. Calvin S. Hall. A Primer of Freudian Psychology.

81. Anderson RN, Smith BL. Deaths: leading causes for 2001. National Vital Statistics Report 2003; 52(9): 1-86.

82. Annenberg Public Policy Center of the University of Pennsylvania. Suicide and the Media.

83. Carney SS, Rich CL, Burke PA, Fowler RC. Suicide over 60: the San Diego study. Journal of American Geriatric Society 1994; 42: 174-80.

84. Centers for Disease Control and Prevention, National Center for Injury Prevention and Control. Suicide Surveillance, 1970-1980. (1985).

85. Centers for Disease Control and Prevention. Regional variations in suicide rates—United States 1990–1994, August 29, 1997. MMWR 1997; 46(34):789-92.

86. Centers for Disease Control and Prevention, National Center for Injury Prevention and Control.

87. Department of Health and Human Services. The Surgeon General's call to action to prevent suicide. Washington (DC): Department of Health and Human Services; 1999.

88. Dorpat TL, Anderson WF, Ripley HS. The relationship of physical illness to suicide. In: Resnik HP, editor. Suicide behaviors: diagnosis and management. Boston (MA): Little, Brown, and Co.; 1968:209-19.

89. Krug EG, Dahlberg LL, Mercy JA, Zwi AB, Lozano R, editors. World report on violence and health.

90. Lubell KM, Swahn MH, Crosby AE, Kegler SR. Methods of suicide among persons aged 10-19 years—United States, 1992- 2001. MMWR 2004; 53:471-473.

91. McCleary R, Chew K, Hellsten JJ, Flunn-Bransford M. Age-and Sec-Specific Cycles in United States Suicides, 1973-1985. American Journal of Public Health 1991; 81: 1494-7.

92. Warren CW, Smith JC, Tyler CW. Seasonal Variation in Suicide and Homicide: A Question of Consistency. Journal of Biosocial Sciences 1983; 15:349-356.

93. Warren Gawalack MG., Historic Theologian Studies Seminary: Seventh day Adventists studies, 1988.

94. 2007, 2016 NIH Funded Reports

95. NIMH 2000 - 2016, funded Reports

BIBLIOGRAPHY

Esta Carini, Dorothy M. Douglas, Lois D. Heck and Marguerite Pearson: The Mentally Ill In Connecticut (Changing Patterns Of Care And The Evolution Of Psychiatric Nursing 1972).

Judith B. Krauss and Ann T. Slavinsky: The Chronically Ill Psychiatric Patient and the Community, 1982.

Abelson D. Willa: A Clinic in the Community, 1913-1963, Half A Century of Psychiatric Service, Clifford W. Beers Guidance Clinic, Inc., 1965, New Haven.

Abrason, Marc F.: The criminalization of mentally disordered behavior: Possible side-effect of a new mental health law, Hospital and Community Psychiatry. 101-105, April 1972.

Abroms, Gene M.: The open-door policy: A rational use of controls. Hospital and Community Psychiatry: 8 1-84, February, 1973.

Albee G. W.: Mental Health Manpower Trends, Basic Books, 1959, New York.

Alexander Franz and Selesnick Sheldon: The History of Psychiatry: An Evaluation of Psychiatric Thought and Practice From Prehistoric Times To Present, Harper and Row, Publishers, 1966, New York.

Altman Stuart H.: Present and future supply of registered nurses, U.S Department of Health, Education & Welfare, Publication, No. (NIH) 73-134, 1972, Bethesda.

American Hospital Association: Mental Health Services and the General Hospital Association, 1970. Chicago.

American Hospital Association and National League for Nursing: Statement on Hospital Diploma Programs in Nursing, Approved by NLA Board of Directors, on Feb, 2, 1967 and by AHA Board of Trustees February 10, 1967.

ANA Conference Group on Psychiatric Nursing Practice: Facing Up To Changing Responsibilities, ANA, 1964. New York.

ANA Research and Statistics Dept.: Facts about Nursing. A Statistical Summary 1970-1971 Edition. ANA 1971, New York.

Arafeh M.K.: Linking Hospital and Community Care for Psychiatric Patients, Amer. Journal of Nursing, 68:1050-1056, May, 1968.

Atlantic States Conference on Mental Health: Legal issues in the patient rights to treatment. October 9, 1972. Williamsburg, Virginia.

Barton Walter.: Trends in community mental health programs. Hospital and Community Psychiatry. 17: 253-258. September 1966.

Bates Barbara and Kern, M. Sue: Doctor-Nurse Teamwork. The American Journal of Nursing. 67: 2066-2071, October 1967.

Hon. David L. Bazelon: The right to treatment: The court's role, Community Psychiatry. 20: 1 29-135, May. 1969.

Allan Beigel.: Law Enforcement, the Judiciary and Mental Health: A growing partnership, Hospital and Community Psychiatry 24: 605612, September, 1973.

Belknap, Ivan: Human Problems of a State Mental Hospital. McGraw Hill Book Co., 1956, New York.

Bennett and Hargrove: The Practice of Psychiatry in General Hospitals, Univ. of Calif. Press, 1956, Berkeley.

Bloomberg, Wilfred: A proposal for a community-based hospital as a branch of a state hospital. The American Journal of Psychiatry, 116: 8l4-817, March 1960.

Board of Examiners for Nursing: Rules and Regulations of the Board of Examiners for Nursing and requirement for registration of professional nurses and certification of licensed practical nurses, State of Connecticut, Effective March 12, 1968, Hartford.

Braceland Francis J.: Comprehensive Psychiatry and Mental Hospitals. 2 – 6, 1957. Changes in the Treatment of involutional melancholia. Hospital and Community Psychiatry. 20: 136 – 140, May 1969. The Institute Of Living. 1822–1972, Connecticut Printers Inc. 1972, Hartford.

Brand Jeanne: The National Mental Health Act of 1946: A Retrospect Bulletin of Medical History. 39: 231,245, 1965.

Bromberg Walter: The Mind of Man, Harper & Bros., Publishers, 1937, New York.

Brown Esther Lucile: Nursing reconsidered. A study of change Part 2. The Professional Role in Community Nursing, J.B. Lippincott Co., 1971, Philadelphia.

Brown Martha M. and Fowler Grace R.: Psychodynamic Nursing, a Biosocial Orientation. 3rd edition. W.B. Saunders Co., 1966, Philadelphia.

Bruch Hilda: 100 Years of Psychiatry

Kraepelin.: 50 years later, Archives General Psychiatry. 21: 257-261. September 1969.

Bureau of Health Professions Education and Manpower Training Division of Nursing: Nursing personnel in hospitals - 1968, USDHEW, PHS-NIH, May 1970. Bethesda.

Busse. Ewald W.: The origins of priorities and the effect of pressure on mental health services. Hospital and Community Psychiatry. 22. 357-361, December 1971.

Cameron. D. Ewen: In General Hospitals, The psychiatric unit must open the doors. The Modern Hospital. 87: 51-54. 144. 146 148. 150. September 1956.

The Psychiatric Unit of the General Hospital. Mental Hospital. 8: 2-7, March. 1957.

Carini Esta: A Study of the Attitudes of 293 Nursing Students at the Outset and the Completion of the Basic Psychiatric Nursing Experience in five Hospitals in the State of New York. Unpublished Doctoral Dissertation. 1958. Fordham University, New York City. Factors in state programs that facilitate or hinder in-service training. Paper presented at Regional Conference on Planning In-Service Training Programs for Mental Health, October 8-11. 1963. Swampscott. Mass. 5, pages.

Report on the selection, performance and attrition of 486 psychiatric aide trainees enrolled in training programs at three state hospitals for the two-year period. July 1, 1961-June 30, 1963. Connecticut Department of Mental Health, 1964, Hartford, 13 pages.

Nurses and mental health: paper presented at workshop on Mental Health and Problems of Contemporary Society. University of Connecticut, July 6, 1964, Storrs.

Report on the selection, performance and attrition of 323 psychiatric aide trainees enrolled in training programs at three state hospitals for the eighteen month period, July 1ˢᵗ 1963-December 31, 1964. Connecticut Department of Mental Health. 1965, Hartford. 21 pages.

Report on the selection, performance and attrition of 376 psychiatric aide trainees enrolled in training programs ~t three state hospitals for the two year period. January 1, 1965- December 31, 1966, Connecticut Department of Mental Health, 1967 Hartford.

Caudill William: The psychiatric hospital as a small society. Harvard University Press, 1958, Cambridge.

Chen Ronald, Healey James and Williams Howard: Problems Purchases and Changing Objectives. Report of a Forum on Partial Hospital, held in Topeka, Kansas, June, 1967.

Claps Joseph A.: Outpatient psychiatric clinic termination, numbers, age, specific rates and age-adjusted rates per 10,000 population. 1960-1972. Statistics Section, Connecticut Department of Mental Health. State Mental Hospital Admissions, numbers specific rates and age-adjusted rates per 10,000 population. Connecticut: 1963-1972, Statistics Section, Connecticut Department of Mental Health, Hartford.

Commission on Hospital Care: Hospital Care in the United States. The Commonwealth Fund. Stone Book Press. 1947, New York.

Commission on Nursing: A Report on Nursing Needs and Resources in Connecticut, 1966, Hartford.

Committee on Hospital Services for the Mentally Ill: A Survey of psychiatric Services in the United States, American Association for Mental Health, Inc., 1958, New Haven.

Cowan, M. Cordelia: The Yearbook of Modern Nursing, 1956, G.P. Putnam's Sons, 1956, New York.

Cowen E. Gardner. L. and Zax: Emergent Approaches to Mental Health Problems, Appleton Century-Crofts, 1967, New York.

Cumming, Elaine: Unsolved problems of prevention, Canada's Mental Health, Supplement No.56, 3-12, January-April, 1968.

Dam, Norman: Concepts of insanity in the United States, 1789 –1865, Rutgers University Press, 1964, New Brunswick, N.J.

Detre, Thomas and Jarecki, Henry: Modern Psychiatric Treatment, J.B. Lippincott Co., 1971, Philadelphia.

Deutsch, Albert: The Mentally Ill in America. A History of Their Care and Treatment from Colonial Times, Doubleday, Doran & Co., Inc. 1937, Garden City, N.Y.

The Mentally Ill in America, Columbia University Press. 1946, New York. The Shame of the States, Harcourt, Brace & Co., 1948.

DeYoung, Carol and Tower, Margene: The role of the nurse in community mental health center: Out of Uniform and Into Trouble, The CV Mosby Co., 1971, St. Louis.

DHEW Publication No. (HSM) 72-9046: Experiments in Mental Health Training. Project Summaries, U.S. Government Printing Office, 197 1, Washington., D.C.

Dietz, Lena Dixon: History and Modern Nursing, F.A. Davis, 1963, Philadelphia. Dodge, Bertha S.: The *Story* Of Nursing, Little, Brown and Company 1954, Boston.

Earl B.V.: Doctor Tucker's mental hospital Odyssey, Hospital and Community Psychiatry, 18: 345-348, November, 1967,

Ginsberg Eli.: Men, Money and Medicine Columbia University Press, 1969, New York. Joseph Giordano and Grace: Overcoming Resistance to Change in Custodial Institutions, Hospital and Community Psychiatry, June 1972.

Goldston, Stephen E. and Padilla, Elena: Mental Health Training and Public Health Manpower, NIMH, U.S. Government Printing Press, July, 1971, Rockville, Md.

Goodnow, Minnie: Nursing History, 7th ed., Whittlesey House, Division of W.B. Saunders Co., 1943, Philadelphia

Gorman, Mike: Every other bed, World Publishing Co., 1956, Cleveland.

Greenblatt, Milton: From custodial to therapeutic care in mental hospitals, Russell Sage, 1955, N.Y.

Hall, S. Calvin: A Primer of Freudian Psychology. Mentor Book, 1982

Hartog, Joseph: Nonprofessionals as mental health consultants, Hospital and Community Psychiatry. 18: 223-229, August 1967.

Hecker. Arthur:: The demise of large state hosPitals. Traditional facilities will be renew kinds of treatment units, Hospital and Community Psychiatry. 21: 261-263, August, 1970.

Hogarty, Gerard E.: The plight of schizophrenics in modern treatment programs, Hospital and Community Psychiatry. 22:197-203, July 1971.

Marie: Current concepts of positive mental health, Basic. New York.

James Arthur W.: Three and a half centuries of the care of the insane in Virginia from a governmental point of view, Mental Health in Virginia, August, 1958.

Jones Donald, Seernan Carolynne, and Taube Carl: Staffing Patterns in Mental Health Facilities 1968, National Institute of Mental Health U.S. Government Printing Office, 1970, Wash. D.C.

Ledney Donna M.: Psychiatric nursing; Breakthrough to independence, RN 34:29-35, August, 197 1.

Losee, Garry and Altenderfer Marion: Health Manpower in Hospitals, U.S. Dept of Health, Education and Welfare, NIH, Bureau of Health Manpower Education, 1970, Wash., D.C.

The Psychiatric Aide In The State Mental Hospital. Washington. D.C. Public Health Service, U.S. Government Printing Office. 1965.

Marshall, Helen E.: Dorothea Dix, Forgotten Samaritan, University of North Carolina Press, 1937, Chapel Hill.

Martin, Morgan: Behavior Modification in the Mental Hospital. Hospital and Community Psychiatry 23: 287-289.

National Committee Against Mental Illness, Inc.: What are the facts about mental illness in the United States? National Committee Against Mental Illness, Inc. 1966, Washington. D.C.

Peplau. Hildegard: Interpersonal Techniques: The Crux of Psychiatric Nursing, Amer. J. Nursing. 62: 50-54 June, 1962.

Peters. James S. and Dorothy S.: Vocational Rehabilitation in Connecticut, 1947-1971. Bulletin 119. State Dept. of Education. 1974. Hartford,

Pitcher. Charles W.: Abstracted Material on Dorothea Lynd Dix. Unpublished, New Jersey State hospital, 1953, Trenton.

Pope. Jane: The changing scene of psychiatric nursing in a State hospital, Perspectives in Psychiatric care 5:163-173, 1967.

Pottle. Clarence H.: From custodial care to modern therapy, Mental Hospitals 9: 26-22 May, l959.

Public Health Service Publication No. 1345: Mental illness and its treatment past and present, U.S. Government Printing Office, 1965, Washington. D.C.

Public Health Service Publication No. 165: 1966 Final Reports State Mental Health Planning, U.S. Dept. of Health, Education and Welfare. NIMI Ill, Nov.1966, Chevy Chase. Md.

Richards, Linda: Early Days in the First American Training School For Nurses. American Journal of Nursing. 73:1574-1575. September l973.

Robinson Alice: Working with the Mentally Ill, 4th edition 1971, Philadelphia.

Roche Report: Psychosurgery called Resurging Menace of Brain Mutilation. Frontiers of Psychiatry 2:1-2, 8-9, Oct. 1, 1972.

Elvin and Stambrook: A History of Psychiatric Nursing in the Nineteenth Century, Part 1, History of Medicine and Allied Science pp.48-74. Winter, 1949.

Shepard, Odell: Connecticut Past and Present, Alfred A. Knopf, 1939, New York.

Sobey, Francine: The Nonprofessional Revolution in Mental Health, Columbia University. Press. 1970, New York.

Solomon Harry: Some historical perspectives, Mental Hospitals. 9: 5-7. February 1958.

Somers, A.R.: Health Care In Transition: Directions for the Future. Research and Educational Trust. 1971 Chicago.

Stanton, A. H. and Schwarts. M. S.: The Mental Hospital. Basic Books. 1954, New York.

Stokes. (;ertrude (ed.): The Roles of Psychiatric Nurses in Community Mental Health Practice. A Giant Step, Faculty Press. 1969 Brooklyn, New York.

Suchotliff Leonard, Steinfeld George: The struggle for patients' rights in a State hospital. Mental Hygiene 54: 230-240, April 1970.

Siasi, Thomas: Ideology and Insanity: Essays on the Psychiatric Dehumanization of Man. Anchor, 1970. Garden City.

Talkington, Percy C.: Critical issues in psychiatry: A call for reassessment of our nation's mental health care, Hospital and Community Psychiatry. 24:17-22, January 1973.

Taylor, Florence R.: Annual statistical review: Connecticut State Hospitals for the mentally ill and Mental Hygiene Clinics, Conn. State Dept. of Mental Health, July. 1956 Hartford.

Title II, Public Law 88 - l64, Regulations: Community Mental Health Act of 1963, U.S. Dept. Health, Education and Welfare, Federal Register, May 6, 1964,

SAMHSA's Health Information Network at 1-877-SAMHSA7 TDD: 1 800-487-4889 http://www.samhsa.gov/grants/2008/ti_08_001.aspx.

Conference on Transforming Mental Health Systems for the 21st Century.

Pilot Programs for National Survey on Drug Use and Health

SAMHSA's Co-Occurring Center for Excellence (COCE)

February issue of the *Journal of the American Medical Association*, Lee Cohen, M.D. *Massachusetts General Hospital*

August 2006 issue of *Archives of General Psychiatry*, Thomas Insel, M.D. Director National Institutes of Health's *NIH*, National Institute of Mental Health *NIMH*.

C. Barr Taylor, M.D., of Stanford University, *First study to show that eating disorders can be prevented among high-risk groups.*

Susan Bryson, MS, MA of Stanford University; Kristine H. Luce, PhD of Stanford University; Darby Cunning, MA of Stanford University; Angela Celio, PhD of the University of Chicago; Liana B. Abascal, MA of San Diego State University; Roxanne Rockwell of San Diego State University;

Pavarti Dev, PhD of Stanford University; Andrew J. Winzelberg, PhD of Stanford University; and Denise E. Wilfley, PhD of Washington University Medical Center study on eating disorders

Archives of General Psychiatry, August 2006. Taylor CB, et al. Prevention of Eating Disorders in At-risk College-age Women.

Karen Berman, M.D., chief of the NIMH Section on Integrative Neuroimaging.

Intramural Research Program report on their functional magnetic resonance imaging *FMRI.* Study posted in the online *Proceedings of the National Academy of Sciences* report January 29, 2007. Drs. Berman, Dr. Jean-Claude Dreher, Dr. Peter Schmidt, *NIMH*

Drs. Philip Kohn and Daniella Furman of the *NIMH,* section on Integrative Neuroimaging, Dr. David Rubinow of the *NIMH* Behavioral Neuroendocrinology Branch

Archives of General Psychiatry, March 2007. Drs. Elizabeth Jane Costello, Dr. Adrian Angold, Duke University, study on *optimized survival under adverse conditions and stress-triggered illness of indicative adaptations in the womb.*

NIMH and *NIH* National Institute of Diabetes and Digestive and Kidney Diseases *NIDDK,* study on (*Osteoporosis As A Silent Disease*) by Drs. Giovanni Cizza, MD, PhD, MHSc, Farideh Eskandari, MD, MHSc, and NIMH Deputy Director Richard Nakamura, PhD. NIH and NIMH, Clinical Center and the National Center for Complementary and Alternative Medicine, study on Depression.

Latino Behavioral Health Institute's Conference on Mental Health, Los Angeles California. September 2007

Study of evaluation on depression and treatment among young, predominantly minority women. July 2 issue of the *Journal of the American Medical Association,* Dr. Jeanne Miranda, Ph.D. University of California at Los Angeles Neuropsychiatric Institute.

Research in Human Development, published in June 2007, *NIMH* Organized Workshop and IV Family Research Consortium. *NIMH* research scientists, Drs. Cheryl Boyce, PhD, and Andrew Fuligni, PhD, University of California, Los Angeles.

Reaching Home NASW-CT Conference, Lisa Mazzeo, LCSW, Clinical Director, Operation Hope, Inc. and Kate Kelly. Reaching Home Supportive Housing for People with Mental Illness and Substance Abuse Disabilities Promotion Specialty Conference, Cromwell Connecticut. http://www.naswct.org

Lecture on mental health conducted at Charles Sturt University School of Humanities and Social Sciences, Australia. Janki Shankar, PhD.

Lecturer in Sociology, University of Sydney, Australia. Fran Collyer, PhD, Lecture on social policy and sociology, University of Sydney School of Social Work, New South Wales, Australia. Margaret Alston Associate Professor of the School of Humanities and Social Sciences, Charles Sturt University

The 2007 *state-wide point in time count,* co-sponsored by the CT Coalition to End Homelessness *CCEH,* Corporation for Supportive Housing *CSH,* and the Partnership for Strong Communities summit.

Research collected for the Asian Americans studies National Latino and Asian American Study *NLAAS,* David Takeuchi, PhD, University of Washington,

Research studies on the interactions between culture, race, and ethnicity with depressive symptoms. Harold Neighbors, PhD, University of Michigan,

Research study on differences in risk for mental disorders based on ethnicity among Native American middle school students, funded by the Substance Abuse and Mental Health Services Administration *SAMHSA.* Teresa LaFromboise, PhD, Stanford University, Robert Roberts, PhD, and Catherine Ramsay Roberts, MPH, PhD, both at the University of Texas. Boyce CA, Fuligni AJ. Issues for Developmental Research Among Racial/Ethnic Minority and Immigrant Families. Research on Human Development, *Jun 4 2007 (1&2):1-17.*

Study on Treating Asian Americans With Depression, Drs. Albert Yeung MD, ScD and Raymond Kam, MD, MS, combined studies funded by the National Institute of Mental Health (NIMH) and National Institute on Alcohol Abuse and Alcoholism (NIAAA) In the August 3, 2005 edition of the *Journal of the American Medical Association (JAMA),* the RAND Corporation's Grant Marshall, Ph.D., Drs. Terry Schell, Marc Elliott, Megan Berthold, Rand Corporation; and Dr. Chi-Ah Chun, California State University.

Dr. Sean Joe, M.S.W., Ph.D. University of Michigan, at Ann Arbor.

National Survey of American Life *NSAL* studies, funded by *NIMH* and published in the November 1, 2006 issue of the *Journal of the American Medical Association.*

Research study *Prevalence of Risk Factors for Lifetime* Suicide Attempts Among Blacks in the United States, Baser RE, Breeden G, Neighbors HW, Jackson JS. Published *Nov 1 2006, JAMA; 296 (17):2112-2123.*

Suicide attempts in the Epidemiologic Catchment Area Study. Moscicki EK, O'Carroll P, Rae DS, Locke BZ, Roy A, Regier DA. Yale J Biol Med. 1988 May-Jun; 61(3):259-68.

Kessler RC, Borges G, Walters EE. Prevalence of and risk factors for lifetime suicide attempts in the National Comorbidity Survey. *Archives of General Psychiatry,* 1999 Jul; 56 (7):617-26.

Research studies of Prevalence and distribution of major depressive disorder in African Americans, Caribbean Blacks, and Non-Hispanic Whites. *Archives of General Psychiatry, March 5, 2007.* David R. Williams, PhD, University of Michigan and Wayne State University, Williams DR, Gonzalez HM, Neighbors H, Nesse R, Abelson JM., Sweetman J, Jackson JS.

Real Men Real Depression Campaign, National Institute on Mental Health *NIMH,* director, Thomas R. Insel, M.D., Dr. Sergio Aguilar-Gaxiola M.D., Ph.D., visiting Professor of Clinical Internal Medicine and the Director of the Center for Reducing Health Disparities, University of California, Davis.

Research study to examine the effect of foreign nativity on the prevalence of mental disorders within Latino immigrant populations, with information gathered from the National Latino and Asian-American Study *NLAAS.* Published in the issue of *Social Science and Medicine, July 2007.* Dr. Margarita Alegria, Harvard University.

Research study on Familias Unidas, Parent-Preadolescent Training for HIV Prevention *PATH,* English for Speakers of Other Languages *ESOL,* Heart Power for Hispanics and the American Heart Association program. Published in the issue of the *Journal of Consulting and Clinical Psychology,* December 2007. Dr. Guillermo Prado, PhD., University of Miami,

Research on randomized controlled trial of parent-centered intervention in the prevention of substance use and HIV risk behavior among Hispanic adolescents. Published in the December issue of the *Journal of Consulting and Clinical Psychology, 2007; 75(6): 914-926.* Dr. Guillermo Prado, PhD., University of Miami, Pantin H, Briones E, Schwartz SJ, Feaster D, Huang S, Sullivan S, Tapia MI, Sabillon E, Lopez B, Szapocznik J.

Epidemiology of Mental Illness, section on Mental Health: A Report of the Surgeon General

Fact Sheets from Culture, Race, and Ethnicity: A Supplement to Mental Health: A Report of the Surgeon General

The Global Burden of Disease study, conducted by the World Health Organization, the World Bank, and Harvard University

ChildStats.gov: Access to statistics and reports on children and families

Research conducted on the Substance Abuse and Mental Health Services Administration *SAMHSA's*, Communities that Care *CTC* and *CSAP* toolkit. A system developed to empower communities to use advances in the preventive science to guide their preventive efforts, J. David Hawkins and Richard F. Catalano.

Understanding Differences in past year psychiatric disorders for Latinos living in the United States: Alegria, M., et al. *Social Science and Medicine, July 2007; 65 (2):214-30.*

Printed in the United States
By Bookmasters